D1139838

Counseling about Cancer

BLACKPOOL, FYLDE AND WYRE
NHS LIBRARY

TV10346

Counseling about Cancer
Strategies for Genetic Counseling

Second Edition

Katherine Schneider

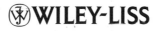
WILEY-LISS

A JOHN WILEY & SONS, INC., PUBLICATION

This book is printed on acid-free paper. ∞

Copyright © 2002 by Wiley-Liss, Inc., New York. All rights reserved.

Published simultaneously in Canada.

While the authors, editors, and publisher believe that drug selection and dosage and the specification and usage of equipment and devices, as set forth in this book, are in accord with current recommendations and practice at the time of publication, they accept no legal responsibility for any errors or omissions, and make no warranty, express or implied, with respect to material contained herein. In view of ongoing research, equipment modifications, changes in governmental regulations and the constant flow of information relating to drug therapy, drug reactions, and the use of equipment and devices, the reader is urged to review and evaluate the information provided in the package insert or instructions for each drug, piece of equipment, or device for, among other things, any changes in the instructions or indication of dosage or usage and for added warnings and precautions.

No part of this publication may be reproduced, stored in a retrieval system or transmitted in any form or by any means, electronic, mechanical, photocopying, recording, scanning or otherwise, except as permitted under Sections 107 or 108 of the 1976 United States Copyright Act, without either the prior written permission of the Publisher, or authorization through payment of the appropriate per-copy fee to the Copyright Clearance Center, 222 Rosewood Drive, Danvers, MA 01923, (978) 750-8400, fax (978) 750-4744. Requests to the Publisher for permission should be addressed to the Permissions Department, John Wiley & Sons, Inc., 605 Third Avenue, New York, NY 10158-0012, (212) 850-6011, fax (212) 850-6008, E-Mail: PERMREQ@WILEY.COM.

For ordering and customer service information please call 1-800-CALL-WILEY.

Library of Congress Cataloging-in-Publication Data:

Schneider, Katherine A.
    Counseling about cancer : strategies for genetic counseling / Katherine A. Schneider.—2nd ed.
        p. ; cm.
    Includes bibliographical references and index.
    ISBN 0-471-37036-3 (pbk : alk. paper)
    1. Cancer—Genetic aspects. 2. Cancer—Patients—Counseling of. 3. Genetic counseling. I. Title.
    [DNLM: 1. Neoplasms—genetics. 2. Genetic Counseling. 3. Neoplasms—nursing. 4. Neoplasms—psychology. QZ 200 S359c 2002]
    RC268.4 .S355 2002
    616.99'4042—dc21

BARCODE No. 456884 3

CLASS No. 616.994 SCH

13 MAY 2002 2001026919

LOAN CATEGORY N/L

Printed in the United States of America.

10 9 8 7 6 5 4 3 2 1

This book is dedicated to my mother,
Patricia E. Daviau,
and my grandmother,
Edith A. Mara,
for their encouragement, love, and support.

Contents

FOREWARD

Seven years ago the first edition of this book appeared. It was the first comprehensive book of cancer genetics written expressly for genetic counselors. At that time, very few counselors had begun to do cancer counseling. Genetic counseling curricula did not yet encompass cancer genetics as a focus. The volume opened the door to an emerging field for a group whose involvement was essential to the ultimate success of that field. Kathy Schneider wrote the book alone.

Seven years later, the landscape has been transformed. Every cancer center has a cancer genetics program. Cancer genetics is taught in genetic counseling training programs, medical genetics programs, and oncology training programs. Genetic counselors have been integrated into oncology and developing area of cancer risk assessment, and have been part of every formal process evaluating cancer genetics, and every process evaluating its potential impact on privacy, family and health. Some geneticists consider cancer genetics to be the paradigm for genetics care of the future, in which subspecialty providers will partner with genetic counselors to provide care in the genetics of their organ system. Whatever the setting, genetic counselors will continue to educate providers, to translate complex information to patients, and to assist in decision making. They are also conducting more independent research.

This volume is twice the size of its predecessor, reflecting the explosion of information over the past 7 years. It includes information about internet-based resources, now invaluable tools for genetic counselors, who must keep track of the plethora of available genetic tests, laboratories, mutation databases, genetic privacy laws, and more. There are many more genes, more detailed information about the genes, more discussion of the medical and psychological implications of genetic testing for individuals and their families. As a single-author text, it complements Kenneth Offit's comprehensive volume. The writing style makes it uniquely suited to genetic counselors and other seeking a clear, readable, insightful approach to a complex field.

Kathy Schneider has done it again. Given the pace of the field, she may not be able to wait seven years for the next edition.

Judy Garber

PREFACE

Health care providers working in oncology repeatedly hear two questions from patients: "Why did I get cancer?" and "Are my children now at higher risk?" This book describes how to determine if patients have a hereditary cancer syndrome and, perhaps even more importantly, what to tell them if a cancer syndrome is present in their family. Although written primarily for genetic counselors, this book should useful to any health care provider working in oncology or genetics.

Cancer genetic counseling is a fairly new medical specialty. In some aspects, it is similar to other genetic counseling specialties, but there are some important differences. The purpose of this book is twofold: to help new cancer genetic counselors get started and to provide an updated resource for those already in the field. This book contains a basic review of cancer genetics terminology and facts as well as practical information about providing cancer genetic counseling and testing. Detailed case examples help illustrate the many complexities of cancer genetic counseling.

Chapter 1 starts with cancer epidemiology. The basic—and sobering—statistics of cancer incidence and mortality create an important foundation for cancer counselors. As this chapter demonstrates, in contrast to other genetic conditions, everyone has at least some risk for developing cancer. In fact, because cancer is such a common disorder, almost everyone has at least one relative who has developed cancer. Now, it is true that only a subset of these people will turn out to have inherited susceptibilities to cancer but that does not mean they are not thinking, and worrying, about the possibility.

The detection and treatment of cancer require a dedicated team of providers that includes oncologists, surgeons, radiologists, and pathologists. The intersecting specialties has created a daunting vocabulary all its own. Chapter 2 discusses the ways in which tumors are detected and treated so that counselors can become more comfortable with the terminology used in clinical oncology. Cancer prevention strategies are also discussed in this chapter.

For the majority of cancer risk counselors, cancers of the breast, colon, and ovary will make up the majority of referrals. For this reason, Chapters

1 and 2 each have special sections discussing these specific malignancies, which includes risk factors, normal anatomy, cancer staging, standard treatments, and prevention options.

Cancer has long been recognized as a disorder of aberrant growth caused by genetically mutated cells. Chapter 3 discusses cancer cell biology, the process of carcinogenesis, the three major classes of cancer predisposition genes, and even epigenetic influencers. Given how quickly the field is moving, counselors are more likely to learn about new scientific discoveries from peer-reviewed journal articles than a textbook. Therefore, this chapter has been designed as an overview of the topic and can be considered a primer to genetic counselors who not only need to have a fundamental understanding of cancer biology but will also be called on to simplify this information for clients.

In terms of genetic syndromes, cancer syndromes are the new kid on the block, meaning that the diagnostic features and associated cancer risks continue to evolve. Keeping this caution in mind, Chapters 4 and 5 provide detailed information about the major cancer syndromes that have been described to date. Chapter 4 describes the clinical and molecular features of 30 specific hereditary cancer syndromes with emphasis on associated cancer risks. Chapter 5 contains lists of cancer syndromes by specific sites of cancer. For example, one table in this chapter lists the cancer syndromes associated with specific skin lesions. Both Chapters 4 and 5 have been designed to be easy-to-use references for counselors and other providers working in the field.

Then there is the provision of cancer counseling itself. This process begins with the collection of a comprehensive cancer history. Chapter 6 discusses how to collect and interpret cancer histories.

The components of the cancer genetic counseling session are described in Chapter 7, with particular attention to the cancer risk assessment. This chapter also discusses issues relevant to specific counseling situations, including newly diagnosed patients, terminally ill patients, and survivors of childhood cancer.

Cancer genetic counseling combines both education and counseling. Chapter 8 details the psychological aspects of cancer risk and the counseling encounter itself. As is discussed in this chapter, the emotional side of risk pervades every aspect of the counseling interaction and requires special skill and tact on the part of the counselor.

Chapter 9 details the role of the genetic counselor in dealing with predisposition testing and counseling. Genetic testing has entered the clinical domain and counselors and other providers with whom they work need to develop comprehensive testing programs. This chapter discusses the important programmatic elements and the challenges that go hand in hand when providing genetic testing for cancer susceptibility.

The complexities of genetic testing are further illustrated in Chapter 10, which discusses the array of ethical dilemmas that can arise. Following a review of the basic ethical principles, five hypothetical cases are presented and thoughtfully discussed.

Clinical cancer genetics has become an important medical specialty and even providers who are not working directly in the field may find themselves in need of the appropriate facts and figures, if only to recognize when to make appropriate referrals. Hopefully, this book will fill a niche in terms of providing up-to-date and practical information about hereditary cancer syndromes and cancer genetic counseling.

The photograph on the cover was taken on June 25, 1937 on the occasion of John and Alice Anderson's 35th wedding anniversary. They are shown with their 7 children, 3 son-in-laws and 4 grandchildren. This picture holds special meaning for me because my great-grandmother, grandmother, and mother are included in it.

Katherine Schneider

Acknowledgments

Although I am the sole author of this book, many, many people helped me along the way. First, I am indebted to my four reviewers, Robin Bennett, Miriam DiMaio, Stephanie Kieffer, and Robert Resta, who provided important feedback for each and every chapter. I am also grateful to my graphic artist, Caroline Woodcheke, who created the figures and tables with such perfection.

I also benefited from the insightful comments from the friends and colleagues who agreed to review one or more chapters. Thank you to Peter Ang, Shari Baldinger, Janice Berliner, Anu Chittenden, Lisa DiGianni, Charis Eng, Heather Gray, Annette Kennedy, Cheryl Medeiros-Nancarrow, Wendy McKinnon, Andrea Patenaude, Beth Peshkin, Robert Pilarski, June Peters, Kristen Shannon, Jill Stopfer, Vickie Venne, Sigitas Verselis, and Cate Walsh-Vockley. Further assistance with checking facts and tracking down references was provided by several genetic counseling interns, notably Tamsen Brown and Kari Brierley.

This book would not have been possible without the wonderful support I received from the colleagues I work with at the Dana-Farber Cancer Institute. From the understanding and support of my supervisors, Drs. Judy Garber and Frederick Li, to the encouragement of my co-workers in Population Sciences—Lisa DiGianni, Lynda Drake, Elaine Hiller, Jeff Johnson, Kathy Kalkbrenner, and Kylie Smith, and the Perini clinic group—Lisa Diller, Cheryl Medeiros-Nancarrow, Christopher Recklitis, and Ellen Casey. And a special thank you to my genetic counseling colleague and friend, Anu Chittenden, who cheerfully took on more than her share of work to provide me with protected time and could always be counted on to track down those elusive references. To all of you—I could not work with a better group of people! I would like to gratefully acknowledge the Jane Engelberg Memorial Fellowship, which supported the development of the first edition of this book in 1993. This special award is available to members of the National Society of Genetic Counselors and I am ever grateful for having received it.

Over the past 9 years, I have had the privilege of providing genetic counseling to numerous individuals and families who were dealing with heightened cancer risks and difficult decisions about genetic testing. I hope you learned as much from me as I learned from all of you.

I am also grateful to John Wiley & Sons, especially my editor, Luna Han, and associate managing editor, Kristin Cooke Fasano who helped walk me through this process and remained encouraging, despite my complete failure to meet deadlines.

Thank you also to my father, Donald Daviau, for his words of encouragement as I was writing this book and to my babysitter and friend, Laura Murray, who kept everything on the home front running so smoothly. Also, thanks to other special people in my life—Elisabeth DePristo, Susan Archer, and Karlen Lyons-Ruth for their emotional support and friendship.

And lastly, I want to acknowledge my three incredibly special sons—Nicholas, Christopher, and Jordan, who took my absences and distractions in stride and only mildly complained at taking more than my share of computer time. I hope they are very proud of "The Book," even though they are as puzzled by my fascination with genetics as I am of their love of alternative rock music.

Cancer Epidemiology

Epidemiologists are aware that cancer strikes neither capriciously nor randomly.
(McKinnell et al., 1998, p. 182)

Cancer epidemiologists seek to answer the question, "Why do certain individuals develop a particular cancer at a particular time?" Cancer epidemiology is the study of the frequency, causation, and distribution of cancer within a population. Chapter 1 provides current cancer statistics and a description of the many known or suspected causes of cancer.

1.1. Cancer Statistics

This section describes the incidence and mortality rates of specific cancers and the differences in cancer rates by ethnic group and geographic location. First, the terminology commonly used in cancer statistics is briefly reviewed:

1. *Incidence*—Incidence refers to the number of new events (i.e., cancer diagnoses or deaths) that have occurred in a defined population during a specified period of time. This term is the most frequently used in reports of cancer statistics. For example, in the fictitious city of Madison, there were 14,000 new cases of lung cancer in 2001. Therefore, the 2001 incidence of lung cancer in Madison is 14,000.

2. *Prevalence*—Prevalence is the number of disease cases (i.e., cancer cases) in a defined population at a designated time. Prevalence includes both individuals newly diagnosed with cancer (incidence) and those who are survivors of the disease. Thus, cancers with high

survival rates will have higher prevalence within a population than malignancies that cause rapid mortality. For example, in Madison, there were 14,000 new cases of lung cancer in 2001 and 5,000 lung cancer survivors. Thus, the 2001 prevalence of lung cancer in Madison is 19,000.

3. *Rate*—Rate is a way of measuring disease frequency that allows comparisons between populations or subsets of populations. Frequently used examples include the incidence rate, prevalence rate, and cancer survival rate. To obtain the incidence rate, divide the number of new cases over a fixed time interval by the number of people in the population during that time. It is also conventional to use a denominator of fixed size in order to compare the rate with other disorders or populations. For example, 14,000 new cases of lung cancer were diagnosed in Madison, which has a total population of 2 million. This means that the incidence rate of lung cancer in Madison is 0.7% or 700 cases per 100,000 people [14,000 (incidence) divided by 2 million (population)].

4. *Relative risk*—Relative risk is a ratio of risk between two populations or groups. A value of 1.0 means that there is no difference in the risks of cancer in two groups, whereas a value above 1.0 means that there is a higher risk in one group. For example, in the neighboring city of Jefferson, the incidence rate of lung cancer is only 300 per 100,000 people. Therefore, the people in Madison (with a lung cancer incidence rate of 700 per 100,000) have a relative risk of lung cancer that is 2.3 times higher than those living in Jefferson.

1.1.1. CANCER INCIDENCE IN THE UNITED STATES

Although often perceived as one disease, [cancer] is a number of diseases subsumed within one diagnostic label. It is often considered more frightening than other equally lethal illnesses. As one patient put it "Cancer is everyone's worst nightmare."

(Burton and Watson, 1998, p. 1)

Almost everyone has a relative or friend who has developed cancer. A glance at Table 1-1 will explain why—cancer is a very common disease. In the United States, women have a one in three chance of developing cancer over their lifetime and men have a one in two chance. Over 1 million new cases of cancer are diagnosed each year.

The risks of certain forms of cancer differ for men and women. In the United States, the most common form of cancer in men is prostate cancer; in women, it is breast cancer (see Table 1-2). For both sexes, lung cancer ranks second and colorectal cancer ranks third.

TABLE 1-1. PROBABILITY THAT MEN AND WOMEN IN THE UNITED STATES WILL DEVELOP INVASIVE CANCER OVER THEIR LIFETIME*

	Birth to 39	40 to 59	60 to 79	Overall
Men	1 in 61	1 in 12	1 in 3	1 in 2
Women	1 in 51	1 in 11	1 in 5	1 in 3

Source: American Cancer Society, 1999, p. 11.

*Excludes nonmelanoma skin cancer.

TABLE 1-2. MOST COMMON FORMS OF CANCER FOR MEN AND WOMEN IN THE UNITED STATES—2000 ESTIMATES

	Cancer	% Cases
Men	Prostate	29
	Lung and bronchus	13
	Colon and rectum	10
	Urinary bladder	6
	Non-Hodgkin lymphoma	5
	Melanoma of the skin	4
	Oral cavity	3
	Kidney	3
	Leukemia	3
	Pancreas	2
	All other sites	19
Women	Breast	30
	Lung and bronchus	12
	Colon and rectum	11
	Uterine corpus	6
	Ovary	4
	Non-Hodgkin lymphoma	4
	Melanoma of the skin	3
	Urinary bladder	2
	Pancreas	2
	Thyroid	2
	All other sites	24

Source: Greenlee et al., 2000, pp. 7–8.

The development of specific cancers peaks at certain ages, as shown in Table 1-3. In general, cancer risk increases with age, with the highest incidence occurring in people over age 65. This may be due to less effective immune responses in the elderly or a lifetime of exposures. Childhood

TABLE 1-3. AVERAGE AGES OF ONSET FOR SELECTED FORMS OF CANCER

	Cancer	Average age (yr)
Adult	Breast	>50
	Colon	67
	Kidney	50–70
	Lung	60
	Ovary	50–75
	Prostate	>65
Childhood	Brain tumor	5–10
	Leukemia (ALL)	4
	Neuroblastoma	2
	Osteosarcoma	16–18
	Retinoblastoma	1–2
	Wilms' tumor	<1

Source: Vogelstein and Kinzler, 1998; and Fromer, 1998.

TABLE 1-4. MOST FREQUENT TYPES OF CANCER FOR CHILDREN 19 YEARS AND YOUNGER (IN DECREASING ORDER OF FREQUENCY)

Leukemia
Brain tumor
Bone (osteosarcoma, Ewing sarcoma)
Non-Hodgkin lymphoma
Hodgkin disease
Soft tissue sarcoma
Wilms' tumor
Neuroblastoma
Rhabdomyosarcoma
Hepatic and endocrine tumors
Retinoblastoma

Source: Fromer, 1998.

cancers are relatively rare and account for less than 1% of all new cancer diagnoses. Table 1-4 lists the most frequent forms of childhood cancer.

1.1.2. CANCER-RELATED MORTALITY AND SURVIVAL IN THE UNITED STATES

As shown in Table 1-5, cancer remains one of the leading causes of death in the United States second only to heart disease. Despite the relative rarity of

TABLE 1 5. TEN LEADING CAUSES OF DEATH FOR TWO SPECIFIC AGE
GROUPS AND FOR ALL AGES (IN DECREASING ORDER OF FREQUENCY)

1–14 years old	25–44 years old	All Ages
Accidents	Accidents	Heart disease
Cancer	Cancer	Cancer
Congenital defects	Heart disease	Cerebrovascular disease
Homicide	Suicide	COPD*
Heart disease	HIV infection	Accidents
Pneumonia	Homicide	Pneumonia and influenza
Cerebral palsy	Chronic liver disease	Diabetes mellitus
Suicide	Cerebrovascular disease	Suicide
COPD*	Diabetes mellitus	Diseases of arteries
HIV infection	Pneumonia and influenza	Chronic liver disease

Source: Friedrich, 1999; Kubetin, 2000; and Greenlee, 2000, pp. 7–8.

*Chronic obstructive pulmonary disease.

cancer in children, it is one of the primary causes of death in this age group
as well. For adults aged 25–44, media attention focuses on violent deaths
(homicides and suicides), yet annual cancer deaths outnumber these two
categories combined.

It is encouraging to note that, over the past two decades, more people
are surviving cancer. The upward trend in cancer survival rates is due, in
part, to the ability to detect cancers at earlier, more treatable stages. Cancer-
related deaths peaked in 1991 and have decreased an average of 0.6% per
year between 1991 and 1996 (Greenlee et al., 2000). The greatest declines in
mortality rates have been among women and among individuals less than
65 years old. Specific mortality rates depend on the site of cancer, how
advanced the cancer is at diagnosis, and how amenable the cancer is to
treatment. As shown in Table 1-6, the highest number of cancer deaths is
from lung cancer, followed by prostate cancer in men and breast cancer in
women.

One commonly used marker in oncology is the 5-year relative survival
rate. This refers to the likelihood that a cancer patient will be alive (with
or without disease) 5 years after diagnosis, after adjustments are made for
normal life expectancy. It is estimated that the overall 5-year survival rate
for cancer is 60%. Because of this, genetic counselors will increasingly encounter clients who have personal histories of cancer. In fact, over 8 million
Americans are cancer survivors, and this number continues to rise.

Table 1-7 lists the 5-year relative survival rates for specific cancers.
Although 5-year survival rates for thyroid, testicular, and prostate cancer
are above 90%, several cancers have rates below 20%, including lung,
esophageal, liver, and pancreatic cancer.

TABLE 1-6. CANCER DEATHS BY SITE AND GENDER—2000 ESTIMATES (IN DECREASING ORDER OF FREQUENCY)

Men	Women
Lung and bronchus	Lung and bronchus
Prostate	Breast
Colon and rectum	Colon and rectum
Pancreas	Pancreas
Non-Hodgkin lymphoma	Ovary
Leukemia	Non-Hodgkin lymphoma
Esophagus	Leukemia
Liver and bile duct	Uterine corpus
Urinary bladder	Brain and other nervous system
Stomach	Stomach
	Multiple myeloma

Source: Greenlee et al., 2000, pp. 7–8.

TABLE 1-7. THE 5-YEAR RELATIVE SURVIVAL RATES OF SPECIFIC CANCERS

Site	% for all Stages
Testis	95
Thyroid	95
Prostate	93
Melanoma	88
Breast (female)	85
Uterine corpus	84
Urinary bladder	82
Uterine cervix	70
Larynx	66
Colon and rectum	62
Kidney	61
Oral cavity	53
Ovary	50
Stomach	21
Lung and bronchus	14
Esophagus	12
Liver	5
Pancreas	4

Source: American Cancer Society, 1999, p. 14.

TABLE 1-8. COMPARISON OF 5-YEAR RELATIVE SURVIVAL RATES FOR
WHITES AND BLACKS LIVING IN THE UNITED STATES, 1989–1994

Form of Cancer	Whites (%)	Blacks (%)
Breast (female)	87	71
Colon and rectum	64	52
Kidney	62	58
Leukemia	44	31
Lung and bronchus	15	11
Melanoma of the skin	88	69
Non-Hodgkin lymphoma	52	41
Oral cavity	55	32
Ovary	50	46
Pancreas	4	4
Prostate	95	81
Thyroid	96	88
Urinary bladder	84	62
Uterine corpus	87	54

Source: American Cancer Society, 1999, p. 16.

Cancer survival rates continue to be significantly lower for non-White Americans. Table 1-8 compares 5-year survival rates for White and Black Americans, which reveals that Black Americans have poorer survival rates for almost all the common cancers. The reasons for this discrepancy are complex but may include poorer access to health care, greater distrust of the medical care system, and less adequate insurance coverage.

1.1.3. INCIDENCE OF CANCER WORLDWIDE

Each year 10 million new cases of cancer are diagnosed worldwide. The estimated risks of cancer vary for different ethnic groups and geographic regions. This is primarily due to different lifestyles and exposures to carcinogens. Of course, genetics play a role as well, but immigrants who move to the United States often have cancer rates indistinguishable from other Americans by the first or second generation.

On the basis of 1985 statistics, the leading cancers worldwide are lung, stomach, breast, colon and rectum, and cervix (Boyle, 1997). Table 1-9 lists the specific countries with the highest and lowest frequencies of specific malignancies. It is important to be aware of the specific population rates of cancer when considering the likelihood of an inherited etiology. For example, the occurrence of breast cancer in two female relatives living in

TABLE 1-9. COUNTRIES OR REGIONS WITH THE HIGHEST AND LOWEST
RATES OF SPECIFIC MALIGNANCIES

Form of Cancer	Highest Rates	Lowest Rates
Breast (female)	United States and Canada, South America (esp. Brazil), Northern Europe	Central & Eastern Europe, Japan, China, Africa (excluding S. Africa)
Cervix	Caribbean, Sub-Saharan Africa, Central and South America	Developed Countries, China, Western Asia
Colon	Australia and New Zealand, United States and Canada, Northern and Western Europe	Asia
Esophagus	Iran, China	Eastern Europe
Liver	Western and Central Africa, China, Eastern and Southwest Asia, Mali	Developed countries
Lung	New Zealand (esp. Maoris), United States (esp. Blacks)	India, Africa and Southern Asia, South America
Melanoma	Australia (esp. Queensland), United States and Canada	Africa (non-Whites), South America (non-Whites)
Prostate	Northern and Western Europe, United States and Canada, Australia/New Zealand, Caribbean, Sub-Saharan Africa, South America	China, Asia, Northern Africa
Stomach	China, Japan, Eastern Europe, Soviet Union, South America	United States and Canada, Africa, South and Southeast Asia

Source: Boyle, 1997; and Parkin et al., 1999.

Japan or China is much more striking than two similarly affected relatives in the United States or Canada. Conversely, a family history of stomach cancer, although rare in North America, is much more commonplace in Asia. One's ethnicity may also play a role in the level of cancer risk: Black Americans, for example, have the lowest rates of melanoma, but the highest rates of lung cancer in the world.

1.2. CANCER ETIOLOGY

Epidemiology provides compelling evidence that many cancers may be avoidable.

(Osborne et al., 1997, p. 27)

TABLE 1-10. THE ESTIMATED AMOUNT OF CANCER CASES ATTRIBUTED TO SPECIFIC RISK FACTORS (IN DECREASING ORDER OF FREQUENCY)

Risk Factors	Cases (%)
Diet	35
Tobacco use	30
Hereditary factors	5–10
Occupational exposures	5
Radiation	1–2
Viruses	1–2
Miscellaneous	16–23

Source: Offit, 1998, p. 34.

In 1883, Sir Percival Potts in London noted that young boys who worked as chimney sweeps developed scrotal cancer at higher than usual rates. This was the first documented report link between an environmental exposure and cancer development. A century later, numerous factors in our environment are known or suspected to cause cancer.

Cancer may develop because of a complex mix of environmental and genetic factors. For some people, environmental factors pose the greatest risk of malignancy; for others, it is their inherited susceptibilities to cancer. In the majority of cases, it is a combination of these factors that leads to cancer development. At this time, the interaction between genetic and environmental risk factors remains poorly understood. For example, the extent to which lifestyle changes can modify the cancer risk in individuals with inherited predispositions to cancer is unclear.

Hereditary factors are the primary underlying source of cancer in only 5–10% of cases. About 65% of cases are thought to be due to either dietary factors or tobacco exposure (see Table 1-10). Other nonhereditary factors may also be important contributors in the occurrence of specific malignancies. Therefore, to calculate a client's cancer risk, genetic counselors may need to consider nonhereditary factors, such as lifestyle risk factors, viral exposures, chronic medical conditions, and occupational exposures.

1.2.1. LIFESTYLE AND ENVIRONMENTAL RISK FACTORS

One's lifestyle and surrounding environment can alter the risks of specific forms of cancer. Table 1-11 lists the cancers associated with dietary, tobacco, radiation, and hormonal exposures.

1. *Diet*—The main dietary risk factor for cancer is alcohol. Moderate or heavy alcohol consumption is associated with a number of cancers,

TABLE 1-11. LIFESTYLE AND ENVIRONMENTAL AGENTS KNOWN OR
SUSPECTED TO BE CARCINOGENIC

Agent	Cancer
Diet	
Alcohol	Mouth, pharynx, larynx, esophagus, liver, breast, colon
Alflatoxins (moldy peanuts)	Colon, rectal
Fat intake	Colon, prostate
Salt	Stomach
Nitate/nitrite (cured/smoked foods)	Stomach
Tobacco (cigarette/pipe smoking, chewing tobacco, or snuff)	Mouth, pharynx, larynx, esophagus, stomach, lung, kidney, pancreas, bladder, cervix
Radiation	
Atomic bomb	Most forms of cancer
Excessive sunlight	Skin, lip
Ionizing radiation	Skin, bone, soft tissue, prostate, ovary, breast, leukemia, lung
Radon	Lung, bronchus
Ultraviolet radiation	Skin, lip
X-rays	Brain, nervous system
Hormones/Medications	
DES	Vagina
Estrogen	Uterus
Testosterone	Prostate
Alkylating agents (chemotherapy)	Leukemia

Source: Tannock and Hill, 1998; and Offit, 1998, p. 34.

including cancer of the mouth, pharynx, larynx, liver, breast, and colon. Variations in diet may account for some of the geographic differences in rates of specific cancer. For example, gastric cancer has been associated with frequent ingestion of foods that have been salt-cured, smoked, or pickled.

2. *Tobacco*—About one-third of cancer deaths worldwide are directly related to cigarettes and smokeless tobacco (chewing tobacco or snuff). This makes tobacco the single most important avoidable cancer-causing agent. Secondhand exposure to tobacco, termed passive smoking, has also been determined to be carcinogenic. The smoking prevalence in the United States has remained steady over the past several years (approximately 25% of all adults). However, rates of smoking continue to rise in other countries, particularly in Japan, China, and Central and Eastern Europe. The most alarming

trend is the increased prevalence of smoking among women world-wide. If this trend continues, lung cancer is expected to surpass breast cancer in terms of cancer-related deaths.

3. *Radiation*—Natural radiation is emitted from cosmic rays (sunlight) and certain rock minerals. Another source of radiation is radon, which emanates from building materials and is associated with poor ventilation. Long-term exposures to natural radiation and radon increase the risks of certain cancers, especially cancers of the skin, lip, and lung. The link between radiation exposure and malignancy was most conclusively demonstrated by the dramatically high rates of malignancy observed among survivors of the atomic bomb attacks in Hiroshima and Nagasaki during World War II. Excessive exposure to ionizing radiation, such as repeated X-rays and radiation therapy, is associated with increased rates of leukemia, bone cancer, and other solid tumors. (See Chapter 2 for more information about radiation therapy.)

4. *Hormones/medications*—In the 1950s, expectant mothers were given a new drug called diethylstilbestrol (DES) to prevent recurrent miscarriages. Twenty years later, it was recognized that women exposed to DES in the womb (so-called DES daughters) have higher rates of clear cell vaginal carcinomas.. Estrogen is a key ingredient in birth control pills and hormone replacement therapy and is associated with increased risks of endometrial cancer. Certain medications may also be carcinogenic. As examples, tamoxifen, an antihormonal agent, is associated with increased risks of uterine cancer and alkylating agents, used for chemotherapy, increase risks of leukemia. (See Chapter 2 for more information about alkylating agents.)

1.2.2. Viruses and Medical Conditions

As shown in Table 1-12, certain viruses and chronic medical conditions are associated with higher rates of malignancy.

1. *Viruses*—At one point, cancer research focused heavily on viruses as cancer-causing agents. As it turns out, only 1–2% of cancer cases can be attributed to viruses, although certain malignancies are more likely to be virally-induced. One example is cervical cancer, which causes about 300,000 deaths annually worldwide. Other examples include hepatitis B (liver cancer), human papilloma virus (genital and skin cancers), and Epstein-Barr virus (lymphoma and nasopharynx cancer). Acquired immune deficiency syndrome (AIDS), which suppresses the immune system response, is associated with lymphoma and Kaposi sarcoma. There are also certain infections linked with

TABLE 1-12. BIOLOGICAL AGENTS AND CHRONIC CONDITIONS KNOWN OR
SUSPECTED TO BE CARCINOGENIC

Agent	Cancer
Virus/infection	
Epstein-Barr virus	Sinus, pharynx, Hodgkin disease, Burkitt's lymphoma
Hepatitis B	Liver
Human papilloma virus	Skin, genital (esp. cervix)
Human T-lymphocytic virus I (HTLVI)	Non-Hodgkin lymphoma, adult T-cell leukemia
Human immunodeficiency virus (HIV)	Non-Hodgkin lymphoma, Kaposi's sarcoma
H. pylori infection	Stomach
Schistosomiasis (a parasitic infection)	Bladder, liver, intestinal
Chronic condition	
Autoimmune disease	Lymphoma
Celiac disease	Colon, lymphoma, small intestine
Crohn's disease	Colon
Diabetes	Uterus, vulva
Gall stones	Gall bladder
Gynecomastia (male)	Breast
Hemachromatosis	Liver
Hypertension	Uterus
Iron deficiency	Esophagus, mouth, pharynx
Nevi (multiple)	Skin (melanoma)
Obesity	Uterus
Pernicious anemia	Stomach
Polycystic kidney disease	Kidney
Polycythemia	Leukemia
Ulcerative colitis	Colon, rectum
Varicose veins	Skin

Source: Tannock and Hill, 1998; and Offit, 1998.

specific cancers, such as *H. pylori* infection (stomach cancer) and schistosomiasis (bladder, liver, intestinal cancers).

2. *Chronic conditions*—Some chronic diseases or medical conditions can over time lead to certain forms of cancer. One such condition is colitis, which is a series of inflammations in the colon that is associated with a 30% lifetime risk of colorectal cancer. There are also conditions that can be triggered by the same mechanisms that lead to malignancy, such as the increased rate of diabetes in families with familial pancreatic cancer.

TABLE 1-13. OCCUPATIONAL EXPOSURES KNOWN OR SUSPECTED TO BE CARCINOGENIC

Agent	Cancer
Arsenic (mines, smelting, pesticide)	Skin, lung, liver
Asbestos (shipyard, insulation workers)	Bronchus, lung, pleura, mesothelioma
Aromatic amines (dye workers)	Bladder
Benzene (varnishes, glue)	Leukemia
Bis-ether (chemical workers)	Lung
Benzidine (dye, rubber workers)	Bladder
Chromium (metal workers)	Lung
Coal tar	Skin, lung
Hardwood manufacture	Nasal, sinus
Hematite mining	Lung
Isopropyl alcohol (furniture making)	Nasal, sinus
Leather dust (boot and shoe workers)	Nasal, bladder
Naphthylamine (dye, rubber workers)	Bladder
Nickel dust (nickel refining)	Nasal, lung
Pesticides	Lymphoma
Polycyclic hydrocarbons (soot, ore)	Lung, scrotum, skin
Radon (mining)	Lung, bronchus
Shoe manufacture	Nasal, sinus
Soot, tar, oil (coal, gas and petroleum workers)	Bladder, lung, skin
Uranium	Lung
Vinyl chloride (PVC manufacturers)	Liver, soft tissue

Source: Tannock and Hill, 1998; Offit, 1998, p. 34; and Cooper, 1992, p. 54.

1.2.3. OCCUPATIONAL RISK FACTORS

About 5% of cancer cases are attributed to occupational exposures (see Table 1-13). Manufacturing and mining are among the most hazardous professions in terms of cancer risks.

1. *Manufacturing*—Factory workers can be exposed to a variety of carcinogenic agents, usually airborne. For example, workers in the dye industry are exposed to aromatic amines, benzidine and napthylamine and, therefore, have higher risks of mesothelioma and cancers of the lung, nasal passages, and sinuses. Manufacturers of shoes, hardwood floors, and furniture have documented increased risks of cancer, particularly lung cancer.

2. *Mining*—Miners are continually exposed to air that is concentrated with minerals and dust, including arsenic, radon, polycyclic

hydrocarbons, and hematite. Miners may be at increased risk for developing lymphoma and cancer of the skin, lung, liver, and nasal sinus.

1.2.4. RISK FACTORS FOR BREAST, COLON, AND OVARIAN CANCER

Individuals at risk for breast, colon, and/or ovarian cancer comprise the largest segment of any high-risk cancer program. This section describes the established risk factors for breast, colon, and ovarian cancer. (See Chapter 4 for information about hereditary breast, colon, and ovarian cancer syndromes.) It remains unclear whether the presence of these risk factors further increase cancer risks in those with inherited susceptibilities.

1. *Breast cancer*—Among women, breast cancer is the most common form of cancer. The lifetime risk for breast cancer in North America is about 12%. Rates of breast cancer have increased steadily from a generation ago especially among premenopausal women. However, the risks of breast cancer substantially increase with age (see Table 1-14). The most important contributors to breast cancer risk, after gender and age, are hormonal and reproductive factors (see Table 1-15). Higher risks of breast cancer are associated with early menarche, late menopause, and delayed childbearing until after age 30 or never having a biological child (nulliparity). Alcohol use has been shown to increase risks of breast cancer, but other dietary factors have not been conclusively shown to increase risk. Family history is an important risk factor. The presence of a first-degree relative with breast cancer increases the risk 1.5- to 4.0-fold, depending on the age of the affected family member. About 1% of breast cancers occur in men. For men, important risk factors are family history, gynecomastia, and Klinefelter syndrome.

TABLE 1-14. ESTIMATED BREAST CANCER RISKS BY AGE

Age	Risk
<25	1/19,608
<35	1/622
<50	1/50
<65	1/17
<85	1/9
Ever	1/8

Source: Feuer et al., 1993.

TABLE 1-15. KNOWN AND SUSPECTED RISK FACTORS FOR BREAST CANCER

Age >40 yr
Alcohol intake (>3 drinks per week)
Benign breast disease (atypical hyperplasia)
Delayed childbearing (>30 yr at 1st birth)
Early menarche (<14 yr)
Estrogen replacement therapy
Family history of breast or ovarian cancer
Female gender
Hormone use (estrogen replacement therapy)
Nulliparity (no biological children)
Late menopause (>55 yr)
Obesity
Previous malignant disease
Proliferative breast disease
Radiation to breasts

Source: Couch and Weber, 1998; and Offit, 1998, pp. 67–69.

TABLE 1-16. KNOWN AND SUSPECTED RISK FACTORS FOR COLON CANCER

Age > 50
Alcohol
Cigarettes
Colorectal polyps (adenomatous polyps)
Chronic disease of the bowel (Crohn's disease, inflammatory bowel disease, ulcerative colitis)
Family history of colon or other related cancers
High fat intake (>40% total intake)
High red meat intake
Low fiber intake
Obesity
Radiation to pelvic area
Ulcerative colitis

Source: Kinzler and Vogelstein, 1998; and American Cancer Society, 1999, p. 20.

2. *Colon cancer*—Colon cancer is the second most common cancer occurring worldwide. In North America, the risk of colon cancer to age 90 is about 6%. The incidence of colorectal cancers is higher after age 50 and is somewhat higher in men. The greatest contributors to colon cancer risk are ingested substances, including alcohol, cigarettes, and high intake of fat and/or red meat (see Table 1-16). Having one affected first-degree relative increases the risk of colon cancer by

TABLE 1-17. KNOWN AND SUSPECTED RISK FACTORS FOR OVARIAN CANCER

Daily talcum powder use (due to asbestos particles)
Delayed childbearing
Family history of ovarian, breast, or colon cancer
High lactose intake (dietary galactose)
Infertility
Nulliparity/low parity

Source: Offit, 1998, p. 115.

three- to fourfold and having several relatives with colorectal cancer may be consistent with a hereditary cancer syndrome.

3. *Ovarian cancer*—Ovarian cancer is the fifth most common type of cancer among women in the United States. The lifetime risk of ovarian cancer in North America is about 1-2%. There is a short list of risk factors that can increase the risk of ovarian cancer (see Table 1-17). Reproductive history is important, with risks of ovarian cancer higher in women who have few or no children or who have delayed childbearing. Other exposures that contribute to ovarian cancer risk are long-term daily use of talcum powder (which contains asbestos) and a high lactose intake. Family history of ovarian cancer increases the risk by threefold. Family history of breast or colon cancer may also suggest an increased risk of ovarian cancer.

1.3. REFERENCES

American Cancer Society. 1999. Cancer Facts and Figures—1999. American Cancer Society, Atlanta, GA.
American Cancer Society. 2000. Cancer Facts and Figures—2000. American Cancer Society, Atlanta, GA.
Boyle P. 1997. Global burden of cancer. Lancet 349, Suppl II:23–26.
Burton M and Watson M. 1998. Having cancer: the patient's experience. In Counselling People With Cancer. John Wiley & Sons, New York, NY, 1-13.
Cooper G. 1992. Elements of Human Cancer. Jones and Bartlett, Boston, MA.
Couch F and Weber B. 1998. Breast cancer. In Vogelstein B and Kinzler K (eds) The Genetic Basis of Human Cancer. McGraw-Hill, New York, NY, 537-563.
Feuer E, Wun L, Boring C, et al. . 1993. The lifetime risk of developing breast cancer. J Natl Cancer Inst 85:892–897.
Friedrich MJ. 1999. Report documents causes of child death. JAMA 282:1903–1905.
Fromer M. 1998. What cancer is. In Surviving Childhood Cancer: A Guide for Families. New Harbinger Publishers, Oakland, CA, 47-60.
Greenlee R, Murray T, Bolden S, et al. . 2000. Cancer statistics, 2000. CA Cancer J Clin 50:7–33.

Kinzler K and Vogelstein B. 1998. Colorectal tumors. In The Genetic Basis of Human Cancer. McGraw-Hill, New York, NY, 568.

Kubetin S. 2000. Top 10 causes of death in 25- to 44-year olds. Ob Gyn News 35:21.

McKinnell R, Parchment R, Perantoni A, et al. 1998. Epidemiology. In McKinnell et al (eds) The Biological Basis of Cancer. Cambridge University Press, Cambridge, UK, 181–217.

McLaughlin J and Boyd N. 1998. Epidemiology of cancer. In Tannock I and Hill P (eds) The Basic Science of Oncology, 3rd edition. McGraw-Hill, New York, NY, 6–25.

National Cancer Institute. 1992. Cancer Statistics Review 1973–1989, National Cancer Institute, Bethesda, MD.

Offit K. 1998. Clinical Cancer Genetics. Risk Counseling and Management. John Wiley & Sons New York, NY.

Osborne M, Boyle P, and Lipkin M. 1997. Cancer prevention. The Lancet 349, Suppl. II:27–30.

Parker S, Davis K, Wingo P et al. 1998. Cancer statistics by race and ethnicity. CA Cancer J Clin 48:31–48.

Parkin D, Pisani P, and Ferlay J. 1999. Global cancer statistics. CA Cancer J Clin 49:33–64.

Rees G, Goodman S, and Bullimore J. 1993. General principles. In Cancer in Practice. Butterworth Heinemann, Oxford, UK, 1–97

Vogelstein B and Kinzler K. 1998. The Genetic Basis of Human Cancer. McGraw-Hill, New York, NY.

Cancer Detection, Treatment, and Prevention

[Cancer] is an unseen enemy: it is part of our body, yet not part of our body. We use powerful combative language to describe it. We talk about cancer "victims," about "fighting" cancer and about how cancer "invades" the body. We are none of us wholly immune to the fears.

(Burton and Watson, 1998, p. 1)

A cancer genetic counseling session often begins with hearing the client's "cancer story"—the symptoms that led to the suspicion of cancer, the way in which the diagnosis was finally made, and the success or failure of treatment. It is important for genetic counselors to become familiar with cancer treatment, detection, and prevention strategies in order to be able to understand the stories of our clients. Chapter 2 describes the process of making a cancer diagnosis, the system used to classify tumors, the ways in which cancers are treated, and current prevention strategies. The focus will be on cancer in general, although whenever possible, issues unique to inherited cancers will be described. Chapter 2 ends with a special section detailing the detection, treatment, and prevention of breast, colon, and ovarian cancers.

2.1. THE DIAGNOSIS OF CANCER

This section provides the information necessary to understanding a cancer diagnosis, from how cancer is diagnosed to the nomenclature used to describe the tumor.

2.1.1. CANCER DETECTION

Initial detection of a tumor is often made through a routine clinical exam or screening test. A physical exam may reveal a palpable growth, swollen lymph gland, or other sign of cancer. A routine screening test, such as a urine test, cervical Pap smear, or blood test, may identify the presence of atypical cells, tumor markers, or a heightened immune response. For example, a blood specimen that shows a dramatically high count of "blasts" (immature white blood cells) in a young child may point to the presence of acute lymphoblastic leukemia.

In many cases, the patients themselves have noticed symptoms suggestive of cancer. They may have noticed a new physical finding, such as an unusual mole or lump, that leads them to seek medical attention, or they may be experiencing health problems that are either not abating over time (such as flu-like symptoms) or are continuing to worsen (such as gastrointestinal upset).

A malignant tumor can be present for months, even years, before it is detected. The reasons why cancer detection can be so difficult include the following:

1. *There may be no signs or symptoms*—There may be no physical symptoms that signal the presence of early-stage cancer. Observable signs of cancer are more likely to be noticed as the cancer progresses. Unfortunately, this means that the earliest signs of cancer detected by a patient, such as a lump, excessive bruising, blood in stool, or unexplained pain, often means the malignancy is already in an intermediate or advanced stage. In fact, it is not unusual for clients to report that their early somatic complaints were ignored or "misdiagnosed" by their physicians. Although it is important to validate the client's experience, counselors must recognize that a delay in diagnosis generally reflects the insidious nature of cancer rather than medical malpractice.

2. *Screening methods are imperfect*—Screening tests need to be easy to perform, be cost-effective, be accurate in detecting disease cases, and have the potential to reduce mortality rates. To have an impact on mortality rates, the tests must be able to detect the cancers at earlier stages. Screening tests are justifiable when the malignancy is fairly common and early diagnosis can clearly make a difference in survival. Routine screening is not always recommended for commonly occurring cancers because it may not improve survival rates. For example, cigarette smokers are no longer recommended to obtain annual chest X-rays because detection of lung tumors by X-rays versus waiting until symptoms develop (typically weeks later) does

not seem to alter lung cancer mortality rates. Screening tests for the less common types of cancer, such as retinoblastoma, are offered only to children known to be at high risk because the screening procedure, which occurs under general anesthesia, is not without its own risks. Clients may not understand why certain monitoring tests are not routinely offered. For example, women with personal or family histories of ovarian cancer may argue that all women should be screened with vaginal ultrasounds and CA-125 blood tests. Although counselors can explain the limited utility of these screening tests, they need to also recognize and acknowledge the clients' underlying sources of frustration (and fear).

3. *Premalignant cells are rarely identifiable*—The understanding that cancer is a multistep process has created optimism that it will someday be possible to identify cancer cells before a malignant tumor has formed. At this point, early stages of tumor development have been well-characterized for only a few types of cancer, including cancers of the colon and cervix, and the currently available tumor marker screening tests continue to be plagued with unacceptable levels of false positives and false negatives. One exception might be the alpha-fetoprotein test, used in China and Southeast Asia to detect hepatoma, which has high sensitivity and specificity.

2.1.2. MAKING THE DIAGNOSIS OF CANCER

The workup for cancer typically begins when other more likely explanations have been ruled out. For example, the differential diagnosis of frequent headaches includes flu, allergies, and stress. More serious possibilities, such as a brain tumor or a neurological problem, are less likely to be entertained at the outset because of their relative rarity. Unfortunately, a common complaint among members of families with hereditary cancer syndromes is that signs of cancer were initially ignored or downplayed by their health care providers.

The method by which the cancer will be identified depends on the tumor type. Diagnostic tests include imaging studies (X-ray, CT scan, or MRI), specialized blood tests (tumor markers, chromosome studies), invasive procedures (endoscopy, laproscopy), and biopsy (of bone marrow, lymph node). For example, the diagnosis of renal cell carcinoma typically involves a urine test and either an abdominal X-ray or CT scan. (See Section 2.5 for specifics about breast, colon, and ovarian cancer.) There may be a delay of several days or longer from the time of the diagnostic procedures to the final confirmation of the diagnosis.

Individuals are referred to an oncologist either when the suspicion of cancer has been raised or after the initial diagnosis. As with most medical specialties, clinical oncology is divided into many subspecialties. Individuals may also be referred to a surgical oncologist and/or radiation therapist; the care of individuals with cancer requires a multidisciplinary team. The team of providers may not always be located at the same institution which may cause clients to feel as though their care is fragmented.

Cancer can be a high-burden disease on both patients and their families. Learning that one has cancer can engender feelings of shock, anger, intense sadness, and extreme anxiety. As patients enter cancer treatment, they often need to make major adjustments in terms of their family and work responsibilities. At many cancer centers, patients and their families have the opportunity to meet with a social worker or psychologist. Patient support groups may also be helpful.

2.1.3. CANCER TERMINOLOGY

> It is not naming as such that is pejorative or damning, but the name "cancer." As long as a particular disease is treated as an evil, invincible predator, not just a disease, most people with cancer will indeed be demoralized by learning what disease they have. The solution is hardly to stop telling cancer patients the truth, but to rectify the conception of the disease, to de-mythicize it.
>
> *(Sontag, 1977, p. 7)*

Hippocrates named the hard, gray tissue extending from a tumor to normal tissue "karkinoma" for its crab-like appearance. The Latin word for crab is "cancer," which continues to be used to describe all malignant tumors.

The terminology used to describe specific tumors can be daunting, and it may be helpful to consider how these names are derived. Tumor nomenclature provides information about where in the body and in what type of tissue and cell the cancer originated.

1. *Site of origin*—The medical term for a tumor is a neoplasm, which literally means new growth. Neoplasms can develop in almost every tissue of the body. The name of a neoplasm will first indicate the site in the body where the cancer has originated. As examples, a hepatocellular carcinoma is a liver cancer and a rhabdomyosarcoma is a tumor of the striated muscle. For a list of the names of different tumors for the major organs and systems of the body, see Table 2-1.

2. *Tissue type*—The type of tissue in which the neoplasm has occurred will also be indicated within the name of the tumor. The major types of neoplasms are carcinomas, sarcomas, leukemias, and lymphomas.

TABLE 2-1. SELECTED LIST OF CANCER TYPES BY ORGAN SYSTEM

Organ System	Tissue Type	Name of Tumor
Breast		Ductal, lobular, medullary, comedo, colloid, papillary carcinomas
Circulatory/ lymphatic systems	Blood vessels	Hemangiosarcoma and Kaposi sarcoma
	All blood cells	Chronic myelogenous leukemia
	Erythrocytes	Acute erythrocytic leukemia
	Granulocytes	Acute myelo- and acute promyelocytic leukemias
	Lymphocytes	Acute lymphocytic and chronic lymphocytic leukemias, Hodgkin's and non Hodgkin lymphomas
	Monocytes	Acute monocytic leukemia
	Megakaryocytes	Acute megakaryocytic leukemia
Connective tissue	Fibrous tissue	Fibrosarcoma
	Fat	Liposarcoma
	Bone	Osteo- and Ewing's sarcomas
	Cartilage	Chondrosarcoma
Digestive system	Esophagus	Adeno- and squamous cell carcinomas
	Stomach	Adenocarcinoma and mesothelioma leiomyosarcoma and lymphoma
	Liver	Cholangio-, hemangio-, and heptocellular carcinomas
	Gall bladder	Adenocarcinoma
	Pancreas	Duct cell adeno-, cystadeno-, giant cell, and colloid carcinomas
	Colorectum	Adenocarcinoma
	Anus	Squamous cell carcinoma
Head and neck	Oral cavity (lip, Tongue, mouth)	Squamous cell carcinoma
	Tonsils	Squamous cell carcinoma
	Nasal cavity	Squamous cell carcinoma
	Nasopharynx	Adenocarcinoma
	Sinuses	Adenocarcinoma
	Eye	Retinoblastoma
Muscle	Smooth	Leiomyosarcoma
	Striated	Rhabdomyosarcoma
Nervous system	Brain	Astrocytoma, glioblastoma, and medulloblastoma
	Nerve cells	Neuroblastoma and neurofibrosarcoma
Reproductive tract (male)	Prostate	Adenocarcinoma
	Testis	Seminoma; chorio-, embryonal, and yolk sac carcinomas, Teratoma
	Penis	Squamous cell carcinoma
Reproductive tract (female)	Ovary	Adeno-, chorio-, and yolk sac carcinomas, teratoma and Brenner tumor
	Endometrium	Squamous cell carcinoma
	Cervix	Squamous cell carcinoma
	Vulva	Squamous cell carcinoma
Respiratory system	Larynx	Squamous cell carcinoma
	Lung	Adeno-, squamous cell, small cell, and large cell carcinomas

Source: Cooper, 1992.

TABLE 2-2. EMBRYONIC ORIGIN OF TISSUE DETERMINES TUMOR TYPE

Embryonic Tissue	Tissue Type	Cancer
Ectoderm	Skin, nervous system	Carcinoma
Mesoderm	Bone, muscle	Sarcoma
	Blood, lymphatic system	Leukemia, lymphoma
Endoderm	Lining of internal organs	Carcinoma

- *Carcinomas* occur in the epithelial cells covering the surface of the body and lining the internal organs. Carcinomas account for about 90% of all cancer.
- *Sarcomas* are the rarest form of neoplasm. Sarcomas are solid tumors occurring in connective tissues, muscle, and bone.
- *Leukemias and lymphomas* are cancers occurring in the circulatory or lymphatic systems and comprise about 8% of all cancer.

As shown in Table 2-2, the rationale underlying the classification of tumors into these three subgroups can be found in embryology. In the early embryo, there are three layers of germ cells termed the ectoderm, the mesoderm, and the endoderm.

- The *ectoderm* gives rise to the skin and nervous system.
- The *mesoderm* gives rise to supporting tissues, such as bone, muscle, and blood.
- The *endoderm* gives rise to the epithelial lining of the internal organs, such as the liver, stomach, and lungs.

Carcinomas are neoplasms that have occurred in tissues of ectodermal or endodermal origin, whereas sarcomas occur in tissues of mesodermal origin. Leukemias and lymphomas are considered a subset of sarcomas, since they also arise in tissues of mesodermal origin. Leukemias (which literally means "white blood") are actually sarcomas of leukocytes, whereas lymphomas are sarcomas of reticuloendothelial cells.

3. *Cell type*—The name of a tumor will often describe the type of cell that has transformed into a cancer cell. Tissues of the body are generally composed of more than one type of cell. Solid tumors can arise from adenomatous cells that are glandular or ductal or squamous cells that are flat. Tumors containing cells with features of both glandular and squamous cells are called transitional cell carcinomas. Leukemias can arise from any of the various cells derived from myeloid or lymphoid

lineages. Lymphomas occur in lymphocytes or macrophages, which are two types of cells from the lymphoid branch.

4. *Exceptions*—Not all tumors are classified by these cell and tissue types. For example, cancers that resemble embryonic tissue are called blastomas. Examples include neuroblastomas and retinoblastomas. Another exception are teratomas, which arise in tissues derived from all three germ cell layers. To further complicate matters, some tumors have been named after the physicians who discovered them. These include Ewing sarcoma, Hodgkin disease, Kaposi sarcoma, and Wilms' tumor.

2.1.4. PRIMARY CANCER OR RECURRENCE

How should the cancers in the following scenario be categorized?

Your client explains that her mother was successfully treated for osteosarcoma at age 9 and was well until age 53 when she was diagnosed and treated for invasive breast cancer. Two years later, cancer cells were found in her liver and she died a few months later at age 55.

In deciphering a pattern of cancer in the family, it is important to determine whether a malignancy represents a primary cancer or is a recurrence of the initial tumor. In the above scenario, the mother's primary cancer is osteosarcoma, her breast cancer is a second primary, and the liver cancer most likely represents metastatic breast cancer .

1. *Primary cancer*—A newly arisen tumor is considered a primary tumor. Individuals can develop more than one primary cancer, although this is uncommon. These second (or third) primaries may occur as a consequence of treating the initial cancer. For example, women with Hodgkin disease who are treated with radiation therapy have higher rates of breast cancer. Multiple primary cancers are also more likely in those with hereditary cancer syndromes. For example, one individual referred to our center reported an uncle with Muir-Torre syndrome who had developed a total of nine separate primaries!

2. *Recurrence*—A recurrence is the reappearance of cancer cells, either at the site of origin (local recurrence) or elsewhere in the body (metastasis). Metastasis can be defined as discontinuous tumor growth. Metastatic cancers generally have a poorer prognosis than cancers that recur locally.

2.2. TUMOR CLASSIFICATION

The tumor classification system helps dictate treatment regimens, predict prognosis, and provide a systematic approach that can be universally recognized and understood. Tumors are assessed for malignant properties or potential and, if malignant, are graded and staged.

2.2.1. BENIGN OR MALIGNANT

The word "tumor" conjures up an image of cancer, yet not all tumors are cancerous. Thus, a lipoma (benign tumor of fat cells) may not be clinically significant, whereas a liposarcoma (malignant tumor of fat cells) represents a serious cancerous tumor. One of the initial steps in cancer diagnosis is to send a tumor specimen to a pathologist, who will determine whether the tumor has any malignant characteristics.

There are several differences between benign and malignant tumors. The most significant difference is that benign tumors do not spread to other sites of the body, whereas all malignant tumors have at least some metastatic potential. Benign tumors tend to be slow growing and innocuous. They are usually enclosed in a fibrous capsule and are not considered cancerous. Malignant tumors, in contrast, can proliferate rapidly and will, over time, spread to neighboring tissues.

Despite the name, "benign" tumors are not always innocuous and can in fact cause significant risks of morbidity and mortality due to the following factors:

1. *Location and size*—As a benign tumor grows, it may press against the normal surrounding tissue. This compression of the normal cell parenchyma can cause the normal cells to atrophy due to insufficient blood supply. In some sites of the body, there is sufficient space to tolerate a benign tumor. One example is the female uterus, in which fibroid tumors can grow to be quite large. In other sites, notably the brain and spine, there is little room for expansion, and even moderately sized tumors can cause significant morbidity and mortality.

2. *Excretion of hormones*—Benign tumors typically resemble their normal cell counterparts, which can be problematic if the cell type is hormone-secreting. The benign tumor, not constrained by normal cell regulatory systems, may begin to produce additional amounts of hormones. Although benign tumors are generally less efficient at hormone production than normal cells, the sheer volume of tumor cells can result in massive—and toxic—levels of hormone being produced. For example, a pheochromocytoma is a benign tumor of the adrenal gland that produces the hormone epinephrine that triggers the "fight or flight" response. Excess levels of epinephrine caused by the pheochromocytoma can result in alarmingly high blood pressure and, if untreated, can result in stroke or myocardial infarction.

TABLE 2-3. Benign and Malignant Tumors for Specific Sites or the Body

Site of Origin	Benign Tumor	Malignant Tumor
Blood vessels	Hemangioma	Angiosarcoma
Bone	Osteoma	Osteosarcoma
Fat	Lipoma	Liposarcoma
Glandular or ductal epithelium	Adenoma	Adenocarcinoma
Lymph vessels	Lymphangioma	Lymphangiosarcoma
Melanocytes	Nevus	Malignant melanoma
Nerve cells	Ganglioneuroma	Neuroblastoma
Smooth muscle	Leiomyoma	Leiomyosarcoma
Squamous cells	Papilloma	Carcinoma
Striated muscle	Rhabdomyoma	Rhabdomyosarcoma
Transitional cells	Papilloma	Carcinoma

Source: Pfeifer and Wick, 1991, p. 8.

In some cases, a benign tumor can be considered a precancerous tumor, i.e., a tumor with malignant potential. Cells proceed through multiple steps before reaching a malignant state, and some benign tumors may actually be malignant precursors. This has been shown to be the case for several types of cancer, such as pigmented moles (nevi) that can evolve into malignant melanoma and adenomas of the colon, which can eventually transform into adenocarcinomas.

Examples of benign and malignant tumors are listed in Table 2-3. Note that benign tumors typically end in the suffix *oma*, which means "a tumor of." Examples are meningioma and glioma (two types of benign brain tumors). As with all rules in cancer nomenclature, there are exceptions to this, notably melanoma, which is a highly malignant skin cancer. It is also of interest to note that, although many sarcomas and carcinomas have benign counterparts, leukemias and lymphomas do not.

2.2.2. Tumor Grading

Once a tumor has been identified as being malignant, a pathologist then determines the extent of the malignancy by grading the tumor. Tumors are graded on their degree of malignancy on a scale of 1 to 4, with 4 being the most advanced (i.e., worst). Grade 4 tumors are generally associated with the poorest prognosis, although this is not always the case. The truest indicator of prognosis is how far the cancer has spread, which is considered when the cancer is staged (see the next section).

Tumor grading involves analyzing the histological appearances and biological properties of the tumor to determine the extent to which the tumor

resembles normal tissue. Histology is the study of the structure and composition of cells, tissues, and organs. A tumor that shows only subtle differences from normal tissue will be considered low grade, whereas a tumor that
bears little or no resemblance to its normal counterpart will receive a high
grade.

Tumor grading is also based on the degree of cell differentiation that is
present. Cell differentiation is the process by which newly formed (immature) cells evolve into different kinds of mature cells. For example, myeloid
progenitor cells in the bone marrow are immature blood cells, which will
then differentiate into platelets, erythrocytes, granulocytes, monocytes, or
macrophages. The majority of cells in normal tissue are differentiated; this
is in contrast to tumors, which have few differentiated cells. Thus, tumors
are graded as to whether their cells appear well-differentiated, moderately
differentiated, or poorly differentiated (see example in Fig. 2-1).

Tissues containing a few cells that are not well-differentiated are considered to be dysplastic, which is a premalignant state. Low-grade tumors
will have well-differentiated cells, whereas higher grade tumors will have
moderate or poor differentiation. Tumors with a complete loss of normal differentiation are described as being anaplastic. In some cases, the cancer
cells are so poorly differentiated that it is impossible to determine the type
of cell from which the tumor originated. This is termed metastatic cancer of
unknown origin.

It is important to realize that the specific criteria used to grade a tumor
has subjective components and depends on the pathologist's skills and

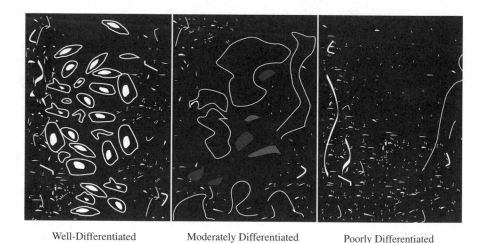

Well-Differentiated   Moderately Differentiated   Poorly Differentiated

FIGURE 2-1. Cellular differentiation. The differences between a well-differentiated
tumor cell (left), a moderately differentiated cell (middle), and a poorly differentiated cell (right) are shown. [Source: Pfeifer and Wick, 1991, p. 11.]

expertise Specialized tumor studies, such as cytogenetics or flow cytometry, may also be performed during the staging process. In cases of rare and/or unusual tumors, it may be useful to have the tumor slides reviewed by a second pathologist.

2.2.3. CLINICAL STAGING

The natural course of a malignancy is to grow and spread to other organs of the body. The purpose of clinical staging is to determine the severity of the extent of disease progression in a specific patient. Staging is an important part of clinical oncology and has implications for both prognosis and treatment recommendations.

The staging system most commonly used in both the United States and internationally for solid tumors is the TNM system. The TNM system was developed by the American Joint Committee on Cancer Staging (AJCCS) and the International Union Against Cancer (IUAC) in an effort to standardize the staging criterion. The premise of this staging system is that cancers having the same site and histology will follow a similar pattern of disease progression. Staging occurs after the initial assessment of the tumor; it is an integral part of diagnosis.

The TNM system classifies cancer into stages 0–IV, with stage IV disease being the most serious. Staging is made by assessing the size of the primary lesion, degree of invasion, and presence or absence of metastases. The more advanced the cancer, the higher each variable is graded. For solid tumors, the three variables in TNM are specifically defined as follows.

1. *T = condition of the primary tumor.*—This considers the overall size and appearance of the tumor. Tumors are classified as being: TIS (in situ), T1, T2, or T3. In situ tumors are those that are confined to the site of origin and have not spread to the surrounding normal tissue.

2. *N = extent of lymph node involvement.*—This is an important variable because cancer cells typically travel to other sites of the body via the lymphatic or circulatory systems. Thus, the greater the lymph node involvement, the greater the likelihood of metastases. Nodes can be classified as N0, N1, N2, or N3.

3. *M = extent of distant metastases.*—Metastases are either absent (M0) or present (M1). The presence of distant metastases indicates an advanced stage of cancer.

Most cancers are staged using the TNM system, but the specific criteria used to define each variable depend on the organ involved. Table 2-4 describes the TNM system for medullary thyroid carcinoma. Note that a particular stage of cancer can be composed of different TNM combinations.

TABLE 2-4. TNM STAGING SYSTEM FOR MEDULLARY THYROID CARCINOMA

Stage	T[1]	N[2]	M[3]
I	T1 (tumor <1 cm, limited to thyroid)	N0	M0
II	T2 (tumor 1–4 cm, limited to thyroid)	N0	M0
II	T3 (tumor >4 cm, limited to thyroid)	N0	M0
II	T4 (tumor of any size, extends beyond thyroid capsule)	N0	M0
III	Any T	N1	M0
IV	Any T	Any N	M1

Source: American Joint Committee on Cancer, 1998, pp. 61–64.

[1] T = primary tumor.

[2] N = regional lymph nodes: 0 = no regional lymph node metastasis; 1 = metastasis in 1–3 regional lymph nodes; 2 = metastasis in 4 or more regional lymph nodes.

[3] M = distant metastases: 0 = no distant metastases; 1 = distant metastases.

2.3. CANCER TREATMENT

> There are more things in heaven and earth than are dreamed of in a contemporary oncologist's philosophy.
>
> *(Rees et al., 1993, p. 88)*

A mother whose child had a recurrent brain tumor once joked that she had learned enough about cancer to get an M.D. degree. With a diagnosis of cancer, patients and their families are thrust into a world with its own vocabulary and often complicated treatment decisions. There are two overall aims of cancer treatment: to prolong life with radical therapy and to relieve suffering with palliative care.

Treatment of cancer falls into the following categories: surgery, radiation, chemotherapy, and transplantation.

2.3.1. SURGERY

Surgery as a mode of cancer treatment is considered local therapy. Surgical resection (removal) is the preferred strategy for eradicating solid tumors. The aim of surgery is to remove the entire tumor as well as a "margin" of surrounding healthy tissue. Surgical resection is most successful if the tumor is slow growing and confined to a single organ. Surgical risks include the small possibility of death related to the procedure (or anesthesia), short- or long-term disabilities, and disfigurement. Surgery is often followed by radiation treatments and/or chemotherapy.

There are four major types of surgery used in treat cancer:

UNIVERSITY OF CENTRAL LANCASHIRE LIBRARY BLACKPOOL SITE

1. *Exploratory surgery*—This initial surgery may be used to assess the extent of cancer present and, in some cases, help determine where the cancer has originated.

2. *Radical surgery*—Radical surgery is used to completely eradicate the tumor. This procedure may involve removing a fair amount of healthy tissue and may cause significant morbidity and disfigurement depending on the site of the cancer.

3. *Conservative surgery*—In conservative surgery, only the tumor and a small margin of surrounding healthy tissue is removed. Thus, it is a far less mutilating procedure than radical surgery. In the case of breast cancer, lumpectomies, used in conjunction with radiation and chemotherapy, have survival rates similar to mastectomy procedures.

4. *Palliative surgery*—The purpose of palliative surgery is to reduce pain or symptoms, not to cure. For example, a spinal cord tumor can cause difficulty walking and excruciating pain; removing even part of the tumor may alleviate these problems.

2.3.2. RADIATION THERAPY

The aim of radiation therapy is to destroy tumor cells before they have had a chance to metastasize. Radiation therapy is considered regional therapy and can be used to treat most solid tumors; it is not used to treat leukemia. Radiation therapy can be used before surgery to shrink tumors or after surgery to destroy remaining local cancer cells. Chemotherapy often follows a course of radiation therapy. Radiation can also be used for palliative care to relieve symptoms of pain or discomfort caused by a large tumor.

Radiation therapy involves targeting selected doses of ionizing radiation to the tumor site. The field of radiation can be compared with the beam of a flashlight. The radiation beam will be strongest at the center of the targeted site, but the "scatter" beam can also inflict damage to cells. This is actually a key benefit of radiation therapy because it can destroy cancer cells that have begun to spread locally. Tumor cells outside the field of radiation will not be affected, so radiation therapy is not an effective curative strategy for cancers that have metastasized, but may be used as a palliative measure.

How does radiation therapy work? The ionizing radiation causes tumor cells to further mutate, leading to programmed cell death. Cells will either die immediately on exposure or when they later attempt to undergo mitosis. Cancer cells that are actively dividing at the time of the radiation exposure are most vulnerable to radiation; higher doses of radiation are needed to destroy quiescent cells (ones that are not actively dividing) and slowly growing tumors with infrequent cell divisions. The radiation energy molecules are often delivered into the cells via the oxygen transport system. Thus, oxygen-poor tumors have some protection against radiation and require higher doses of radiation.

Radiation doses used to be measured in rads but is currently measured in units of Gray (Gy); a centiGray (cGy) is equivalent to a rad. The daily dosages and total radiation exposure will differ depending on the tumor's location and size and the patient's tolerance to the treatments.

The effectiveness of radiation therapy depends on many factors, including the energy of the beam, length of radiation exposure, density of the absorbing tissue, and distance it is from the radiation source. Even in the best of scenarios, only a proportion of cancer cells will be destroyed by a single course of radiation. For example, if a single radiation dose kills 99% of a tumor that consists of one million cells, then 10,000 tumor cells will still remain after treatment.

Unfortunately, a proportion of normal cells within the field of radiation are also destroyed by the exposure to radiation. This is the major downside of radiation therapy, and the doses must be monitored throughout the course of treatment. To determine the optimal radiation dose, radiation oncologists will consider the estimated number of tumor cells present and the maximum amount of radiation that will be tolerated by the normal tissue. Normal cells generally recover faster than their malignant counterparts unless the damage to the tissue is overwhelming or unless there are insufficient stem cells remaining to rebuild the tissue. Because normal stem cells divide infrequently, they are generally less vulnerable to radiation damage.

There are multiple side effects of radiation, including alopecia, cystitis, dermatitis, diarrhea, and lethargy, and radiation can also cause permanent damage to the irradiated organ. Long-term effects can include cataracts (irradiated eyes) and sterility (irradiated gonads). The lungs and kidneys are also sensitive to radiation damage. Radiation can also lead to premature athrosclerosis. Radiation therapy in children can cause damage to bone and soft tissues, leading to reduced growth or deformity. Brain irradiation in young children can also lead to increased learning difficulties. Radiation therapy can also cause a second cancer, most commonly leukemia, lymphoma, or sarcoma.

2.3.3. CHEMOTHERAPY

Chemotherapy is systemic therapy that has the capability of destroying cancer cells throughout the body. It is usually given orally or intravenously. The aims of chemotherapy are twofold: to further increase the probability that the tumor is eradicated and to prevent or delay metastases.

Chemotherapy can effectively destroy actively dividing cells but is much less effective against quiescent cells. A course of chemotherapy can consist of a single drug but often involves a combination of drugs. Most chemotherapy agents target cells that are in a particular mitotic phase; however, using combinations of agents can target all phases of the cell cycle. Regimens of chemotherapy may need to be altered during treatment because the remaining tumors cells are more likely to be the ones resistant to the agents that have been used. Because these remaining cells continue to actively divide to replenish the tumor, chemotherapy agents will eventually cease to be effective in slowing tumor growth.

The total number of chemotherapy courses administered to a patient will depend on the drug's effectiveness and toxicity. Typically, each course is spaced out in 1- to 3-week intervals to give the normal blood cell population a chance to recover.

Because of the cumulative toxicities, it is not possible for patients to remain indefinitely on chemotherapy. Most types of chemotherapy cause bone marrow toxicity, leading to a decrease in neutrophils or platelet production. This can lead to short-term and long-term immune system compromise and severe anemia and thrombocytopenia. Chemotherapy drugs can also cause permanent damage to nonrenewing tissues, including the heart and nervous system, and can cause sterility and, in women, premature menopause.

The first clinical use of chemotherapy was in 1942 when highly toxic nitrogen mustard was used to treat lymphoma. Today, there are numerous chemotherapeutic agents available, and chemotherapy regimens are increasingly designed to target a tumor's specific histological properties. Types of chemotherapy include the following:

1. *Cytoxic agents*—Cytoxic drugs includes antimetabolites, alkylating agents, and vinca alkaloids. Antimetabolites (for example, methotrexate or 5-fluorouracil) work by interfering with the production of DNA. Alkylating agents (for example, adriamycin and cyclophosphamide) directly damage the DNA, and vinca alkaloid agents (for example, vincristin and vinblastinc) damage the mitotic spindle. Cytoxic drugs target rapidly dividing cells; this explains their devastating effect on hair follicles and bone marrow production.

2. *Hormonal agents*—Steroid and nonsteroid hormones are actively involved in cellular proliferation and differentiation. Many tumors have hormonal features, including cancers of the prostate, breast, endometrium, thyroid, ovary, and kidney. These types of tumors have surface hormonal receptors that can be targeted by hormonal therapy. Hormone (or trophic) therapy aims to shrink tumors by reducing the amount of available hormone and/or by inhibiting the binding of the hormone to the receptor. These agents cannot eradicate a malignant tumor but can greatly increase the cure rate if given in combination with other chemotherapy drugs. For example, tamoxifen is an example of an anti-hormonal agent that successfully reduces breast

cancer recurrences. One advantage to hormonal agents is that they rarely cause organ toxicity.

3. *Immunotherapy*—Immunotherapy agents stimulate both the body's immune response to more effectively fight the tumor and cellular differentiation, which impairs the tumor's ability to grow. Examples include interferon-alpha, which is used in the treatment of melanoma and hairy cell and myelogenous leukemia, and interferon-2, which is used to treat metastatic renal cell carcinoma and hairy cell leukemia. Short-term side effects may include fatigue and flu-like symptoms.

4. *Retinoid agents*—All trans-retinoic acid induces differentiation of epithelial cells, thus impairing the tumor's ability to grow. Retinoic acid has been found to be quite effective in treating a few types of cancer, including basal cell carcinomas, bladder cancer, and promyelocytic leukemia. Side effects include soreness of the skin, general malaise, and liver toxicity.

2.3.4. STEM CELL TRANSPLANTATION

Stem cells arise in the bone marrow and differentiate into mature cells in the circulatory and lymphatic systems. A stem cell transplant can rejuvenate a compromised immune system, keep chemotherapy schedules on track despite low blood counts, and allow higher doses of chemotherapy and/or radiation than would otherwise be possible.

The main source of stem cells is the bone marrow. Bone marrow transplantation is an extreme form of therapy that involves treatment of high dose chemotherapy followed by the injection of healthy marrow, that is, stem cells, into the cancer patient, which, when successful, can achieve cure. However, there are many potential complications of the transplant procedure, including organ toxicity, bleeding, mouth sores, and hair loss.

The two major types of bone marrow transplants are described below.

1. *Allogeneic transplant*—In an allogeneic transplant, the transplanted bone marrow is from a human leukocyte antigen (HLA)-matched donor, typically a sibling or parent. If there are no matches among family members, donor registries can be searched. Such registries have increased the number of potential matched donors, although minority ethnic groups remain underrepresented. Cancer patients who undergo allogeneic transplants are at risk for developing graft versus-host disease, which can lead to the rejection of the foreign tissue and potentially lethal side-effects. Allogeneic transplants have been successfully used to treat leukemias and lymphomas. As an aside, allogeneic transplants are also used to treat other genetic conditions in which the primary genetic defect is in the bone marrow,

including severe combined immune deficiency syndrome and sickle cell disease.

2. *Autologous transplant*—In an autologous transplant, a sample of the patient's own bone marrow is removed and then returned to the patient after he or she has been given chemotherapy and/or radiation. Autologous transplants allow higher doses of treatment to be given, while sparing the critical population of the individual's stem cells. The transplanted stem cells have been spared exposure to toxic treatments and may also be able to mount a more effective immune system response. Autologous transplants are performed for many types of hematological and solid tumors, although its efficacy in treating some malignancies, such as breast cancer, remains unproven.

Stem cells can also be obtained in the peripheral bloodstream by using growth factor to artificially stimulate stem cell growth in the bone marrow. This causes the crowded bone marrow to release some of the immature stem cells into the bloodstream. These cells can then be removed from the bloodstream through a process called apherisis. The stem cells are then returned to the patient following treatment similar to bone marrow transplant. In some centers, peripheral stem cell transplantation is replacing bone marrow transplantation as the procedure of choice. This is because the cells are so much easier to obtain and peripheral cells are more likely to be disease-free than bone marrow cells. However, the associated morbidity is similar for both procedures.

Another source of stem cells is the umbilical cord. Cord blood is rich in stem cells that can potentially be used in allogeneic or autologous transplants. There are now facilities that, for a fee, will store cord blood specimens indefinitely; an option that might be of interest to families at high risk for cancer.

2.4. CANCER PREVENTION

In 1971, President Richard M. Nixon declared a "war on cancer" and signed into law the National Cancer Act, which made funding for cancer research a national priority. The ambitious goal of the National Cancer Act was to reduce the incidence of cancer in half by the year 2000. Unfortunately, as we enter into the next century, we remain far from this goal. However, there are several strategies that effectively reduce the risks of specific forms of cancer.

2.4.1. LIFESTYLE CHANGES

Making specific lifestyle changes can modify generalized cancer risks, although it is less clear that these strategies will reduce risks of inherited

TABLE 2-5. LIFESTYLE RECOMMENDATIONS TO MINIMIZE CANCER RISK*

Avoid tobacco
Avoid alcohol
Avoid sun exposure (especially from 10 am–3 pm)
Reduce fat intake (<30% daily calories)
Reduce cholesterol (300 mg daily)
Increase carbohydrates (55–65% daily calories)
Reduce protein (15% daily calories)
Increase dietary fiber intake (20–30 g daily)
Eat 5 fruits/vegetables daily
Avoid obesity
Minimize alcohol consumption (<1 oz daily)
Minimize salt intake (<6 g daily)

* These guidelines are endorsed by the American Cancer Society, National Cancer Institute, and American Heart Association.

forms of cancer. However, given the high rates of cancer in the general population (refer to Tables 1-1 and 1-2), it makes sense for everyone to follow the American Cancer Society's guidelines for healthy living. (see Table 2-5). Modifying lifestyle in three general areas—smoking, sun exposure, and diet—would substantially reduce the rates of cancer-related morbidity and mortality. There is also interest in exploring prevention strategies outside of traditional Western medicine termed homeopathic or alternative strategies.

1. *Smoking*—The American Cancer Society estimates that one-third of cancer deaths could be prevented if cigarette smoking were eliminated. Prevention strategies related to tobacco use comprise a large public health effort, and for good reason. Even long-term heavy smokers can sharply reduce their cancer risks by quitting smoking.

2. *Sun exposure*—One consequence of the thinning ozone layer is an increased exposure to radiation, which has led to higher rates of skin cancer, including melanoma. Screening programs emphasize the importance of avoiding excessive sun exposure. Individuals who have fair skin and repeatedly sunburn are at particularly high risk to develop skin cancer. To reduce risks of skin cancer, individuals are recommended to avoid sun exposure at peak hours and use sunscreen and protective clothing. Excessive use of tanning booths may also increase skin cancer risks.

3. *Diet*—The American Cancer Society dietary recommendations (refer to Table 2-5) include increasing the intake of fiber, fruits, and vegetables and limiting the intake of salt, red meat, and alcohol. Most links

between dietary factors and specific malignancies remain tenuous. However, one clear association is that the ingestion of pickled and cured foods increases the risk of gastric cancer. Alcohol is another well-established cancer risk factor. Cancers associated with heavy alcohol use include liver, stomach, bladder, and breast. The level of cancer risk associated with light or moderate use of alcohol is not yet established.

4. *Homeopathic strategies*—There seems to be a recent surge of interest in "alternative" strategies to prevent (as well as to treat) cancer. Concerns about homeopathic strategies are twofold: the efficacy of most substances has never been proven in rigorous clinical trials and people might use such strategies instead of seeking medical attention, which could result in a delay in the diagnosis of cancer. However, the tension between traditional Western medicine and the homeopathic community appears to be lessening. Certain homeopathic substances, such as vitamin E and black tea, may lower risks of cancer by boosting the body's immune system. Other popularly ingested substances, such as shark's tooth and garlic, have not been proven to be effective and are in need of further study.

2.4.2. EARLY DETECTION

Cancer survival rates tend to be closely linked to the stage of the cancer at diagnosis. To increase the possibility that cancers are detected at an early stage, it is recommended that high-risk individuals have regular physician visits, undergo special cancer monitoring tests, and pay attention to any possible signs of cancer.

1. *Regular physician visits*—People at increased risk for cancer should maintain a regular schedule of physician visits. At the visit, the physician can take a history of symptoms, perform a careful physical examination, and order specific screening tests. Of course, it is useful if the physician has been made aware of the family history of cancer and is cognizant of the features associated with the hereditary cancer syndrome. Although physicians are beginning to ask more questions about family history, high-risk individuals should be encouraged to bring up the topic themselves. It is also advantageous for an individual to be followed by one physician who can track symptoms and review results of screening tests. It is also recommended that high-risk individuals be monitored by specialists in addition to their primary care physicians. In fact, it may be prudent for all providers to be aware of the heightened cancer risks. As an example, one woman was first detected to have an osteosarcoma of the jaw by her dentist.

2. *Cancer monitoring*—For several types of cancer, there are established screening tests. The purpose of these screening tests is to detect signs of cancer at an early stage. Individuals at increased risk of specific forms of cancer are often recommended to undergo specific screening tests at regular intervals (often annually). For example, siblings of a child with retinoblastoma are recommended to have careful eye exams (under anesthesia) every year until at least age 3. In adult-onset cancer syndromes, the monitoring recommendations may be similar to those for the general population but initiated at a much younger age. This is true for breast, colon, and prostate cancer. Although high-risk individuals should adhere to cancer monitoring recommendations, most of the screening tests are suspected rather than proven to be effective in reducing cancer morbidity and mortality.

3. *Warning signs*—It is important to educate high-risk individuals about potential signs or symptoms that they could have cancer. Early-stage cancer may cause few physical ailments; however, patients are usually the ones to first detect a problem. Physicians rely on their patients' knowledge of their bodies and recognition that something is not right. Individuals at high risk for cancer should be encouraged to seek prompt medical attention when experiencing any of the warning signs of cancer (see Table 2-6 for a general list). A warning sign of cancer includes any somatic complaint that is of increased severity or duration. For example, complaints of "growing pains" in the limbs of an active 10-year old are fairly common; however, if the pain is unremitting for several days or seems more intense than usual, the child's pediatrician should be consulted (especially if the family has Li-Fraumeni syndrome).

High-risk individuals may need to be reassured that frequent telephone calls to their physicians will not cause them to be viewed as pests or hypochondriacs. If their physicians are not appropriately responsive, then

TABLE 2-6. COMMON WARNING SIGNS OF CANCER

C — Change in bowel or bladder habits
A — A sore that does not heal
U — Unusual bleeding or discharge
T — Thickening or lump
I — Indigestion or difficulty in swallowing
O — Obvious change in wart or mole
N — Nagging cough or hoarseness

Source: American Cancer Society.

patients should further educate them about the features of the hereditary cancer syndrome in their family or consider switching their care to physicians who will recognize the potential seriousness of their complaints.

2.4.3. PREVENTION STRATEGIES

The search for prevention strategies represents the "holy grail" of oncology; such strategies are assumed to exist but, for the most part, have remained frustratingly elusive. Given the high risks of cancer associated with hereditary cancer syndromes, there is a great deal of research into strategies for preventing cancer beyond avoidance of carcinogens and other lifestyle changes. Although gene therapy may one day be available to individuals with inherited predispositions to cancer, at this time, prevention strategies fall into two major categories: chemoprevention and prophylactic surgery.

1. *Chemoprevention*—Chemoprevention involves taking a medication, often daily, to reduce tumor formation. Examples include tamoxifen, an anti-hormone that reduces risks of breast cancer, and sulindac, which appears to reduce the risk of colon polyps. Chemopreventive agents are rigorously studied for efficacy and safety in large, randomized clinical trials. Given the interest in identifying effective agents, it is likely the number of chemoprevention trials will increase. Individuals at high risk for cancer may be ideal candidates for such trials, and they may be especially motivated to participate.

2. *Prophylactic surgery*—Another strategy is to remove the tissue at highest risk of becoming malignant. Surgical removal of healthy tissue as a form of cancer prevention is termed prophylactic surgery. Obviously, this strategy is limited to tissues that are not crucial to survival. However, it is a reasonable option for individuals at high risk for developing breast, colon, ovarian, or gall bladder cancer. Prophylactic surgery dramatically reduces, but does not generally eliminate, the risk of cancer, an important point for clients to understand. There are also short-term and long-term consequences of surgery that must be considered beforehand. For example, contemplating bilateral prophylactic oophorectomies can raise several different medical and psychological issues, including potential complications with surgery, the prospect of early menopause, the safety of hormone replacement therapy, the anticipated changes in body image or sexuality, and the end of being able to have a biological child. Discussions about prophylactic surgery should involve the client, surgeon, primary care physician, and mental health professional. Genetic counselors can also play an important role in facilitating or participating in these discussions.

2.5. BREAST, COLON, AND OVARIAN CANCER

Genetic counselors will frequently be asked to assess family histories of breast, colon, or ovarian cancer. Thus, it is important to have a basic understanding of the medical management of these three cancers. This includes information about normal anatomy, detection, and prevention strategies as well as tumor types and treatment options.

2.5.1. BREAST CANCER

1. *Normal anatomy*—The female breast is a network of fat, glands, muscles, and ligaments. Each breast consists of 15–20 lobes and 20–40 lobules (see Fig. 2-2). These lobules lead to ducts (milk sinuses) that lead to the nipple placed in the center of the areola. The breasts are held in place by mammary ligaments (also called Cooper's ligaments) that extend from the bottom layer of breast tissue to the pectoralis muscle of the chest wall. Breast tissue also extends toward the underarm. Lymphatic vessels lead to axillary nodes under the arms.

2. *Detection and prevention strategies*—The primary early detection strategies are clinical breast examinations and mammograms. Women are

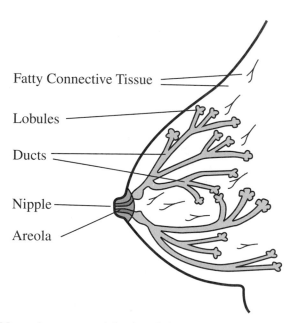

FIGURE 2-2. Normal anatomy of the female breast. [Source: Runowicz et al., 1999, p. 20.]

TABLE 2-7. COMMON WARNING SIGNS OF BREAST CANCER

Lump in breast or underarm
Ill-defined area of thickening
Skin dimpling
Deformity or asymmetry
Ulceration
Hot, swollen, or reddened
Nipple discharge

Source: Rees et al., 1993, p. 143.

also encouraged to perform monthly self-breast examinations. Breast ultrasonography can be used during pregnancy or as follow-up for a suspicious mammogram finding. Breast MRIs are also being studied to determine their potential usefulness at detecting early-stage cancer. Warning signs of breast cancer are listed in Table 2-7. Prevention strategies include the use of tamoxifen, an anti-hormonal agent that appears to reduce the risk of breast cancer by 50%, and prophylactic mastectomies, which may reduce breast cancer risks by 90% (Hartmann et al., 1999). Surgical removal of the ovaries also seems to reduce the risk of breast cancer. Lifestyle suggestions include reducing alcohol intake and increasing exercise, but it is not clear how effective these strategies are in women at risk for inherited forms of breast cancer.

3. *Types of cancer*—About 80% of breast cancers are ductal adenocarcinomas. Other types of breast cancer include lobular, medullary, mucinous, and tubular carcinomas. Inflammatory disease and sarcomas represent rare forms of breast cancer. Paget's disease is an inflammatory pre-cancerous condition of the nipple and areola. Breast cancers associated with *BRCA1* and *BRCA2* mutations are most commonly ductal carcinomas, but other forms of invasive breast cancer have also been reported. It remains unclear whether ductal carcinoma in situ (DCIS) is a feature of the *BRCA1/2* phenotype. Lobular carcinoma in situ (LCIS) is a precancerous condition that does not appear to be associated with *BRCA1* or *BRCA2* mutations. Breast sarcomas have been reported in Li-Fraumeni syndrome families.

4. *Cancer staging*—As shown in Table 2-8, breast cancers are staged from stage 0 (DCIS) to stage IV (metastatic disease), and, predictably, survival rates vary according to stage (see Table 2-9). Cancer staging is based on the presence, size, and features of tumor cells obtained from the breast biopsy and the presence or absence of metastases to lymph nodes or other organs. The underarm lymph nodes are routinely dis-

TABLE 2-8. TNM STAGING SYSTEM FOR BREAST CANCER

Stage	T[1]	N[2]	M[3]
0	Tis (carcinoma in situ or Paget's disease of the nipple with no tumor)	N0	M0
I	T1 (tumor <2 cm)	N0	M0
IIA	T0 (primary tumor cannot be assessed) T1 (tumor <2 cm) T2 (tumor between 2–5 cm)	N0	M0
IIB	T2 (tumor between 2–5 cm) T3 (tumor >5 cm)	N0	M0
IIIA	T0 (primary tumor cannot be assessed) T1 (tumor <2 cm) T2 (tumor between 2–5 cm) T3 (tumor >5 cm) T3 (tumor >5 cm)	N0	M0
IIIB	T4 (tumor of any size extended to chest wall or skin)	Any N	M0
	Any T	N3	M0
IV	Any T	Any N	M1

Source: American Joint Committee on Cancer, 1998, pp. 159–170.

[1] T = primary tumor.

[2] N = regional lymph nodes: 0 = no regional node involvement; 1 = metastasis to movable ipsilateral axcillary lymph node(s); 2 = ipsilateral axcillary lymph node(s) fixed to one another or other structures; 3 = metastasis to ipsilateral internal mammary lymph node(s).

[3] M = distant metastases: 0 = no distant metastases; 1 = distant metastases.

TABLE 2-9. PROGNOSIS FOR BREAST CARCINOMA BY STAGE OF DISEASE

Stage Grouping	5-Year Survival (%)
0	92
I	87
IIA	78
IIB	68
IIIA	51
IIIB	42
IV	13

Source: American Joint Committee on Cancer, 1998, p. 164.

sected and examined for the presence of tumor cells except when the tumor is stage 0. Other tests include estrogen receptor status (ER-positive tumors carry a better prognosis) and presence of the *Her-2/neu* oncogene, which is indicative of a more aggressive tumor. The most common sites of breast cancer metastases are bone, lung, liver, and brain.

5. *Cancer treatment options*—The major treatment decision for newly diagnosed breast cancer patients is whether to have a mastectomy, which removes most of the breast tissue, or a lumpectomy, which is less disfiguring. Patients who choose the tissue-sparing lumpectomy procedure are also recommended to undergo radiation treatments. Survival rates appear similar for patients who undergo mastectomy versus those who choose lumpectomy and radiation, although it is not clear whether this is the case for women with inherited breast cancers. Chemotherapy is recommended if there is any evidence that the cancer has spread beyond the initial site or if the tumor pathology suggests aggressive disease. Chemotherapy regimens may include cyclophosphamide, methotrexate, 5-fluorouracil, and/or taxol. Once the cancer is in remission, female breast cancer patients with estrogen receptor (ER)-positive tumors are usually given the drug tamoxifen as a way of reducing the risks of recurrence.

2.5.2. COLON CANCER

1. *Normal anatomy*—The large intestine extends from the terminal ileum of the small intestine to the anal canal. The adult colon is about 150 cm, and the rectum is about 12 cm. As shown in Figure 2-3, the large intestine is divided into the following sections: the cecum, ascending (right) colon, transverse (middle) colon, descending (left) colon, sigmoid colon, and rectum. The large intestine is composed of both muscle and epithelial cells. Most of the rectum is sheathed in a layer of peritoneum, which contain cells that are similar to ovarian epithelial cells.

2. *Detection and prevention strategies*—The primary early detection strategies are the rectal exam, the sigmoidoscopy, which assesses the sigmoid colon and rectum, and the colonoscopy, which assesses most of the large intestine. Another detection strategy is to analyze stool samples for the presence of occult blood. Warning signs of colorectal cancer are listed in Table 2-10. Sigmoidoscopy and colonoscopy can also be considered prevention strategies because precancerous polyps can be removed during the procedures. The cyclooxygenase (COX) inhibitors are non-steroidal anti-inflammatory drugs (NSAIDs) that, in limited studies, have been shown to reduce the number of polyps in people with familial adenomatous polyposis (FAP) (Richter et al., 2001). Further studies are needed but early data is encouraging that COX-inhibitors could potentially reduce the risk of colorectal cancer in people at high risk. Individuals at risk for FAP are recommended

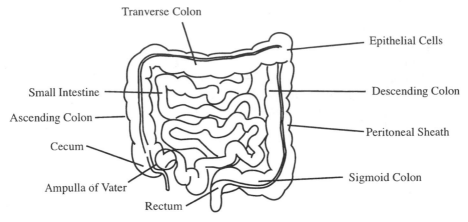

FIGURE 2-3. Normal anatomy of the colon. [Source: Cooper, 1992, p. 297.]

TABLE 2-10. WARNING SIGNS OF COLORECTAL CANCER

Abdominal discomfort
Blood in the stool
Constipation
Diarrhea
Severe nausea and vomiting
Significant weight loss
Weakness
Anemia
Change in bowel habits
Feeling that bowel does not completely empty

Source: Rees et al., 1993, p. 126.

to have their colon and rectum removed prophylactically. Lifestyle suggestions include increasing the intake of fiber, fruits, and vegetables and reducing the consumption of red meat, although it is not clear how effective these strategies are in reducing risks of inherited forms of colorectal cancer.

3. *Cancer types*—Colorectal cancers are adenocarcinomas of various histologies. About 70% of sporadic cancers occur in the sigmoid or rectum. This is in contrast to hereditary nonpolyposis colon cancer (HNPCC) syndrome tumors, which are frequently found in the ascending colon. Adenocarcinomas almost always arise from benign growths (polyps) in the lining of the intestine, although not all polyps have the same malignant potential. Adenomatous (flat) polyps carry

TABLE 2-11. TNM Staging System for Colorectal Cancer

Stage	T[1]	N[2]	M[3]	Dukes[4]
0	Tis (carcinoma in situ)	N0	M0	
I	T1 (tumor invades submucosa)	N0	M0	A
	T2 (tumor invades muscularis propria)			
	T3 (tumor invades through muscularis propria into subserosa or into nonperitonealized pericolic or perirectal tissues)			
II	T3 (tumor invades through muscularis propria into subserosa or into nonperitonealized pericolic or perirectal tissues)	N0	M0	B
	T4 (tumor directly invades other organs or structures)	N0	M0	
III	Any T	N1	M0	C
	Any T	N2	M0	
IV	Any T	Any N	M1	

Source: American Joint Committee on Cancer, 1998, pp. 81–88.

[1] T = primary tumor.

[2] N = regional lymph nodes: 0 = no regional lymph node metastasis; 1 = metastasis in 1–3 regional lymph nodes; 2 = metastasis in 4 or more regional lymph nodes.

[3] M = distant metastases: 0 = no distant metastases; 1 = distant metastases.

TABLE 2-12. Prognosis For Colorectal Carcinoma by Stage of Disease

Dukes Stage	5-Year Survival (%)
A (localized)	91
B (regional)	66
C (distant)	9

Source: American Cancer Society, 1999, p. 22.

the highest risks of undergoing neoplastic transformation. It is estimated that 40% of villous adenomatous polyps and 5% of tubular adenomatous polyps will eventually become malignant.

4. *Cancer staging*—Table 2-11 shows the different stages of colon cancer by the older Dukes classification system and the current TNM system. Survival rates per stage are listed in Table 2-12. The staging process involves biopsing the tumor and sampling neighboring lymph nodes. Each section of the colon has its own regional lymph nodes, and, thus, the exact location of the primary tumor dictates which regional nodes

will be sampled. For example, a "right-sided" colon cancer would involve sampling the ileocolic, middle colic, and right colic lymph nodes. Colorectal metastases can be present in any organ but most frequently occur in the liver or lungs.

5. *Cancer treatment options*—The colon cancer treatment of choice is surgery, followed by chemotherapy, if there is evidence that the cancer has spread through the intestinal wall. Small lesions can be removed without disturbing the colorectum. The presence of a larger lesion may necessitate removing a portion of colon and then reconnecting the remaining sections. Surgical removal of the entire colon and sometimes rectum (colectomy) is performed if the colon is carpeted with polyps or the tumor size or location makes it impossible to save enough of the colon to reconnect it together. Ileostomy is a surgical procedure that involves connecting the small intestine with the anal canal. This may result in having a colostomy bag or pouch. Colon cancers that have metastasized will be treated with adjuvant chemotherapy, such as 5-fluorouracil and levamisole. Radiation is sometimes used to treat tumors in the rectum or anus but is not usually recommended for tumors in the colon because the gut poorly tolerates radiation.

2.5.3. OVARIAN CANCER

My body turned a cold back on me, at less than
forty-three
It started a war
whatever for
in the middle of the middle of my life
it rose a black dividing mass
in my ovaries alas . . .

(Gilda Radner, from "Gilda's Poem", 1989)

1. *Normal anatomy*—The ovaries are almond-shaped organs which lie on either side of the uterus and are held in place by several ligaments (see Fig. 2-4). Each ovary houses thousands of follicles, each of which contains an oocyte in various stages of maturity. At ovulation, a single mature oocyte bursts from the ovary. The outer lining of the ovary must then repair itself by creating a new epithelial wall.

2. *Detection and prevention strategies*—The only way to truly diagnose ovarian cancer is to surgically remove the ovaries and evaluate them. Transvaginal ultrasound can detect a tumor that has altered the shape or size of the ovary; however, this procedure may miss some early-stage cancers. Pelvic examinations may be able to detect palpable

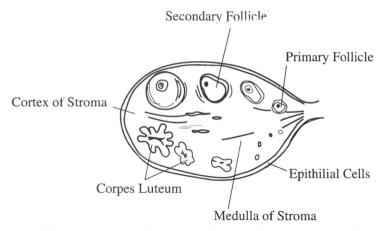

FIGURE 2-4. Normal anatomy of the ovary. [Source: Runowicz et al., 1999, p. 206.]

TABLE 2-13. WARNING SIGNS OF OVARIAN CANCER

Pelvic pain
Generalized abdominal discomfort
Low back pain
Persistent bloating
Frequent urination
Feeling of fullness
Severe vomiting
Significant weight loss
Post-menopausal bleeding

Source: Runowicz et al., 1999, p. 215.

tumors of a more advanced stage. Warning signs are usually subtle and are listed in Table 2-13. The most effective prevention strategy for women at high risk is to surgically remove the ovaries prophylactically. Women who undergo prophylactic oophorectomy continue to have a small risk of developing cancer of the peritoneum, the sheath surrounding the abdominal organs, whose cells resemble that of ovarian epithelium. Prophylactic oophorectomy is complicated by the fact that it causes surgical menopause, often at an earlier age than normal menopause would have been and yet there are concerns that hormone replacement therapy might increase breast cancer risks. Birth control pills constitute a form of chemoprevention, and even 3 months of use appears to reduce risks of ovarian cancer by 50% in the general population (Narod et al., 1998). The daily use of talcum powder should be avoided as it is an established risk factor for ovarian cancer.

3. *Cancer types*—About 90% of ovarian cancers are carcinomas that have arisen in the frequently dividing cells of the epithelium. The tumors typically contain cysts that are further characterized as serous, endometriod, or mucinous. Mucinous carcinomas carry the best prognosis. So-called borderline tumors demonstrate malignant properties, but there is no evidence of tumor in the stroma; the tumor is completely confined to the epithelium. Other types of ovarian tumors cancer arise in the stroma (granulosa cell tumors) or within the germ cells themselves (dysgerminomas). Granulosa cell tumors and dysgerminomas generally occur at younger ages than do carcinomas but are rarely hereditary. Ovarian carcinomas are a recognized feature of breast-ovarian cancer syndrome and HNPCC. Because ovarian cancer is often bilateral at diagnosis, this is a less useful indicator that a patient has an inherited form of cancer. Also note that an ovarian tumor may not represent a malignant tumor; about 75% of ovarian tumors turn out to be benign. In addition, a malignant tumor may actually represent metastatic disease. As examples, cancer of the breast and stomach can metastasize to the ovary.

4. *Cancer staging*—Ovarian cancers are staged from stage IA to stage IV, as shown in Table 2-14. Overall 5-year survival rates are only 25%, although this rate climbs to 80% for granulosa cell and dysgerminoma tumors. Survival rates per stage at diagnosis are presented in Table 2-15. About two-thirds of patients are found to have peritoneal metastases at diagnosis. Even patients with no overt signs that the cancer has spread may later be found to have distant metastases. This phenomenon coupled with the few physical warning signs that accompany early-stage disease has earned ovarian cancer its terrible nickname "the silent killer." Ovarian cancer commonly spreads to the liver and lungs.

5. *Cancer treatment options*—The treatment of choice for ovarian cancer is surgery. Surgery typically involves removal of the ovaries and fallopian tubes (bilateral salpingo-oophorectomy) and uterus (hysterectomy). The surgeon will also carefully examine the abdominal organs for signs of cancer and will collect lymph node specimens and peritoneal fluid samples. If the cancer is in an advanced stage, there may be cancer cell deposits throughout the omentum (the tissue that holds the abdominal organs in place). Scraping the tumor cells from the omentum is called debulking, and this procedure can be performed more than once. The intent of debulking is palliative rather than curative; when successful, it can reduce symptoms and prolong life. Given the insidious nature of ovarian carcinomas, chemotherapy is fre-

TABLE 2-14. TNM STAGING SYSTEM FOR OVARIAN CANCER

Stage	T[1]	N[2]	M[3]
IA	T1a (limited to 1 ovary)	N0	M0
IB	T1b (limited to both ovaries)	N0	M0
IC	T1c (capsule ruptured, tumor on ovary surface or cells in ascites or peritoneal washings)	N0	M0
IIA	T2a (tumor also in uterus or tube)	N0	M0
IIB	T2b (tumor also in other pelvic tissues)	N0	M0
IIC	T2c (tumor in other pelvic tissues and malignant cells in ascites or peritoneal washings)	N0	M0
IIIA	T3a (microscopic peritoneal metastases beyond pelvis)	N0	M0
IIIB	T3b (macroscopic peritoneal metastasis <2 cm beyond pelvis)	N0	M0
IIIC	T3c (peritoneal metastasis >2 m beyond pelvis)	N0	M0
	Any T	N1	M0
IV	Any T	Any N	M1

Source: American Joint Committee on Cancer, 1998, pp. 187–190.

[1] T = primary tumor.

[2] N = regional lymph nodes: 0 = no regional lymph node involvement; 1 = regional lymph node involvement.

[3] M = distant metastases: 0 = no distant metastases; 1 = distant metastases.

TABLE 2-15. PROGNOSIS FOR OVARIAN CARCINOMA BY STAGE OF DISEASE

Stage	5-Year Survival (%)
IA & IB	91–98
IC	90
II	80
III	15–20
IV	<5

Source: Runowicz et al., 1999, pp. 228–230.

quently recommended. A typical course of chemotherapy is six cycles, and it is usually administered intravenously. First-line treatment drugs may include cisplatin or carboplatin and paclitaxol. Second-line treatments include topotecan, doxorubicin, cyclophosphamide, etoposide, and 5-fluorouracil. Low levels of radiation may also be used if the tumor has spread into the pelvis or abdominal cavity. In cases of borderline or germ cell tumors, removing the one affected ovary may be the only treatment necessary.

2.6. REFERENCES

American Cancer Society. 1999. Cancer Facts and Figures 1999. American Cancer Society, Atlanta, GA.

American Joint Committee on Cancer. 1998. AJCC Cancer Staging Handbook, 5th edition. Lippincott Williams and Wilkins, Philadelphia, PA.

Boyer, M and Tannock, I. 1998. Cellular and molecular basis of chemotherapy. In Tannock I and Hill R (eds) The Basic Science of Oncology. Eds.: Tannock IF, and Hill RP. McGraw-Hill, New York, NY, 350–369.

Bristow, R and Hill, R. 1998. Molecular and cellular basis of radiotherapy. In Tannock, I and Hill, R (eds) The Basic Science of Oncology. McGraw-Hill, New York, NY, 295–321.

Burton, M and Watson, M. 1998. Counselling People With Cancer. John Wiley & Sons, New York, NY.

Cooper, G. 1992. Elements of Human Cancer. Jones & Bartlett, Boston, MA, 297.

Hartmann, L, Schaid, D, Woods, J et al. 1999. Efficacy of bilateral prophylactic mastectomy in women with a family history of breast cancer. NEJM. 340:77–84.

McKinnell, R, Parchment, R, Perantoni, A et al. 1998. The Biological Basis of Cancer. Cambridge University Press, Cambridge, UK.

Narod, S, Risch, H, Moslehi, R et al. 1998. Oral contraceptives and the risk of hereditary ovarian cancer. NEJM. 339:424–428.

Pfeifer, J and Wick, M. 1991. The pathologic evaluation of neoplastic diseases. In American Cancer Society Textbook of Clinical Oncology. Eds.: Holleb A, Fink D, and Murphy G. American Cancer Society, Atlanta GA.

Radner, G. 1989. It's always something. Avon Books, New York, NY.

Rees, G, Goodman, S, and Bullimore, J. 1993. Cancer in Practice. Butterworth Heinemann, Oxford, UK.

Richter, M, Weiss, M, and Weinberger, I et al. 2001. Growth inhibition and induction of apoptosis in colorectal tumor cells by cyclooxygenase inhibitors. Carcinogenesis. 22:17–25.

Runowicz, C, Petrek, J, and Gansler, T. 1999. Women and Cancer. American Cancer Society.

Sontag, S. 1977. Illness as metaphor. Farrar, Straus, and Giroux, New York, NY.

CANCER BIOLOGY

If there were no errors in DNA, cancer would not occur. On the other hand, it is hard to imagine copying 10^{27} nucleotides over a lifetime without making many, many errors. Why don't cancerous cells arise every few minutes? The extremes—no cancer at all and cancer occurring so often as to not permit human life—are philosophical boundaries that we can only contemplate.

(Ross, 1998, p. 57–58)

3.1. THE MALIGNANT CELL

The process by which a normal cell becomes malignant can be simplistically summed up as "cell replication gone awry." In preparation for a discussion of carcinogenesis, this section provides an overview of the changed features and functional properties of cancer cells.

3.1.1. FEATURES OF MALIGNANT CELLS

Cancer cells are both anatomically and biochemically altered from normal cells. These differences are described below.

1. *Anatomic features*—Diagnosis of a tumor is based on several features including an abnormal size and shape of cells, abnormal mitoses, abnormal nuclear content, and misshapen tissue architecture. It is not always easy to distinguish cancer cells from their normal counterparts. For example, follicular thyroid cancer cells and low grade lymphomas may contain only subtle changes from normal tissue. In cancer cells, changes are present in each major component of the cell,

but occur most significantly within the nucleus. Nuclear changes include abnormal and unstable karyotypes. Chromosomal aneuploidy is common, as are all types of structural rearrangements. The cells within the tumor population are heterogeneous, meaning that that individual cells have varying features. For example, tumor cells proliferate and gain metastatic potential at varying rates and have differing sensitivities to chemotherapy or radiation.

2. *Biochemical features*—As shown in Table 3-1, cancer cells can have biochemical requirements different from normal cells. Some cancer cells require lower concentrations of growth factors or hormones to replicate than normal cells. There are also biochemical features and secretory changes that are lost or gained in cancer cells. For example, cancer cells lose fibronectin (a protein important for cell-to-cell adhesion) and gain the ability to produce their own growth factors.

3.1.2. FUNCTIONAL PROPERTIES OF CANCER CELLS

The fingers of a newborn child or the pattern of a butterfly's wing represent what we normally admire in biological systems: form, control; a unity of design and function that favors the survival of the organism. In cancer, all of these virtues are lost. Cancer cells divide without restraint, cross boundaries they were meant to respect and fail to display the characteristics of the cell lineage from which they were derived.

(Varmus and Weinberg, 1993. p.1)

Carefully regulated cellular processes, such as differentiation, proliferation, and programmed cell death, are greatly changed in cancer cells. The impact

TABLE 3-1. MAJOR BIOCHEMICAL FEATURES OF CANCER CELLS

Compared with normal cells, cancer cells
  Require lower concentrations of growth factors to reproduce
  Require less oxygen to reproduce and function
  Lose complex cell surface glycolipids (interferes with cell-to-cell
    communications)
  Lose extracellular fibronectin (increases mobility)
  Lose cyclic adenine monophosphate (causes loss of cell cohesion and density-
    dependent growth)
  Produce more cell surface enzymes (allows metastatic potential)
  Produce autogenic growth factors. (allows growth without external stimuli)
  Produce more prostaglandins (helps suppress immune system and establish
    tumor metastases)

Source: Lovejoy, 1987.

of mutated cancer susceptibility genes on the cell cycle is shown in Figure
3-1. As discussed below, cancer cells are able to do the following.

1. *Dedifferentiate*—Terminally differentiated cells have been programmed to have specific structures and functions and do not differentiate again under normal circumstances. Losing the characteristics
   of a normal mature cell is termed dedifferentiation. Dedifferentiation
   occurs when a mature cell loses its normal phenotype due to somatic
   genetic changes or epigenetic changes that have occurred during
   replication. It is also possible for an immature stem cell to abnormally
   differentiate into a cancer cell. The failure of a cell to appropriately
   differentiate is termed maturation arrest.

2. *Gain proliferative abilities*—Cell proliferation is the process by which
   new cells are generated. Fully differentiated cells do not typically
   replicate; however, some less differentiated cells may go through
   multiple cycles of growth over their lifespan. For normal cells to
   proliferate, several requirements need to be met, including the presence of sufficient growth factors and appropriate anchoring of the
   cell. One result of the genetic changes that occur in cancer cells is

Cell Cycle

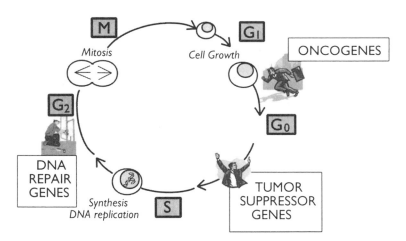

FIGURE 3-1. The cell cycle and placement of major cancer predisposition genes.
These gene types are oncogenes, tumor suppressor genes, and DNA repair genes. See
text in Sections III, IV, and V for further description of these genes. [Printed with
permission from: Offit, 1998, p. 40.]

increased proliferation. Cancer cells divide with greater frequency and for longer periods of time.

3. *Bypass cell cycle checkpoints*—The G_1 and G_2 checkpoints in the cell cycle allow time for DNA replication errors to be detected and the cell to be either repaired or destroyed. In cancer cells, the genes responsible for halting mitosis may be mutated or silenced. This allows the cells to bypass these checkpoints and retain their damaged DNA content.

4. *Dismantle DNA repair*—Cancer cells may continue to halt appropriately at the G_1 and G_2 checkpoints, but the problem may lie with the genes responsible for repairing the replication errors. Thus, the checkpoints may be rendered ineffective by faulty DNA repair genes. This allows cells to survive and replicate despite the presence of numerous DNA mutations.

5. *Avoid apoptosis*—Programmed cell death is termed apoptosis. Apoptosis constitutes an important mechanism for tissues to control the number of growth cycles per cell. Normal cells undergo apoptosis either at a designated time or when perceived as damaged. Tumor cells that are able to dismantle or bypass the apoptosis pathway become "immortal." Immortalized cells have greatly expanded lifespans and will not be targeted for apoptosis. Attaining immortal status confers a huge advantage to tumor cells, and they may be preferentially selected for growth.

6. *Undergo angiogenesis*—A small tumor, less than 2 mm, is usually able to sustain itself with nutrients from the surrounding tissue. However, as the tumor grows, it will require a regular food source. In response to this need, tumors stimulate a process termed angiogenesis. Angiogenesis involves the secretion of angiogenic factors and the differentiation of specific cells into capillaries that can bring blood, i.e., nutrients, directly to the tumor. The tumor is then able to divert the blood supply that was meant for the normal surrounding tissue. Tissues—normal or tumor—that do not have a sufficient blood supply may contain large areas of necrosis (dead tissue).

7. *Gain ability to metastasize*—With the exception of cells in the circulatory and lymphatic systems, normal cells are typically fixed within the highly regimented tissue architecture and are not mobile even within the tissue. In contrast, cancer cells destroy the normal architecture of the tissue and gain the ability to move throughout the tissue. Eventually cancer cells gain the ability to penetrate through the walls of the tissue and spread to other tissues. The ability to metastasize is perhaps the most distinctive feature of malignant cells. (see section 3.2.1 for more information about metastasis.)

3.2. CARCINOGENESIS

A cell goes through multiple steps en route to becoming a fully malignant cell. The development of a tumor begins with a single mutated cell somewhere in the body that multiplies and creates a small colony of cells within the same tissue. Further genetic changes occur within the colony of abnormal cells, leading to cells with enhanced growth potential and other special features, such as increased mobility and angiogenesis. The cascade of events that occur in carcinogenesis occurs randomly, not because a cancer cell is deliberately planning its next move. The phases of carcinogenesis may be completed rapidly or may take a decade or more. Some precancerous cells regress back to normal states, some remain in precancerous states indefinitely, and, in others, malignancy is an inevitable event.

3.2.1. STAGES OF CARCINOGENESIS

The phases of carcinogenesis are termed initiation, promotion, progression, and metastasis. These phases are illustrated in Figure 3-2.

1. *Initiation*—The first stage of carcinogenesis is termed initiation. Typically, the primary event of carcinogenesis is the occurrence of a genetic mutation within a single cell that leads to abnormal proliferation. This mutation may be inherited in the germline, but most occur somatically. Somatic mutations occur because of errors during mitosis or because of exposure to carcinogens termed initiators or initiating agents. The time span from this initial carcinogenic exposure to a detectable tumor is highly variable, even up to several years. This time period is also referred to as the latency period. Initiating agents include tobacco and radiation. An initiated cell can be considered a malignant stem cell that, given the right environment, has the potential of "seeding" or developing into a fully malignant tumor. However, initiated cells do not always lead to a malignant tumor. Some initiated cells will be destroyed before they have proliferated and others will remain fixed in a nonneoplastic state.

2. *Promotion*—Promotion is the second phase of carcinogenesis. Within this stage, cells have acquired a selective growth advantage. This leads to rapid growth within the initiated cells and the formation of a small, pre-cancerous tumor population. Promotion occurs because of a random error during cell division or exposure to certain carcinogens termed promoters or promoting agents. Hormones and dietary fat are two examples of promoters. At this stage, the carcinogenic process is still reversible. If the exposure to the promoting agent is removed, then the cells will cease their growth and begin to die out. However, cells that continue to mutate and divide will continue on the carcinogenic pathway.

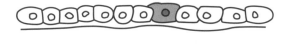

Initiation
Single initial proliferative cell

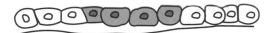

Promotion
Hyperproliferative cells

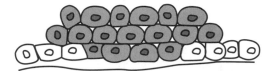

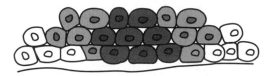

Early Progression
Small Adenoma

Late Progression
Large Adenoma and Carcinoma

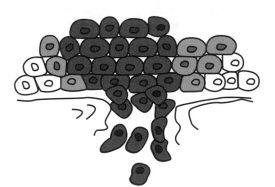

Metastatic Carcinoma

FIGURE 3-2. The stages of carcinogenesis. The major stages of cancer development are termed initiation, promotion, progression, and metastasis. Note that the process begins with a single mutated cell (lightly shaded cell) and ends with many fully carcinogenic cells (darkly shaded cells) breaking away from the tumor and traveling to other sites of the body. [Source: Cooper, 1992, p. 23.]

3. *Progression*—Progression designates the stage at which the tumor characteristics become irreversible. Genetic mutations continue to occur and accumulate as a result of the rapid, continuous cell divisions, and the carcinogenic process is no longer reversible. As the tumor continues to grow, certain mutated cells can be selected to proliferate depending on the needs of the tumor within its current environment. For example, a small subpopulation of cells that does not require hormones to replicate may eventually outgrow the cells that are hormone dependent. Although tumor growth is stochastic rather than calculated, it does follow a "survival of the fittest" paradigm. Eventually, the tumor will consist of a population of fully malignant tumor cells, many of which will have metastatic capabilities. Due to the highly unstable DNA, tumor karyotypes typically reveal unusual deletions and rearrangements.

4. *Metastasis*—Malignant cells must undergo further genetic changes in order to gain metastatic properties. The metastatic process involves multiple steps, as listed in Table 3-2. One of the initial steps of metastasis is for malignant cells to enter the circulatory or lymphatic system. This is why, regardless of the primary site of the cancer, blood samples and/or lymph nodes are continually monitored. Common sites for metastases are lung, liver, bone, and the central nervous system. Specific tumors will demonstrate different, but somewhat predictable, patterns of spread. However, cancer cells can potentially be carried to any site of the body. The pattern of spread has been compared to scattering seeds over a large patch of ground—only those planted in favorable soil will grow. It is estimated that less than 1 in 10,000 malignant cells successfully metastasizes. However, this statistic is not comforting when considering that large primary tumors shed millions of cancer cells daily into the circulatory or lymphatic system. In fact, more than 90% of cancer-related deaths are caused by metastatic disease.

TABLE 3-2. STEPS INVOLVED IN METASTASIS

The cancer cell must
  Separate from the primary tumor
  Enter into the circulatory or lymphatic system
  Survive journey through the body
  Escape destruction by the immune system
  Enter into the target organ
  Attach to the surface of the new tissue site
  Proliferate cells to create a new tumor
  Provide nourishment for the new tumor mass

Source: Cooper, 1992, p. 23.

3.2.2. KNUDSON'S MODEL OF RETINOBLASTOMA

In 1971, Alfred G. Knudson sought to describe cancer development in a way which explained both inherited and sporadic forms of retinoblastoma. His two-hit theory (illustrated in Fig. 3-3) explained that children with the inherited form of retinoblastoma were born with one working copy of the *RB1* gene and one nonworking, mutated copy. The retinal tumors occurred only if a second genetic event or "hit" destroyed the functional *RB1* gene. In contrast, children with the sporadic form of retinoblastoma develop the eye cancer after two separate events have knocked out both copies of their retinoblastoma genes in a single retinal cell. This explained why 9 of 10 children with an inherited mutant *RB1* gene eventually develop a retinoblastoma tumor, whereas the incidence of sporadic retinoblastoma tumors is about 1 in 20,000.

The Knudson two-hit hypothesis described cancer development as a process rather than the result of a single event or exposure, thus revolutionizing our understanding of carcinogenesis. The two-hit model fits other neoplasms as well; however, this probably should be renamed the multiple-hit model because, as it turns out, most neoplasms require a minimum of four to six separate hits to reach full metastatic potential.

3.2.3. VOGELSTEIN'S MODEL OF COLON CANCER

The model of carcinogenesis in colorectal cancers, first described by Feuron and Vogelstein (1990), elegantly demonstrates that a combination of genetic events leads to malignancy. As shown in Figure 3-4, the initial carcinogenic event may be a germline or somatic mutation in the *APC* tumor suppressor

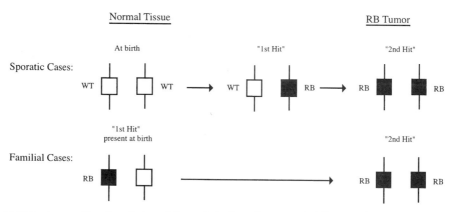

FIGURE 3-3. Knudson's two-hit model of carcinogenesis. This model demonstrates a mechanism that explains both sporadic and familial forms of retinoblastoma. WT, wild type; RB, Mutation in *RB* gene. [Source: Knudson, 1971.]

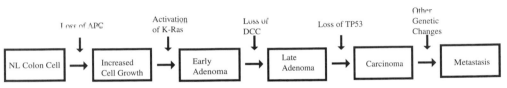

FIGURE 3-4. Vogelstein's multistep process of carcinogenesis. This model demonstrates the cascade of genetic events that need to occur for a colorectal tumor to form. [Source: Fearon and Vogelstein, 1990.]

gene termed "the gate-keeper." Additional genetic mutations (or alterations) of "care-taker genes" then lead to the activation of the K-*RAS* oncogene and loss of the *DCC* and *TP53* tumor suppressor genes. It is the accumulation of genetic events and the order of genetic changes that is important. Certain genetic changes do seem to occur more frequently as early events and other mutations as later events. The series of genetic changes in colorectal cells has been shown to correspond to the development of adenomas (in early, intermediate, and late stages) and metastatic carcinoma.

Other types of tumors have been found to be the result of multiple genetic mutations. In the majority of cases, these genetic events are somatic. While individuals with hereditary cancer syndromes have inherited a predisposition to cancer, other genetic events need to occur for cancer to develop. A better understanding of this chain of events has the potential of leading to improved ways to treat and even prevent cancer.

3.3. ONCOGENES

The discovery of viral oncogenes in the 1960s provided the first evidence that mutations in specific genes could induce cancer. This section describes the normal cellular functions of proto-oncogenes and the processes that can trigger oncogene activation and lead to malignancy. The *RET* oncogene is described at the end of the section.

3.3.1. GENERAL DESCRIPTION

Nearly 100 oncogenes have been described to date and each tumor will contain at least a few activated oncogenes. Oncogenes behave as dominant growth-promoting genes; therefore, only one copy of the gene needs to be mutated to affect a cell's growth or expression. More than one activated oncogene is usually required to cause cancer.

The names of oncogenes are typically composed of three-letter acronyms that can refer to the type of cancer induced by the virus, the species of animal that the virus infects, or the scientist who first isolated the virus. For example, *ABL* is named for the scientist Abelson and the cancer it induces (leukemia), and the *ras* oncogenes were first isolated from a rat sarcoma virus. Table 3-3 describes the origin of selected oncogene acronyms. Standard nomenclature for human oncogenes is written in italicized capital letters, whereas nonhuman oncogenes are written in italicized lower-case letters.

Oncogenes originate from normal cellular genes called proto-oncogenes. Although the name implies otherwise, the primary function of proto-oncogenes is not to give rise to oncogenes. Rather, most proto-oncogenes play crucial roles in the cell's signaling pathway, which maintains normal physiological cell function. Proto-oncogenes have remained highly conserved throughout evolution and appear to be crucial for normal tissue differentiation, particularly during embryogenesis.

The cellular signal transduction pathway is illustrated in Figure 3-5. In simplistic terms, the "sentry" proto-oncogenes recognize that certain external stimuli are present (such as growth signals or perceived "threats" to the cell) and will initiate sending a warning message to the nucleus. The message is given to the nearest messenger gene, which hands it off to the next gene in line and so on until the nucleus is reached. The nucleus will then evaluate the threat and can decide to turn on or off appropriate genes in response. The response messages from the nucleus are also relayed by messenger genes. A breakdown anywhere in the signaling pathway can therefore have major consequences for the function and integrity of the cell and its neighbors.

Proto-oncogenes are classified according to their function and placement in this signaling pathway. The major types of proto-oncogenes are described below.

1. *Growth factors*—The body has several specific growth factors that serve as intercellular signals for cell growth. Some proto-oncogenes encode growth factors that are small proteins active in the cell membrane. Examples of growth factor genes include *HER2/neu, INT-1* and

TABLE 3-3. ORIGIN OF SELECTED ONCOGENE ACRONYMS

Oncogene	Origin of Name
abl	Viral gene discovered by scientist Abelson; found in leukemic cells
C-myc	Gene discovered in a myelocytomatosis virus first isolated in chicken
N-MYC	Found first in human neuroblastomas
ras	First isolated from a rat sarcoma virus
K-ras	Virus discovered by scientist Kirsten
ret	Rearranged transforming gene

Source: Cooper, 1992; and Cooper, 1990.

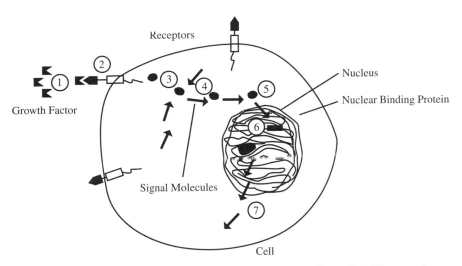

FIGURE 3-5. The cellular signal transduction pathway. Steps 1–7 illustrate how a cell receives a signal, delivers it to the nucleus, and generates a response. [Source: Ross, 1996, p. 133.]

SIS. Mutations in these proto-oncogenes will constantly stimulate adjacent cells to grow and enable them to ignore signals to halt growth.

2. *Growth factor receptors*—The signal transduction pathway begins with the binding of growth factor to a receptor. Many of these growth factor receptors lie in the cellular membrane and most are tyrosine kinases. Examples include *RET*, *MET*, and *ERBB-1*. Mutations in receptor genes can result in the overproduction of receptors or in a continually activated state. The cellular response to an overproduction of receptors is to divide into two cells, a process that will continue as long as the cells sense that extra receptors are present.

3. *Cytoplasmic tyrosine kinases*—Certain proto-oncogenes encode intracellular messengers of growth signals. These genes can be tyrosine kinases or serine-threonine kinases and can be located in the cytoplasm or nucleus. Examples include the *SRC* and *ABL* genes. Mutated messenger genes can send false information to the nucleus that triggers a response of enhanced growth and proliferation.

4. *Signal transducers*—Signal transducer proto-oncogenes also act as intracellular messengers. These gene products bind with GTP and are present in the inner membrane of the cell. Aberrant genes will lead to increased proliferation. The most important signal transducer genes are the *RAS* genes (e.g., K-*RAS*, H-*RAS*); mutated *RAS* genes are present in about one-third of human cancers.

5. *Nuclear transcription factors*—At the end of the cellular signaling pathway are the nuclear factors, which can activate DNA replication or transcription. Nuclear transcription factors include N-*Myc*, *Jun*, and *Fos*. Mutated nuclear transcription factors can perpetuate cell growth indefinitely and do not depend on any extracellular factors.

3.3.2. ONCOGENE ACTIVATION

The transformation of a proto-oncogene to an oncogene is called activation. Oncogene activation can lead to either of two outcomes: (1) deregulation and increased expression of a particular proto-oncogene or (2) a change in the structure and function of the proto-oncogene's protein.

Oncogene activation more typically occurs at the somatic level rather than in the germline. In fact, there are very few examples of oncogenes that are activated in the germline (and are thus the basis of specific hereditary cancer syndromes). Examples include the *RET*, *CDK4* , and *KIT* oncogenes.

At the somatic level, there are four major mechanisms that lead to oncogene activation.

1. *Point mutation*—A simple error in cell replication can result in a hyper-functional oncogene. This is the most common method of oncogene activation. For instance, the *RAS* oncogene in bladder carcinoma has been found to differ from its normal precursor by one base pair change, which results in a single amino acid substitution.

2. *Chromosome rearrangement*—Translocations and insertions can also result in oncogene activation. This appears to be a common cause of hematological malignancies. For example, the *ABL* oncogene, located on chromosome 9, becomes activated when fused to the middle of a gene on chromosome 22 called *BCR* (named for breakpoint cluster region). If the *ABL* gene is translocated at a major breakpoint, the fused *ABL/BCR* gene produces a P210 protein, which is a hybrid protein with growth-promoting properties. This rearrangement, known as the Philadelphia chromosome is present in about 90% of chronic myelogenous leukemias. If the *ABL* translocation occurs at a minor breakpoint, the *ABL/BCR* gene product is a P190 protein, which also has growth-promoting properties and is associated with acute lymphocytic leukemias.

3. *Gene amplification*—Errors in replication or reproduction can also result in multiple copies of an oncogene. The presence of multiple copies of an oncogene within a cell confers clonal advantages to the cell. Several cancers have been noted to contain specific oncogene amplifications. Neuroblastoma, for example, often contains multiple copies of the N-*Myc* oncogene.

4. *Viral insertion*—Oncogenes were first discovered within viruses. In fact, almost all human oncogenes are thought to have viral counterparts. Viruses can insert themselves into the machinery of a human proto-oncogene and convert it into a viral oncogene. This has been reported to occur with DNA tumor viruses, such as Epstein-Barr virus and human papilloma virus and also retroviruses, such as HIV. Viral exposures have been implicated in about 5% of human cancers.

3.3.3. THE *RET* ONCOGENE

The underlying cause of multiple endocrine neoplasia (MEN), type 2, is a germline mutation in the *RET* oncogene. The mutated *RET* oncogene is dominantly inherited and individuals with MEN 2 have increased risks for developing endocrine tumors. (See Chapter 4, entry 18 for the clinical features of MEN 2)

The *RET* proto-oncogene is one of the receptor genes in the signaling pathway. Specifically, it is a tyrosine kinase gene that encodes a receptor for GDNF (glial cell-derived neurotrophic factor).

The *RET* gene lies on chromosome 10q11.2 and is one of the few cancer susceptibility genes in which specific germline mutations lead to distinct phenotypes. As shown in Figure 3-6, specific *RET* mutations cause MEN 2A or 2B, whereas other mutations can lead to familial medullary thyroid carcinoma (FMTC) or Hirschsprung disease.

The *RET* Gene

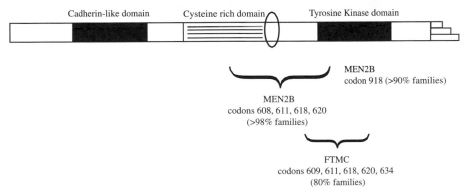

FIGURE 3-6. Phenotype-genotype correlations of *RET* mutations. As shown in this diagram, mutations in specific codons predicts the disease pattern. [Source: Hansford and Mulligan, 2000.]

3.4. TUMOR SUPPRESSOR GENES

The majority of hereditary cancer syndromes are due to a germline muta-tion in a dominantly inherited tumor suppressor gene. This section describes tumor suppressor genes and their role in cancer development and ends with a description of the *TP53* gene.

3.4.1. GENERAL DESCRIPTION

One of the major roles of tumor suppressor genes is to halt growth in damaged cells. Tumor suppressor genes encode proteins that negatively regulate the growth of cells. This family of genes plays important roles in both the signal transduction pathway and cell cycle regulation. More than a dozen tumor suppressor genes have been characterized and several more have been localized.

In contrast to oncogenes, it is the inactivation of tumor suppressor genes that leads to cancer development. In a target cell, the presence of a single functional tumor suppressor gene can maintain cell growth control and sup-pression of cancer. Loss of both copies of a tumor suppressor gene results in deregulated growth and potentially tumor growth in a target cell (for example, loss of both copies of the *RB* gene in a retinal cell). Thus, tumor suppressor genes can be said to behave in both a dominant and recessive manner, dominant in terms of its inheritance pattern and recessive at the cellular level.

3.4.2. TUMOR SUPPRESSOR GENE INACTIVATION

The inactivation of the initial tumor suppressor allele can occur at either the germline or somatic level. Inactivation of the second tumor suppressor allele always occurs at the somatic level. As described below, there are five major ways for the second allele to become inactivated.

1. *Point mutation or deletion*—A simple error in cell replication can cripple the tumor suppressor gene. If a DNA nucleotide is a missense mutation, then it is important for the laboratory to determine whether the change is a functional mutation or a polymorphism of no clinical significance. For example, a deleterious point mutation or a deletion in the *TP53* gene may lead to a number of neoplasms.

2. *Chromosome rearrangement*—Translocations or insertions can also result in the inactivation of a tumor suppressor allele.

3. *Mitotic nondisjunction*—Mitotic nondisjunction causes the loss of the entire chromosome containing the normal tumor suppressor gene. During mitosis, nondisjunction occurs, resulting in one daughter cell with three copies of a chromosome and one daughter cell with a

single abnormal copy. The daughter cell, lacking a functional tumor suppressor gene, will divide further, leading to a small colony of abnormal cells.

4. *Mitotic recombination*—Mitotic recombination leads to the loss of the normal tumor suppressor gene. Recombination between the maternal and paternal alleles followed by mitosis will lead to one daughter cell with both maternal alleles and one daughter cell with both paternal alleles. One cell, therefore, may have two abnormal tumor suppressor genes.

5. *Gene amplification*—The overexpression of certain proteins can result in the inactivation of a tumor suppressor protein. For example, overexpression of certain proteins (such as mdm-2) can lead to the binding and subsequent inactivation of TP53 protein products.

3.4.3. THE *TP53* TUMOR SUPPRESSOR GENE

The *TP53* gene has been nicknamed "the guardian of the genome." It has three important functions: controlling the cell cycle, initiating apoptosis, and maintaining the integrity of the genome. The *TP53* gene monitors the accumulation of DNA damage and will mediate a G_1 cell cycle arrest so that DNA repair can be initiated. If the damaged cell is deemed beyond repair, *TP53* will induce apoptosis. Dismantling the *TP53* regulatory system is the main way in which malignant cells attain immortality. The loss of normal TP53 protein also appears to lead to overall genomic instability. It is estimated that over 50% of all tumors contain damaged or absent *TP53* genes—by far the most common genetic error that occurs in neoplasms.

The *TP53* gene lies on chromosome 17p13 and its product is a 53-kDa protein that binds to DNA in the nucleus. Normal cells express low levels of TP53 protein, whereas higher levels are present in damaged cells. When mutated, the *TP53* gene can act like a growth-promoting oncogene, thus conferring a clear advantage to the cell.

3.5. DNA REPAIR GENES

DNA repair genes represent a third category of cancer susceptibility genes. This section describes the different types of DNA repair genes that, when nonfunctional, can contribute to cancer development.

3.5.1. GENERAL DESCRIPTION

The major function of DNA repair genes is to identify and fix DNA nucleotide errors made during replication. As shown in Figure 3-7, successful DNA repair requires multiple steps:

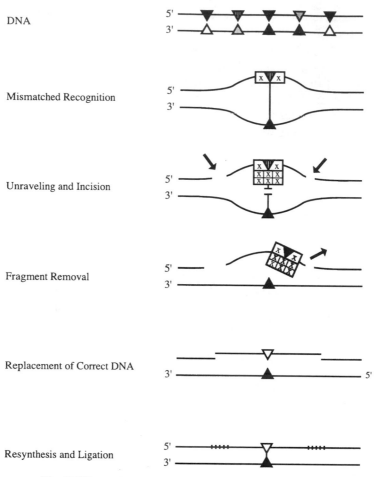

DNA

Mismatched Recognition

Unraveling and Incision

Fragment Removal

Replacement of Correct DNA

Resynthesis and Ligation

FIGURE 3-7. The DNA repair system. This illustration depicts the five major steps involved in DNA repair. [Source: Squire et al., 1998, p. 66.]

1. recognition of the sequence error,
2. recruitment of the appropriate proteins,
3. incision of the DNA and excision of the mistaken nucleotide(s),
4. resynthesis of the correct nucleotide(s), and
5. reattachment of the DNA strand.

Inactivation of any of the genes involved in the repair process will make the system less efficient, leading to the accumulation of DNA errors within a cell. If these DNA mutations occur in proto-oncogenes or tumor suppressor genes, then this could eventually result in the formation of a tumor. Therefore, cancer occurs as a secondary effect of faulty DNA repair genes.

This is in contrast to oncogenes and tumor suppressor genes, which have a more direct role in tumorigenesis.

3.5.2. MISMATCH REPAIR GENES

Several mismatch repair genes have been implicated in hereditary nonpolyposis colon cancer, including *MLH1*, *MSH2*, *MSH6*, *PMS1*, and *PMS2*. Homologues of these human mismatch repair genes were initially characterized in *E. coli* and yeast. Germline mutations in the mismatch repair genes follow a dominant pattern of inheritance.

Mismatch repair genes have the important function of correcting DNA errors that occur during replication. This process has been compared with the spell-checker function on a computer. At multiple sites in the genome, there are sequences of repeated DNA nucleotides, such as, $TT(T)_n$ or $CACA(CA)_n$ called microsatellite DNA. These sequences appear susceptible to errors during DNA transcription. Cells with faulty mismatch repair genes will cause "stutters" in the microsatellite DNA and can result in altered lengths of repeated DNA sequences. This phenomenon is termed microsatellite instability (MSI). The presence of MSI is suggestive of a faulty mismatch repair gene, although the correlation is not perfect. It is estimated that 80%–90% of HNPCC-related colorectal tumors demonstrate MSI, whereas less than 10% of sporadic colorectal tumors do so.

3.5.3. OTHER DNA REPAIR GENES

Some of the DNA repair genes concentrate on fixing the DNA in cells that have been damaged from an external source, such as radiation. These genes are also termed DNA damage response genes. Exposure to ultraviolet or ionizing radiation can cause extensive DNA damage to cells, which must either be excised and repaired or destroyed and replaced. If these DNA repair genes are not working properly, cells with chromosomal instability will be allowed to function and further divide.

Examples of hereditary cancer syndromes caused by a faulty DNA damage response gene include Fanconi anemia, Bloom syndrome, ataxia-telangiectasia, and xeroderma pigmentosum. These rare syndromes are characterized by increased rates of several types of cancer, particularly leukemias and skin cancers. In contrast to HNPCC, these cancer syndromes follow an autosomal recessive pattern of inheritance.

3.6. EPIGENETIC MECHANISMS

As discussed earlier in this chapter, germline mutations in growth regulating genes can detrimentally affect gene expression and trigger or hasten the development of a tumor. Another important mechanism that can affect gene expression is the activation or silencing of specific growth regulatory genes due to epigenetic changes (Epi means "upon" or "in addition to"). An epigenetic modification of gene expression is one that does not involve an alteration of the gene's DNA sequence. Thus, the altered expression is potentially reversible. Because this process can be reversed, it is hoped that a better understanding of epigenetic mechanisms will ultimately lead to improved cancer treatment strategies.

A high percentage of sporadic tumors, particularly those of embryonic origin, have undergone epigenetic changes. In fact, this may represent one of the most common alterations in human cancers. The most widely recognized epigenetic modifier is that of gene silencing. This section describes the role of gene silencing in tumorigenesis.

3.6.1 GENE SILENCING MECHANISMS

Epigenetic "gene silencing" refers to processes that render genes nonfunctional without disturbing the DNA of the gene. Therefore, if the gene silencing mechanism is repaired or lifted, then the gene would be functional. If growth regulatory genes are the ones that are inappropriately silenced, then this potentially acts as a carcinogenic "hit" that could ultimately lead to a neoplasm.

Several mechanisms can lead to inappropriate gene silencing, including the following:

1) *a defect in the imprint organizing center*—Abnormal imprinting can result from a deletion or mutation in any of the genes that comprise one of the imprint organizing centers. This type of defect can cause a failure of the initial "locking in" of which parental-origin alleles are to be silenced.

2) *separation of the imprint organizing center from target genes*—In chromosome rearrangements, such as translocations, a gene might become separated from its imprint organizing center. This could lead to abnormal gene expression patterns.

3) *uniparental disomy*—The presence of two alleles derived from the same parent is termed uniparental disomy (UPD) and results in abnormal imprinting due to the excess of one allele and absence of the other. In paternal UPD, for example, the maternal alleles are lost (silenced) and the paternal alleles, which are duplicated, will be amplified. The majority of hereditary paragangliomas in the Netherlands are associated with paternal UPD involving the *SDHD* gene (Taschner, 2001). Paternal UPD is also associated with some cases of Wilms' tumor, rhabdomyosarcoma, and osteosarcoma. Maternal UPD has been reported in cases of neuroblastoma and acute myelogenous leukemia.

4) *abnormal methylation of CpG islands*—Alleles that are generally active might be abnormally silenced by the methylation of the promoter regions. Conversely, there could be a loss of methylation, leading to the activation of normally silent genes. The abnormal methylation could affect a single gene, a few neighboring genes, or multiple chromosomes.

5) *the loss of trans-acting factors*—Little is known about *trans*-acting factors except that they appear to play an important role in maintaining normal patterns of gene expression. Mutations in or loss of these *trans*-acting factors could result in relaxed or abnormal imprinting or methylation.

The two major mechanisms of gene silencing, genomic imprinting and methylation, are described below:

1. *Genomic imprinting*—As demonstrated by genomic imprinting, the maternal and paternal copies of each gene and chromosome are required for normal development. In addition to having the full complement of 46 chromosomes, it is important to have an equal balance of maternal and paternal alleles. Thus, contrary to Mendel's theory, maternal and paternal alleles are not always equivalent and 2 copies of an allele, without attention to parental origin, are not sufficient to assume normal function. An extreme example of this can be observed when an "embryo" is erroneously formed with 2 sets of paternally-derived chromosomes or 2 sets of maternally-derived chromosomes. A paternal-only genome results in the formation of a hydatiform mole and a maternal-only genome forms a complete ovarian teratoma Thus, an imbalance of maternal and paternal alleles has the potential of causing neoplastic growth.

   Genomic imprinting is an epigenetic modification of a specific parental allele of a gene or chromosome that leads to differential expression of the two alleles in the offspring's cells. In other words, this process silences one copy of each allele and in many cases, the inactivation of an allele is not random but rather based on the allele's parent of origin and the specific needs of the tissue. The most important imprinting event occurs during embryogenesis when the allelic expression of different tissue types is "locked into place" by use of imprint organizing centers. Genomic imprinting is then maintained, at least in part, through a process termed methylation. Thus, normal genomic imprinting is a continuous, developmental process not a single event.

   Beckwith-Weidemann (BWS) is a classic example of a genetic condition that can be caused by abnormal genomic imprinting. BWS is an overgrowth syndrome that is associated with increased risks of embryonic tumors (see Chapter 4, entry 3). Various genomic imprinting errors can result in the BWS phenotype including:

- switched imprinting (the maternal allele is erroneously silenced, paternal allele is erroneously activated),
- a rearrangement in the maternal allele that disrupts the function of the normally activated genes, or
- paternal UPD that causes the over-expression of the paternal allele and loss of the maternal allele.

2. *Methylation*—The process of methylation effectively silences an allele of a gene or chromosome. DNA methylation is a carefully programmed process based on the potential of DNA methyl groups to act as a "5th basepair." This 5th basepair can be formed and maintained at any cytosine-guanine (CpG) dinucleotide effectively blocking or silencing the gene. DNA methylation generally occurs in the CpG islands of the genes. CpG islands are regions that have a high number (200+) and concentration of CpG dinucleotides. CpG islands are frequently present in the promoter region or first exon of the so-called housekeeping genes (including growth regulatory genes). It is estimated that 80% of CpG islands within genes are methylated. During a person's lifetime, methylation can only be removed during the replication process or by enzymatic action. For example, over-expression of the enzyme methyltransferase, can "flag" a gene for silencing. The methylation status of particular genes is generally permanent and is somatically inherited. However, the pattern of methylated genes is reversed in many tumors.

Abnormal methylation can result in switching allele activation from the maternal to the paternal allele or vice versa, or can lead to the activation or silencing of both alleles. This process can lead to neoplastic growth if it has activated normally silent copies of growth-promoting genes or has silenced normally functional copies of tumor suppressor genes. For example, in Wilms' tumor, the maternal allele can be abnormally silenced (which results in the loss of two tumor suppressor genes, *H19* and *CDKN1C*) and/or the paternal allele can be activated (which retains the advantageous growth factor, IGF2).

Specific tumors that have demonstrated abnormal methylation include Wilms' tumor, neuroblastoma, rhabdomyosarcoma, osteosarcoma, hepatoblastoma, and acute myelogenous leukemia. Colorectal tumors with microsatellite instability may have germline *MLH1* mutations, if familial, and promoter hypermethylation and loss of expression of *MLH1* if sporadic (due to hypermethylation). Other genes that are sensitive to methylation include *RB1*, *VHL*, *TP16*, and possibly *BRCA1*.

The contribution of imprinting or methylation in the development of cancer is still poorly understood. Future research may demonstrate that epigenetic mechanisms play an important role in heritable and non-heritable malignancies.

3.7 REFERENCES

Benchimal, S and Minden, M. 1998. Viruses, oncogenes, and tumor suppressor genes. In Tannock, I and Hill, R (eds) The Basic Science of Oncology. McGraw-Hill, New York, NY, 79–105.

Cooper, G. 1990. Oncogenes. Jones & Bartlett Publishers, Boston, MA.

Cooper, G. 1992. Elements of Human Cancer. Jones & Bartlett Publishers, Boston, MA.

Fearon, E and Vogelstein, B. 1990. A genetic model for colorectal tumorigenesis. Cell 61:759–567.

Fineberg, A. 1998. Genomic imprinting and cancer. In Vogelstein, B and Kinzler, K (eds) The genetic basis of human cancer. McGraw-Hill, New York, NY 95–107.

Hansford, J and Mulligan, L. 2000. Multiple endocrine neoplasia type 2 and RET: from neoplasia to neurogenesis. J Med Genet 37:818.

Hodgson, S and Maher, E. 1999. Molecular genetics of cancer. In A practical guide to human cancer genetics, 2nd edition. Cambridge University Press. Cambridge, UK, 11–21.

Kinzler, K and Vogelstein, B. 1996. Lessons from hereditary colorectal cancer. Cell. 87:159–170.

Knudson, A 1971. Mutation and cancer: statistical study of retinoblastoma. Proc Natl Acad Sci USA 68:820–823.

Lovejoy, N. 1987. Alterations in cell biology. In Ziegfield, C (ed) Core Curriculum for Oncology Nursing. WB Saunders, Philadelphia, PA, 3–17.

Malik, K and Brown, K. 2000. Epigenetic gene deregulation in cancer. Br J Cancer 83:1583–1588.

Offit, K. 1998. Cancer as a genetic disorder. In Clinical Cancer Genetics. John Wiley & Sons, New York, NY, 39–65.

Ponder, B. 2001. Cancer genetics. Nature. 411:336–341.

Ross, D. 1996. Introduction to Molecular Medicine, 2nd edition. Springer-Verlag. New York, NY.

Ross, D. 1998. Introduction to Oncogenes and Molecular Cancer Medicine. Springer-Verlag. New York, NY.

Squire, J, Whitmore, G, and Phillips, R. 1998. Genetic basis of cancer. In Tannock, I and Hill, R (eds) The Basic Science of Oncology. McGraw-Hill, New York, NY, 48–78.

Taschner, P, Jansen, J, Baysal, B et al. 2001. Nearly all hereditary paragangliomas in the Netherlands are caused by two founder mutations in the SDHD gene. Genes Chromosomes Cancer 38:274–281.

Varmus, H and Weinberg, R. 1993. Genes and the Biology of Cancer. Scientific American Library, New York, NY.

HEREDITARY CANCER SYNDROMES

The question, "Is cancer hereditary?" has been answered with a resounding "Yes." . . . However, a litany of vexing questions emanates from these discoveries."

(Lynch, 1998)

Over 200 hereditary cancer syndromes have been described, although most are quite rare. It is estimated that 5–10% of cancers have a hereditary component . Hereditary cancer syndromes are characterized by substantial but not absolute risks of specific cancers. Associated cancer risks can vary widely, ranging from a 5% risk of cancer with Neurofibromatosis to the 2,000-fold increased risk of skin cancer with xeroderma pigmentosum. Most hereditary cancer syndromes have lifetime risks of cancer that far exceed the cancer risks due to noninherited factors. There is also widely variable expressivity in hereditary cancer syndromes. Some individuals have severe phenotypes and others are more mildly affected. Even among members of the same family, the occurrences of cancer may differ greatly in terms of age of onset, site of cancer, tumor grading, clinical staging, and survival rates.

Section 4.1 of this chapter describes the clinical features and underlying genetic basis for 30 major hereditary cancer syndromes. Section 4.2 provides a description of the cancer risks associated with the following three chromosomal aneuploidies:

1. Down syndrome
2. Klinefelter syndrome
3. Turner syndrome

4.1. HEREDITARY CANCER SYNDROMES

This section provides general information about 30 hereditary syndromes in which cancer is a prominent feature. The syndromes are listed in alphabetical order and cross-referenced where appropriate. Primary references used to compile this section are listed at the end of the chapter.

1. AUTOIMMUNE LYMPHOPROLIFERATIVE SYNDROME
(also Canale-Smith syndrome)

Incidence:	Rare
Penetrance:	100%
Inheritance:	Autosomal dominant
Genes:	*FAS* at 10q24.1
	FASL at 1q23
	CASP10 at locus 2q33–q34
Cancer risks:	Increased, but not quantified
Clinical features:	Autoimmune lymphoproliferative syndrome (ALPS) is an autoimmune disorder that is usually diagnosed in childhood. Individuals with ALPS often present with very enlarged lymph nodes and spleen and may be aggressively worked up for cancer. The lymphadenopathy and splenomegaly are caused by hemolytic anemia and thrombocytopenia. Affected individuals have an increased number of DNT lymphocytes (double negative T cells), which can lead to an abnormally heightened immune system response. Adults with ALPS appear to be at risk for Guillain-Barré syndrome and panniculitis; both of which are autoimmune disorders.
	Individuals with ALPS are at increased risk for developing B-cell lymphoma. Hepatocellular carcinoma and other solid tumors have been reported in a few cases. Although it is less common, ALPS can also present in adulthood.
Diagnostic criteria:	The cardinal features of ALPS are hemolytic anemia, thrombocytopenia, and lymphadenopathy during childhood or adolescence.
Cancer monitoring:	Individuals with ALPS are followed carefully by a hematologist, who will also monitor them for signs of lymphoma.
Molecular findings:	The *FAS* gene (also called *TNFRSF6* or *CD95*) plays an important role in programmed cell death of lymphocytes. The failure of apoptosis mediated by the FAS protein causes an accumulation of lymphocytes, which

leads to a damaged immune response and an increased risk of lymphoma. The underlying cause of ALPS may also be a mutation in the FAS ligand (FASL), also termed TNFSF6 or CD95L. Other genes along the *FAS* pathway, such as the Caspase-10 gene (*CASP10*), can also cause the ALPS phenotype.

ALPS can be subdivided into four subtypes based on the molecular findings: ALPS 1A: mutation in *FAS* gene; ALPS 1B: mutation in *FAS* gene; ALPS 2: mutation in *CASPASE 10* gene; ALPS 3: no defined genetic cause.

Genetic testing: Available on a research basis only

2. ATAXIA-TELANGIECTASIA

Incidence: 1 in 30,000 to 1 in 100,000
                  Frequency of heterozygous carriers is about 1%
Penetrance: 100% in homozygotes
Inheritance: Autosomal recessive
Gene: *ATM* at 11q22.3
Cancer risks: 30–40%
Clinical features: A young child with ataxia-telangiectasia (AT) walks with an unsteady, lurching gait, the hallmark feature of the syndrome. Cerebellar ataxia, which occurs before age 10, is present in 100% of cases, and choreoathetosis/dystonia and dysarthria is present in 90%. Most affected individuals are wheelchair bound by adolescence and develop degenerate spinal muscular atrophy in their twenties and thirties. Other features of AT include slurred speech, disturbed eye movements, endocrine dysfunction, immunodeficiency, vitiligo, café au lait spots, premature aging and graying of the hair, and telangiectasia. Telangiectases, which are red marks caused by the abnormal dilation of capillaries, become noticeable after age 7 in skin exposed to the sun. Mental retardation and/or dementia are not typical features of AT . Although affected individuals often live into their thirties, they rarely live past age 45.

Infection is one of the major causes of death for individuals with AT, followed by cancer. About one-third of all individuals with AT will develop cancer at some point in their lives. The most common malignancies are non-Hodgkin lymphomas (typically B-cell, but also T-cell) and leukemias (typically chronic lymphocytic, but also acute promylocytic). Lymphomas and leukemias account for over 80% of the AT-associated cancer diagnoses and can occur in early adolescence or adulthood. Other malignancies associated with AT include melanoma and cancers of the breast, stomach, pancreas, and ovary. Leiomyosarcomas, medulloblastomas and gliomas have also been reported. Cancer treatment is complicated by the fact that radiation treatments are contraindicated, given the frequency of chromosomal breakage in radiation exposed cells.

Diagnostic criteria: Diagnosis of AT is typically based on clinical features, but there are two laboratory tests that can be used: the serum alphafetoprotein test, because values are consistently elevated among individuals with AT, and radioresistant DNA synthesis. This test analyzes the frequency of spontaneous chromosomal aberrations, particularly at T-cell and B-cell receptor sites. Such breakpoints may be seen in 10% of mitoses in individuals with AT. Radioresistant DNA synthesis does not appear to be a reliable screen for heterozygous carriers, hence the interest in refining the genetic test.

Cancer monitoring: Individuals with AT are suggested to undergo periodic blood counts, careful skin examinations, and upper gastrointestinal imaging if symptoms are reported. It is unclear whether X-rays, with their exceedingly low rates of radiation, can be harmful to people with AT , but concerns have been raised. To be cautious, X-rays should be used for diagnostic purposes rather than as a screening tool. Mammograms are still recommended, although there is some controversy about offering mammography to young female AT carriers. The benefits of cancer screening in people with AT have not yet been established.

AT heterozygotes: There was quite a stir among high risk breast cancer clinics when it was first reported that women who were heterozygous *ATM* carriers had increased risks of breast cancer, perhaps fivefold higher than that of the general population. However, subsequent studies have failed to corroborate excess breast cancer rates among AT heterozygotes, particularly in cases of premenopausal breast cancer. As a precaution, mothers of an affected child are still advised to initiate breast cancer surveillance programs beginning in their thirties. AT heterozygotes (male and female) may also be at increased risk for other forms of cancer, including leukemia, stomach cancer, and lung cancer.

Molecular findings: The *ATM* gene is expressed in all organs tested to date, but its function remains unclear. Preliminary studies suggest that it may be a protein kinase that interacts with proteins upstream from TP53 in intracellular signaling pathways. The *ATM* gene contains 61 exons and consists of four complementation groups: A, C, D, and E, with A being the most common worldwide. Of the hundreds of reported *ATM* mutations, over 85% result in a truncated protein.

Genetic testing: Available on a research basis only

BANNAYAN-RILEY-RUVALCABA syndromes—see *Cowden syndrome*

3. BECKWITH-WIEDEMANN SYNDROME (also EMG syndrome)

Incidence: 1 in 14,000
Penetrance: May be 100% in familial cases
Inheritance: Autosomal dominant; most cases are isolated occurrences
Gene: *BWS* at 11p15
Cancer risks: 8-20% (higher if hemihypertrophy is present)
Clinical features: Beckwith-Wiedemann syndrome (BWS) is an example of an overgrowth syndrome. BWS (also termed EMG syndrome) is characterized by exomphalos (umbilical hernia), macroglossia, and gigantism. Other features include earlobe grooves, minor facial dysmorphia, enlarged liver, kidney, or spleen, cryptorchidism, and occasionally cardiac defects, neonatal hypoglycemia, and hemihypertrophy. Affected individuals have mild to moderate mental retardation and exhibit compulsive overeating as they become older.

Children with BWS are at increased risk for developing tumors of embryonal origin. The risk of malignancy is between 8-20% but children born with hemihypertrophy may have cancer risks as high as 40%. The following tumors have been seen in children with BWS: Wilms' tumor, adrenocortical carcinoma, hepatoblastoma, rhabdomyosarcoma, neuroblastoma, and gastric teratoma. These malignancies typically

	occur by age 5. Cases of hepatocellular carcinoma have also been reported.
Diagnostic criteria:	Diagnosis is typically based on clinical features. Molecular studies can sometimes be helpful as can chromosome studies.
Cancer monitoring:	Cancer screening in children with BWS consists of frequent physical examinations and abdominal ultrasounds throughout early childhood. Alpha-fetoprotein blood tests may also be used as a screening tool.
Molecular findings:	BWS occurs as a result of failed genetic imprinting of chromosome 11. Instead of being born with one maternally imprinted and one paternally imprinted allele, the individual with BWS has two paternally derived BWS genes. A small subset of BWS cases have duplications of 11p15 as a result of an unbalanced translocation. Risks of disease are higher if the mother rather than the father is the transmitting parent.
Genetic testing:	Clinically available

4. BIRT-HOGG-DUBE SYNDROME

Incidence:	Rare
Penetrance:	Unknown
Inheritance:	Autosomal dominant
Gene:	localized to 17p12-q11.2
Cancer risks:	Increased, but not quantified
Clinical features:	Birt-Hogg-Dube syndrome (BHD) is a dermatological genetic disorder. Affected individuals develop one or more fibrofolliculomas (a raised skin lesion with a central hair). Other associated skin lesions include trichodiscomas, acrochordons (skin tags), papules, and trichilimmomas. Lipomas have also been reported. Onset is usually adulthood. Associated malignancies include renal cell carcinoma and parathyroid adenomas.
Diagnostic criteria:	The triad of features in BHD are fibrofolliculomas, trichodiscomas, and acrochordons. The identification of BHD is based on these three features as well as the associated malignancies listed above.
Cancer monitoring:	Individuals with BHD are at increased risk for developing renal cancer and should be monitored accordingly. Monitoring for renal cancers can include abdominal computed tomography and ultrasonography.

Molecular findings: Families with BHD have tested negative for mutations in the *VHL* and *MET* genes. A novel *BHD* gene has recently been mapped to region 17p12-q11.2 (Khoo et al, 2001).

Genetic testing: None available

5. BLACKFAN-DIAMOND SYNDROME

Incidence: 1 in 5,000,000 births
Penetrance: Unknown
Inheritance: Most cases sporadic, but autosomal dominant and autosomal recessive cases reported
Gene: Unknown
Cancer risks: Increased but not quantified
Clinical features: Blackfan-Diamond syndrome (BDS) is characterized by congenital hypoplastic anemia, although leukocyte and platelet counts are normal. Most children are diagnosed by 3 months of age. Affected individuals have an increased risk of developing acute nonlymphocytic leukemia.
Diagnostic criteria: Diagnosis of BDS is based on the results of a CBC (complete blood count) that reveals hypoplastic anemia, normal leucocytes, and normal platelets. Affected individuals also have an increased number of chromosome breakages.
Cancer monitoring: Children with BDS need to be followed carefully for signs of leukemia.
Molecular findings: The underlying molecular basis for BDS has not been identified. However, some individuals with BDS have been found to carry mutations in a gene encoding ribosomal protein S19 (located at 19q13). Patients were heterozygous for these mutations.
Genetic testing: Not currently available

6. BLOOM SYNDROME

Incidence: Rare in general population; frequency of heterozygotes among Ashkenazi Jews is about 1 in 200.
Penetrance: 100%
Inheritance: Autosomal recessive
Gene: *BLM (RECQL3)* at 15q26.1
Cancer risks: 20%
Clinical features: Bloom syndrome (BS) is characterized by severe growth deficiency, sun-sensitive facial erythema/telangiectasia ("butterfly rash") with malar hypopla-

sia, nasal prominence, small mandible, and dolicho-cephalic skull. Individuals demonstrate hypersensitiv-ity to sunlight and often have patchy skin. Affected individuals are highly susceptible to infection due to a severe immune defect with reduced gamma-globulin (IgA and IgM) levels. They may also be at increased risk for developing diabetes mellitus. Most have normal intelligence, although learning disabil-ities are common. Survival into adulthood is rare.

About 20% of individuals with BS develop cancer, with half the cases occurring before age 20. Individu-als with BS have increased risks of non-Hodgkin lym-phoma, acute leukemia, carcinomas of the mouth, stomach, larynx, lung esophagus, colon, skin, breast, and cervix. A few cases of Wilms' tumor have also been reported.

Diagnostic criteria: Diagnosis is usually based on clinical features. Confir-matory laboratory testing can look for an increased rate of sister chromatid exchanges (SCE) which lead to excess breakage and possibly loss of heterozygosity.

Cancer monitoring: Cancer screening includes routine physical examina-tions and blood counts during childhood and after age 20. Individuals with BS are suggested to undergo sur-veillance for skin and gastrointestinal tract cancers, and affected females should also be monitored for cer-vical and breast cancers. Most importantly, affected individuals are advised to avoid direct sunlight.

Molecular findings: Individuals of Ashkenazi Jewish heritage are at increased risk for having a specific *BLM* founder mutation (6 basepair deletion/7 basepair insertion at nucleotide 2281). Carrier testing is sometimes offered to couples of Eastern European (Ashkenazi) Jewish ancestry as part of a prenatal screening profile. About 20% of children with BS are mosaic for the homozy-gous *BLM* mutations.

The *BLM* (or *RECQL3*) gene is one of the 5 known human *RECQL* helicase genes. The BLM protein is an "antirecombinase" which means that it normally suppresses sister chromatid exchanges during genetic recombination. Some families with Rothmund-Thomson syndrome and Werner syndrome also have mutations in one of the DNA helicase genes.

Genetic testing: Clinically available.

7. BLUE RUBBER BLEB NEVUS SYNDROME

Incidence:	Rare
Penetrance:	Presumed 100%
Inheritance:	Autosomal dominant (some cases are *de novo*)
Gene:	Unknown
Cancer risks:	May not be increased
Clinical features:	There are approximately 200 families worldwide who have been diagnosed with Blue Rubber Bleb Nevus syndrome (BRBNS). It appears as though all individuals with BRBNS develop the characteristic raised lesions that can be blue or green in color. Some people develop only a few of these bladder-like skin hemangiomas, others develop hundreds. The skin hemangiomas may be present at birth, but can continue to appear during childhood and adulthood.
	Individuals with BRBNS can also develop internal hemangiomas, especially in the small intestine or elsewhere along the digestive tract. Hemangiomas can develop in other organs as well, including the eyes, pharynx, and uterus. Medical complications associated with BRBNS are uncommon but can occur secondary to the internal hemangiomas depending on their size and location. This can include severe iron deficiency anemia or hemorrhaging (digestive tract), impaired breathing (pharynx), or impaired vision (eye).
	In early descriptions of BRBNS, childhood medulloblastoma was mentioned as a possible feature. However, no additional cases of medulloblastoma have been reported, which makes it questionable whether it is truly an associated feature of BRBNS.
Diagnostic criteria:	The diagnosis of BRBNS is based on the presence of blue or green bladder-like skin hemangiomas.
Cancer monitoring:	No special cancer monitoring is suggested. However, individuals with BRBNS should be regularly monitored for signs of anemia or respiratory problems. A one time retinal exam in childhood is also suggested.
Molecular findings:	A few families with BRBNS have been localized to chromosomal region 9p, but the exact location and identification of the gene is still being sought.
Genetic testing:	Not available

8. BREAST-OVARIAN CANCER SYNDROME

Incidence: 1 in 800 to 1 in 2,500 in general population; frequency
                        may be as high as 2% in Ashkenazi Jews.
Penetrance: 85% or less
Inheritance: Autosomal dominant
Gene: *BRCA1* at 17q21
                        BRCA2 at 13q12
Cancer risks: 85% or less
Clinical features: Breast-ovarian cancer syndrome (BOCS) is charac-
                        terized by breast adenocarcinomas, either ductal or
                        lobular in origin, and ovarian carcinomas (generally of
                        epithelial origin). The risk of breast cancer in classic
                        BOCS families may be as high as 3% by age 30, 19%
                        by age 40, 51% by age 50, 54% by age 60, and 85% by
                        age 70. For female *BRCA1* mutation carriers, the risk
                        of ovarian cancer is about 26% for most families,
                        although a significant subset exhibits much higher
                        risks, perhaps 85% by age 70 (Easton, 1993).

                        Germline *BRCA1* mutations are associated with
                        cancer in the following organs: breast (50-85% risks),
                        ovary (20-60% risks), prostate, and colon. Females are
                        at small but increased risks for developing papillary
                        serous carcinoma of the peritoneum. Cases of male
                        breast cancer have been reported.

                        Germline *BRCA2* mutations in females are asso-
                        ciated with cancers in the following organs: breast
                        (50-85%), ovary (10-20% risks), fallopian tube, and
                        peritoneum. Males who carry *BRCA2* mutations have
                        increased risks of breast and prostate cancer. The risk
                        of pancreatic cancer is increased for both men and
                        women. *BRCA2*-linked breast cancers tend to occur at
                        older ages (after age 50) compared to *BRCA1*-linked
                        cases. *BRCA2* mutation carriers may also be at small
                        increased risks of developing ocular melanoma, other
                        head and neck cancers, and cancers of the gallbladder,
                        bile duct and stomach.
Diagnostic criteria: Families with BOCS have patterns of cancer that
                        include the following features: early-onset breast
                        cancer; bilateral breast cancer, breast cancer in two or
                        more generations, ovarian cancer, breast and ovarian
                        cancer in the same relative, and breast cancer in a male
                        relative.
Cancer monitoring: Women carrying *BRCA1* or *BRCA2* mutations are sug-

gested to do monthly breast self-examinations beginning by age 21, undergo bi-annual clinical breast examinations beginning at age 25–30, and begin annual mammography at age 25–30. Some providers also suggest that at-risk women undergo annual breast MRI exams, although the efficacy of this imaging technique has not been established. Ovarian surveillance consists of pelvic examination, transvaginal ultrasound beginning at age 25–30, and measurement of serum CA-125 levels in postmenopausal women. Men who carry BRCA1 or BRCA2 mutations are suggested to have annual clinical breast exams and follow standard guidelines regarding screening for prostate cancers, beginning at age 50.

Cancer prevention: Because current surveillance strategies are poor at detecting early stage ovarian cancer, women with BRCA1 or BRCA2 mutations are recommended to have prophylactic oophorectomies. Prophylactic mastectomies are also presented as an option. Women also have the option of considering chemopreventive strategies, such as tamoxifen to reduce breast cancer risk or oral contraceptives to reduce ovarian cancer risk. Although these strategies can lower the risks of specific cancers, no strategy to date can eliminate the risk completely.

Molecular findings: About one-half to two thirds of families with significant histories of breast cancer will be found to have detectable BRCA1 or BRCA2 mutations. About 80% of families with histories of breast and ovarian cancer will have detectable mutations, more frequently in the BRCA1 gene. The BRCA1 gene is 22 exons in length, and the BRCA2 gene is 27 exons. Germline mutations include several hundred distinct deletions, insertions, and point mutations. Large gene mutations, such as the 3 large deletions in the Dutch population, will not be detected by conventional DNA sequencing methods. The three founder mutations in the Ashkenazi Jewish population are 187delAG (also referred to as 185delAG), 5385insC mutations in the BRCA1 gene, and the 6174delT mutation in the BRCA2 gene. Founder BRCA1 and/or BRCA2 mutations have also been reported in other ethnic groups, including French-Canadians, Icelanders, Japanese, Finnish, and Swedish. The BRCA1 and BRCA2 genes are tumor suppressor genes of unknown function. Researchers continue to search for additional breast cancer suscep- tibility genes.

Genetic testing: Clinically available

CANALE-SMITH SYNDROME: *see Autoimmune lymphoproliferative syndrome*

CARNEY COMPLEX: *see NAME syndrome*

9. COWDEN SYNDROME (also multiple hamartoma syndrome and Bannayan-Riley-Ruvalcaba syndromes)

Incidence: 1 in 200,000 to 250,000 in Dutch population
Penetrance: May be 100%
Inheritance: Autosomal dominant
Gene: *PTEN* at 10q23
Cancer risks: About 50%
Clinical features: Cowden syndrome (CS) is thought to be rare but is almost certainly underreported. Women with CS have a 30% lifetime risk of breast cancer and an increased, but unknown risk for endometrial cancer. Affected individuals also have an up to 10% lifetime risk of non-medullary thyroid cancer, especially of the follicular histology. Other cancers thought to be part of the CS phenotype include renal cell carcinoma, melanoma, and glioblastoma.
Diagnostic criteria: The diagnostic criteria for CS is shown in Table 4-1. The hallmark feature of CS are the facial and oral muco-cutaneous lesions, which are often trichilimmomas. Individuals may also have macrocephaly (usually dolichocephaly). Internal hamartomas are present in 60% of affected individuals, typically in the gastroin-testinal or genitourinary tract. Other features include fibrocystic breast disease, thyroid disease, lipomas, fibromas, oral mucosal papillomatosis ("scrotal tongue"), and Lhermitte-Duclos disease. Lhermitte-Duclos disease is characterized by a hamartoma (dysplastic gangliocytoma) in the cerebellum, which causes an altered gait and seizures.
Cancer monitoring: Women with CS should undergo annual mammo-grams and clinical breast exams every 6-12 months beginning about age 30-35 and should undergo annual pelvic exams. Endometrial biopsies every 1-2 years can

TABLE 4-1. DIAGNOSTIC CRITERIA FOR COWDEN SYNDROME

Proband meets at least one of the following:
At least 6 facial papules listed as pathognomonic criteria
*2 major criteria, but must include macrocephaly or Lhermitte-Duclos disease**
1 major criteria and 3 minor criteria
4 minor criteria

Pathognomonic features	Trichilemmomas, facial
	Acral keratoses
	Papillomatous papules
	Musosal lesions
Major criteria	Breast cancer
	Thyroid cancer, especially papillary carcinoma
	Macrocephaly
	Lhermitte-Duclos disease*
	Endometrial cancer
Minor criteria	Other thyroid lesions
	Mental retardation
	Gastrointestinal hamartomas
	Fibrocystic breasts
	Lipomas or fibromas
	Genitourinary tumors (e.g. renal cell carcinoma, uterine fibroids)
	Genitourinary malformations

Source: Eng, 2000, p. 829.
*Lhermitte-Duclos disease is characterized by a glial mass in cerebellum, altered gait, and seizures.

also be considered although the efficacy of this monitoring strategy remains unproven. Men and women with CS should be regularly screened for thyroid cancer.

Molecular findings: Numerous germline mutations in the *PTEN* gene have been identified, including both nonsense and missense mutations. It is estimated that 80% of families with CS will have an identifiable mutation in the *PTEN* gene which is 9 exons in length. The major functions of the PTEN phosphatase are to control cell cycle arrest and apoptosis.

The finding that *PTEN* mutations are also the underlying basis of the Bannayan-Riley-Ruvalcaba syndromes suggests a broad phenotype. *PTEN* mutations have also been found in individuals with proteus-like syndrome (lipomas, exostoses of the skull, bony growth and other dermatological features). It may turn out that there are clear genotype-phenotype differences that explain the wide spectrum of clinical features associated with *PTEN* mutations, although this has not yet been demonstrated.

Genetic testing: Clinically available

DRASH SYNDROME: *see Wilms' tumor, familial*

DYSPLASTIC NEVUS SYNDROME: *see Melanoma, familial*

10. FAMILIAL ADENOMATOUS POLYPOSIS (also attenuated FAP, Gardner syndrome, Turcot syndrome, and hereditary desmoid disease)

Incidence: 1 in 6,000–13,000
Penetrance: Close to 100% (for classic FAP)
Inheritance: Autosomal dominant
Gene: *APC* gene at 5q21
Cancer risks: 100%
Clinical features: Familial adenomatous polyposis (FAP) accounts for less than 1% of colon cancer cases. Affected individuals will develop colorectal cancer by age 40 unless the colon and rectum are surgically removed (colectomy). Other risks include cancer of the ampulla of Vater (which joins the common bile duct to the small intestine), bile duct, thyroid, small intestine, and thyroid (non-medullary type). There is also an association with childhood hepatoblastoma.

In general, the risk of colorectal cancer far exceeds the risks of other cancers. However, in Japan, individuals with FAP are at higher risk for developing gastric cancer than colon cancer.

Diagnostic criteria: The criteria for FAP is the presence of greater than 100 colorectal polyps. Most affected individuals have the characteristic "carpeting" of polyps by age 20. Clinical variants of FAP are described below.

Attenuated FAP: The attenuated form of FAP is associated with fewer colorectal polyps at later ages of onset. This may make it difficult to distinguish from hereditary nonpolyposis colon cancer. Individuals with attenuated FAP have increased risks of colon cancer, but the tumors tend to occur at older ages than for classic FAP and the overall cancer risk may be well below 100%. Individuals with attenuated FAP may present with multiple extracolonic polyps. In fact, they may have more polyps in the upper gastrointestinal tract than in the colon.

Gardner syndrome: Gardner syndrome is characterized by polyposis and FAP-related malignancies plus sebaceous cysts, lipomas, desmoid tumors, and fibromas. Other features include osteomas of the jaw (mandible), epidermoid cysts, extra (supernumery) or unerupted teeth, and an eye finding termed CHRPE (congenital hypertrophy of the retinal pigment epithelium).

Turcot syndrome: Turcot syndrome is characterized by polyposis and FAP-related malignancies plus brain tumors, particularly medulloblastoma. Affected individuals may also have increased risks of developing stomach cancer and basal cell carcinomas. (There is also a form of Turcot syndrome associated with hereditary nonpolyposis colon cancer syndrome.)

Hereditary desmoid disease: In this FAP variant, the affected individual develops multiple desmoid tumors but does not develop colorectal polyposis.

Cancer monitoring: Management of individuals with FAP involve annual sigmoidoscopies or colonoscopies beginning at age 10–12 followed by total colectomy at the onset of polyps. Affected adults are recommended to undergo annual surveillance for the extracolonic tumors, including upper endoscopy procedures and screening for thyroid cancer. The effectiveness of chemopreventive agents, such as sulindac or COX-2 inhibitors, is being assessed in families with polyposis.

Molecular findings: The *APC* gene is a tumor suppressor gene that has earned its place in genetics textbooks as being the gene showcased in Vogelstein's model of carcinogenesis (refer to Fig. 3-4). The APC protein product appears to have many important cellular functions. One of the major functions is to control apoptosis.

Most families with FAP can be identified as having a protein truncating mutation in the *APC* gene. One-fourth to one-third of cases represent *de novo* mutations (thus family history may be negative). The *APC* gene is 15 exons in length. Mutations in the extreme 5′ end of the *APC* gene are associated with the attenuated form and mutations in the extreme 3′ end are associated with hereditary desmoid disease. There do not appear to be specific mutations that predict Gardner or Turcot syndrome. See Figure 4-1.

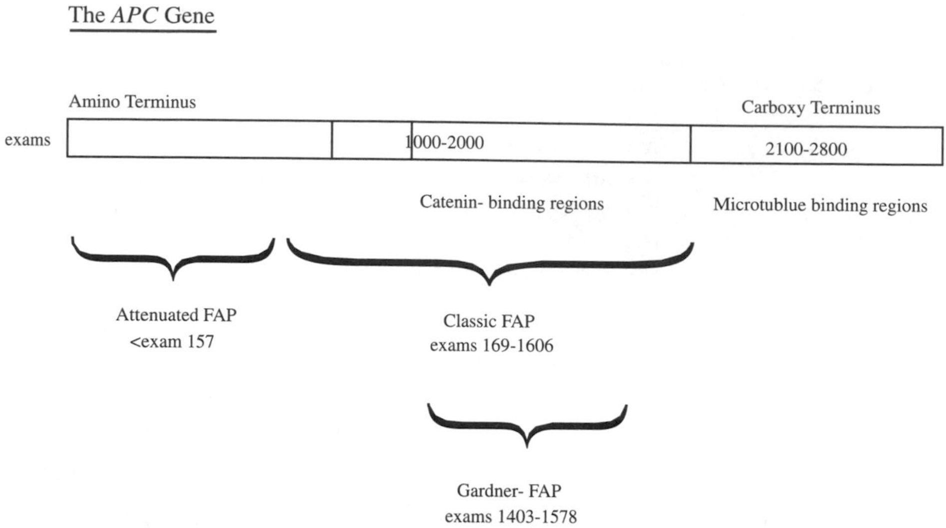

The *APC* Gene

FIGURE 4-1. The genotype-phenotype correlations of mutations in the *APC* gene. Note that mutations in the 5' end of the gene are associated with a milder phenotype. [Source: Offit, 1998, p. 132.]

I1307K mutation:	This mutation was discovered serendipitously and is estimated to be carried by 6% of the Ashkenazi Jewish population. Individuals with the I1307K mutation do not develop polyposis but may have increased risks of colorectal cancer. The magnitude of risk remains uncertain but may be a twofold-increased risk over the general population. This is interesting considering that other mutations in the same region of the gene lead to a more classic FAP phenotype. Genetic testing for the I1307K is clinically available, although it remains controversial, since it is unclear whether the presence of the mutation should alter surveillance recommendations.
Genetic testing:	Clinically available

FAMILIAL MOLE-MALIGNANT MELANOMA SYNDROME: *see Melanoma, familial*

11. FANCONI ANEMIA

Incidence:	1 in 360,000 in general population; carrier frequency is 1 in 300 to 1 in 600 in general population; about 1 in 100 in Ashkenazi Jews

Penetrance:	100%
Inheritance:	Autosomal recessive
Gene:	*FACA* at 16q24.3
	FACB is unmapped
	FACC at 9q22.3
	FACD at 3p25.3
	FACE is unmapped
	FANCF at 11p15
	FANCG at 9p13
Cancer risks:	May be as high as 50%
Clinical features:	Fanconi anemia (FA) is typically diagnosed around age six, because of aplastic anemia, bleeding, and/or easy bruising. The underlying problems are the progressive pancytopenia and chromosome breakage that worsens with exposure to alkylating agents. There is a wide variability of features among individuals with FA. Affected individuals may have abnormalities in any organ system, but frequent features include low birth weight, abnormal skin pigmentation, absent thumbs, skeletal deformities, and renal malformations. About 75% have some dysmorphic features.
	Individuals with FA are at greatly increased risk of developing leukemia, usually acute myelocytic leukemia. There is also a greatly increased risk of developing multiple squamous cell carcinomas. Hepatocellular cancers and brain tumors have also been reported in FA.
Diagnostic criteria:	FA is diagnosed by assessing levels of chromosome breakage that is not visible on a standard karotype. Testing is performed by doing either a mitomycin C chromosome stress test or the DEB test (diepoxybutane). These tests will reliably detect homozygotes but not heterozygotes.
Cancer monitoring:	Individuals with FA are encouraged to undergo serial bone marrow aspirations to screen for hematological cancers. It has also been suggested that affected individuals undergo regular skin exams, liver enzyme assessments, frequent oral scrutiny by a dentist, and imaging of the esophagus, lower pharynx, and stomach. Bone marrow transplants are an option, but individuals with FA may be particularly susceptible to developing graft versus host disease.
Molecular findings:	Individuals with FA have been found to have germline mutations in the *FACA* and *FACC* genes. DNA analy-

sis for the *FACB* and *FACE* genes is proving to be more difficult. Currently, there is no reliable test that will identify FA heterozygotes. Individuals with FA who are of Ashkenazi Jewish ancestry frequently have a founder mutation in the *FACA* gene.

Genetic testing: Clinically available

GARDNER SYNDROME: *see Familial adenomatous polyposis*

GORLIN SYNDROME—*see Basal cell nevus syndrome*

HEREDITARY DESMOID DISEASE: *see Familial adenomatous polyposis*

12. HEREDITARY MIXED POLYPOSIS SYNDROME

Incidence: Rare
Penetrance: May be greater than 90%
Inheritance: Autosomal dominant
Gene: *HMPS* localized to 6q
Cancer risks: May be greater than 90%
Clinical features: Individuals with hereditary mixed polyposis syndrome (HMPS) develop multiple atypical juvenile polyps in the colon. Polyps of other histological types have also been reported, including adenomatous and hyperplastic lesions. Individuals with HMPS are at increased risk for developing colorectal cancer. Carcinoma of the colon or rectum seems to be the predominant cancer risk with HMPS; no extracolonic tumors have been reported to date.
Diagnostic criteria: Individuals with HMPS have characteristic atypical juvenile polyps of the colon.
Cancer monitoring: Affected individuals need to be regularly monitored for benign or malignant polyps in the colon or rectum.
Molecular findings: HMPS may turn out to be a variant form of juvenile polyposis syndrome. The exact location of the *HMPS* gene is still being sought.
Genetic testing: None available

13. HEREDITARY NONPOLYPOSIS COLON CANCER
(also Lynch syndrome)

Incidence: 1 in 200 to 1 in 1,000
Penetrance: As high as 90%

Inheritance:	Autosomal dominant
Genes:	*MSH2* at 2p22
	MLH1 at 3p21
	PMS1 at 2q31
	PMS2 at 7p22
	MSH6 at 2p16
Cancer risks:	May be as high as 75%
Clinical features:	Hereditary nonpolyposis colon cancer (HNPCC) accounts for about 2% of colon cancer cases. Individuals with HNPCC have about 70-75% risks of developing colorectal cancer. These tumors usually arise from a colon polyp, but polyposis is absent. Colon tumors frequently arise in the right-side portion of the colon. Women with HNPCC are estimated to have 30% risks of developing endometrial cancer and lower, but increased risks of ovarian cancer. It is unclear whether women with HNPCC are at increased risk for developing breast cancer.
	Other associated risks for men and women with HNPCC include cancers of the stomach, small intestine, ureter and kidney (usually transitional cell of the renal pelvis). Other tumors in the gastrointestinal or genitourinary tracts have also been reported including renal cell carcinoma.
Diagnostic criteria:	HNPCC is diagnosed on the basis of the pattern of cancer in the family. Table 4-2 delineates the criteria for HNPCC termed the Amsterdam criteria. Families who meet Bethesda criteria (also shown in Table 4-2) should be offered testing for microsatellite instability (MSI) to determine if they could have HNPCC.
Muir-Torre syndrome:	Muir-Torre syndrome is thought to be a variant of HNPCC that is characterized by HNPCC-related malignancies plus sebaceous gland tumors and skin keratocanthomas. The characteristic skin lesions are typically present in adulthood.
Turcot syndrome:	In addition to HNPCC-related malignancies, people with Turcot syndrome are also at risk for developing brain tumors, typically glioblastomas. There is also a form of Turcot syndrome associated with familial adenomatous polyposis.
Cancer monitoring:	Individuals with HNPCC are recommended to have colonoscopies every 1–2 years. Endometrial biopsies are also suggested, although this screening method has not been proven to be effective.

TABLE 4-2. DIAGNOSTIC CRITERIA FOR HEREDITARY NONPOLYPOSIS COLON CANCER (HNPCC) AND MICROSATELLITE INSTABILITY (MSI)

Criteria for HNPCC

Amsterdam Criteria	Family meets all criteria	3 cases of colorectal (CRC) cancer 2 successive generations 2 cases are first-degree relatives 1 CRC diagnosis <40 yrs Familial adenomatous polyposis (FAP) has been ruled out Tumors should be verified by pathology
Amsterdam Criteria II	Family meets all criteria	3 relatives with HNPCC-related cancer* 2 cases are first-degree relatives 2 successive generations 1 diagnosis <50 yrs FAP has been ruled out Tumors should be verified by pathology

Criteria for MSI Testing

Bethesda Criteria	Family or Proband meets at least one criteria	Family fits either Amsterdam criteria Proband has 2 HNPCC-related cancers* Proband has CRC plus 1st-degree relative with CRC or HNPCC-related extracolonic tumor or CRC adenoma <45 yrs Proband has at least 1 of the following Diagnosed prior to <45 yrs: CRC or endometrial cancer Right-sided colon cancer if undifferentiated Signet-ring cell type CRC Colon adenomas

Source: Vasen et al., 1991; Vasen et al., 1999; and Rodriguez-Bigas et al., 1997.

*HNPCC-related malignancies include cancers of the endometrium, small intestine, ureter or renal pelvis.

Molecular findings: About 60% of HNPCC families who meet Amsterdam criteria will be found to carry a mutation in the *MLH1* or *MSH2* gene. One-third of mutations are missense mutations, which do not cause protein truncation of the protein product and may be of uncertain clinical significance. Mutations have been reported throughout the *MLH1* gene (19 exons) and the *MSH2* gene (16 exons). The five genes linked with HNPCC are all mismatch repair genes.

It is conjectured that families with the Turcot or Muir-Torre variants will be found to carry specific mutations. At this point, a few families with Turcot syndrome have been found to carry mutations in the *PMS2* and *MLH1* genes and some with Muir Torre syndrome have *MSH2* mutations.

About 80% of HNPCC colon tumors show microsatellite instability (MSI) compared with only 15% of sporadic colon tumors. Thus, MSI testing can be used as a screening test to determine which families should proceed to *MSH2* and *MLH1* testing. Families with *MSH6* mutations are less likely to demonstrate MSI (at least at mono- and di-nucleotide repeat markers).

Genetic testing: Clinically available

14. JUVENILE POLYPOSIS

Incidence: Rare
Penetrance: May be greater than 90%
Inheritance   Autosomal dominant
Gene: *SMAD4* at 18q21.1
                        BMPRIA at 10q22-23
Cancer risks: About 30%
Clinical features: Juvenile polyposis (JP) is associated with juvenile (inflammatory) hamartomatous polyps in the colon, stomach, and small intestine. Individuals with JP do not have the freckling or hyperpigmentation associated with Peutz-Jeghers syndrome. The major problems are anemia and bleeding due to the size and number of the gastrointestinal polyps. Associated cancer risks include cancer of the colon, stomach, pancreas, and small intestine. Some affected children will have other associated anomalies, such as polydactly, clubbing of feet, heart defects, small head circumference (often below the 10th percentile), and mental retardation.
Diagnostic criteria: Diagnosis of JP is based on the presence of multiple juvenile gastrointestinal hamartomatous polyps and the exclusion of other hamartoma polyposis syndromes. The number of polyps can range from a few to several hundred.
Cancer monitoring: Frequent colonoscopy examinations are recommended. It is also important to screen for upper gastrointestinal tumors with endoscopy.

Molecular findings: Germline *SMAD4* and *BMPR1A* mutations have been
                       identified in about half the families with JP studied.
                       The *SMAD4* tumor suppressor gene (also referred to
                       as *DPC4*) is an important transcription factor that
                       helps regulate the transforming growth factor beta
                       (TGF-β) signaling system within the cell. The *BMPR1A*
                       gene encodes a receptor protein for bone mor-
                       phogenetic proteins (BMPs), which stimulate bone
                       growth.

Genetic Testing: Available on a research basis only

LAMB SYNDROME: *see NAME syndrome*

15. LI-FRAUMENI SYNDROME

Incidence   Rare
Penetrance   May be as high as 90%
Inheritance   Autosomal dominant
Gene: *TP53* at 17p13.1
Cancer risks: May be as high as 90%
Clinical features: Component malignancies of Li-Fraumeni syndrome
                       (LFS) are osteosarcomas, soft tissue sarcomas, breast
                       cancer, brain tumors, adrenocortical carcinomas, and
                       acute leukemias. Individuals with LFS are also at in-
                       creased risk for malignancies in other organ systems,
                       particularly the stomach, colon, and lung. Childhood
                       neuroblastomas have been reported. The risk of mela-
                       noma may also be increased. Most forms of sarcomas
                       have been reported in LFS families, including breast
                       and uterine sarcomas. The one exception is Ewing
                       sarcoma which is not a feature of LFS (and in many
                       ways is not a "true" sarcoma).

                           Malignancies occur in both children and adults.
                       Individuals with LFS have an estimated 90% chance of
                       developing cancer by age 70. About 25% of the cancers
                       occur before 18, with approximately one-half of af-
                       fected individuals presenting with a malignancy by
                       age 40. Lifetime cancer risks are higher for women
                       than men because of the high breast cancer risks. The
                       risk of a second primary tumor may be as high as 50%;
                       radiation exposure appears to increase the risks of
                       additional malignancies.

TABLE 4-3. DIAGNOSTIC CRITERIA FOR LI-FRAUMENI SYNDROME AND LI FRAUMENI-LIKE SYNDROME

Li-Fraumeni syndrome	Family meets all criteria	Proband with sarcoma <45 yr
		1st-degree relative with any cancer <45 yr
		1st-degree or 2nd-degree relative with any cancer <45 yr or sarcoma at any age
Li-Fraumeni-like syndrome	Family meets all criteria	Proband with any childhood cancer or sarcoma, brain tumor, or adrenocortical tumor <45 yr
		1st-degree or 2nd-degree relative with typical LFS cancer at any age*
		1st-degree or 2nd-degree relative with any cancer <60 yr

Source: Li and Fraumeni, 1969; and Birch et al., 1994.

*Typical LFS cancers are soft tissue sarcoma, osteosarcoma, breast cancer, adrenal cortical carcinoma, brain tumor, and acute leukemia.

Diagnostic criteria:	Criteria for LFS and the variant form, called Li-Fraumeni-like syndrome (LFL) are listed in Table 4-3.
Cancer monitoring:	There is no accepted screening for individuals with LFS. Affected individuals are suggested to undergo regular physical examinations and consider having scans of the head and abdomen. Women with LFS should undergo bi-annual clinical breast exams and annual mammography beginning by age 25-30. The use of mammography is somewhat controversial given the increased sensitivity in those with germline *TP53* mutations. Most importantly, individuals with LFS should be worked up carefully if they report any symptoms of unusual magnitude or duration.
Molecular findings:	Germ line *TP53* mutations can be identified in 75% of LFS families and a much lower percentage of families with LFL. The *TP53* gene has 11 coding regions. Many of the germline mutations are within exons 5–9, although as many as 25% of mutations are outside this region. The *TP53* gene plays a crucial role in cell repair, the apoptosis pathways, and maintaining genomic stability.
Genetic testing:	Clinically available

LYNCH SYNDROME: *see Hereditary nonpolyposis colon cancer*

16. MELANOMA, FAMILIAL (Dysplastic nevus syndrome, Familial atypical mole-malignant melanoma syndrome, Melanoma-astrocytoma syndrome)

Incidence:	Unknown
Penetrance:	Close to 100%
Inheritance:	Autosomal Dominant
Genes:	*CMM1* mapped to 1p36
	TP16 (*CDKN2*) at 9p21
	CDK4 at 12q14
Cancer risks:	May be greater than 90%

Clinical features: Everyone is recommended to pay attention to moles (nevi) that change size or color, but individuals with dysplastic nevus syndrome (DNS) or familial atypical mole-malignant melanoma syndrome (FAMM) must remain especially vigilant. Unless suspicious moles are excised early, their risk of becoming malignant is virtually 100%. In fact, affected individuals are at increased risk for developing multiple primary melanomas. The average age of the initial melanoma diagnosis is age 34, which is two decades earlier than the disease is typically seen in the general population. Astrocytomas and pancreatic cancer have also been reported in people with familial melanoma.

Diagnostic criteria: Individuals are considered to have familial melanoma if they have 10–100 dysplastic nevi of varied size, color, and outline, on their upper trunk and limbs and/or have two first degree relatives who have developed melanoma. Individuals who have had multiple primary melanomas may have familial melanoma even if they do not have positive family histories or numerous dysplastic nevi.

Cancer monitoring: Cancer surveillance involves monthly skin self-exams and clinical examinations by a dermatologist every 6 months. For comparison purposes, the entire skin should be photographed and any suspicious lesions promptly excised. Individuals are also advised to use sunscreen daily and avoid becoming sunburned.

Molecular findings: Although at-risk family members are fairly easy to identify, uncovering the basis of the melanoma syndromes has proven to be difficult. The *TP16* gene is a tumor suppressor gene containing 3 exons. Mutations have included nonsense, splice donor site, missense, and insertions; most cause truncation of the protein.

Although some families with dysplastic nevus syn-drome have mapped to 1p36 (the region of the *CMM1* gene), others have not. Only a few families have been found to have germline mutations in the *CDK4* proto-oncogene (8 exons in length). *CDK4* mutations can create a tumor-specific antigen which disrupts cell-cycle regulation mediated by TP16 protein. Researchers continue to search for additional gene(s) responsible for familial melanoma

Genetic testing: Clinically available

MUIR-TORRE SYNDROME: *see Hereditary nonpolyposis colon cancer*

17. MULTIPLE ENDOCRINE NEOPLASIA, TYPE 1
(originally Werner syndrome)

Incidence:	Uncommon
Penetrance:	90%
Inheritance	Autosomal dominant
Gene:	*MEN1* at 11q13
Cancer risks:	Below 10%
Clinical features:	Multiple endocrine neoplasia, type 1 (MEN 1) is characterized by multiple tumors of the parathyroid glands, pancreatic islets, and pituitary glands. Most tumors are benign, but there is an increased risk of parathyroid carcinomas, pancreatic islet cell tumors (gastriomas) and carcinoid tumors. Other benign tumors include facial fibroangiomas, skin collagenomas, adrenal gland adenomas, and lipomas. The first sign of the disorder may be hyperparathyroidism due to parathyroid hyperplasia. MEN 1 has variable expressivity, and childhood onset is rare.

MEN 1 is not associated with medullary thyroid carcinomas or pheochromocytomas, both of which are features of multiple endocrine neoplasia, type 2. Both MEN subtypes are associated with parathyroid hyperplasia and adenomas.

Diagnostic criteria: A diagnosis of MEN 1 should be made if the proband meets one of the following criteria:

1. proband has endocrine tumors in at least two of the three major tissue systems (parathyroid, anterior pituitary, and gastrointestinal);

2. proband has one endocrine tumor and a first-degree relative with MEN 1.

Cancer monitoring:	At-risk individuals are suggested to undergo regular biochemical screening for parathyroid tumors beginning in childhood (before age 10). These screening tests should include the measurement of serum-ionized calcium and prolactin as well as pituitary, parathyroid, and pancreatic hormone levels. Imaging of the pituitary glands can also be performed.
Molecular findings:	MEN1 is a tumor suppressor gene whose product is called menin, which binds to JUND, a transcription factor. Two-thirds of mutations cause premature truncation.
Genetic testing:	Clinically available

18. MULTIPLE ENDOCRINE NEOPLASIA, TYPE 2
(originally Sipple syndrome)

Incidence:	1 in 30,000
Penetrance:	Nearly 100% by biochemical screening
Inheritance:	Autosomal dominant
Gene:	RET at 10q11.2
Cancer risks:	70% by age 70
Clinical features:	Multiple endocrine neoplasia, type 2A (MEN 2A) and multiple endocrine neoplasia, type 2B (MEN 2B) are characterized by medullary thyroid carcinomas (MTC), pheochromocytomas , and benign parathyroid tumors.
Diagnostic criteria:	The diagnosis of MEN 2A and MEN 2B is based on the criteria above plus following specifics:
MEN 2A:	In addition to developing MTCs, about 50% of affected individuals develop one or more pheochromocytomas. The most common presenting symptom in MEN 2A is a neck mass, but can also be hypertension. By age 50, about one-half have developed at least one syndrome-associated feature.
MEN 2B:	Onset of disease typically occurs in childhood. Affected children can also have developmental abnormalities, and have specific physical features including enlarged lips comprised of mucosal neuromas, ganglioneuromatosis of the intestine, and a marfanoid habitus (tall with broad chest and unusually long arms). MEN 2B is associated with MTCs that tend to be more aggressive and occur earlier than those in MEN 2A but appears to have lower risks of clinically apparent hyperparathyroidism.

Familial MTC: Individuals with familial MTC develop MTCs but not pheochromocytomas. The MTC tumors tend to occur at later onset and are generally amenable to treatment.

Cancer monitoring: The standard of care in North America and the United Kingdom is for individuals with *RET* mutations to undergo prophylactic thyroidectomy. Surgery should be performed before age 6 years for children with MEN 2A and before age 3 years for children with MEN 2B. Further, at-risk individuals should undergo annual screening for pheochromocytomas and hyperparathyroidism.

Molecular findings: Mutations in different regions of the *RET* gene can lead to different phenotypes (refer to Fig. 3-6). The *RET* proto-oncogene, 21 exons in length, is a tyrosine kinase receptor. Gain of function mutations of the *RET* proto-oncogene results in constitutive activation of the tyrosine kinase (MEN 2A) or alteration of substrate specificity (MEN 2B).

Genetic testing: Clinically available

19. NAME SYNDROME (also Carney complex and LAMB syndrome)

Incidence: Rare

Penetrance: Unknown

Inheritance: Autosomal dominant

Gene: *PRKAR1A* at 17q23-24
CNC2 at 2p16

Cancer risks: Increased but not quantified

Clinical features: NAME syndrome refers to nevi, atrial myxoma, myxoid neurofibromas, and ephelides (freckles). NAME syndrome also includes two other rare syndromes: Carney complex consists of the following features: cardiac myxoma, spotty pigmentation and cutaneous myxomas, and pituitary and adrenocortical carcinomas. LAMB syndrome consists of the following: lentigines, atrial myxomas, mucocutaneous myxoma, and blue nevi syndrome. Individuals with NAME syndrome are at increased risk for developing multiple benign and malignant tumors. Malignant tumors include large-cell calcifying Sertoli-Leydig cell tumors, liposarcomas, and cancers in the following organs: testes, thyroid, colon, rectum, and pancreas. Benign tumors include pituitary adenomas, cardiac myxomas, myxoid uterine leiomyomas, and thyroid adenomas.

	Other skin findings are common including tiny black-brown macules, café au lait macules, lentigines, blue nevi, dermal fibromas, and myxoid neurofibromata. Pigmentation is spotty, particularly on the face, vulva, glans, penis, hands, and feet. The pigmentation in people with NAME syndrome is more widespread than with Peutz-Jeghers syndrome, and the buccal mucosa is seldom involved. Also, canthal pigmentation is common in Carney complex, but rare in Peutz-Jeghers syndrome.
Diagnostic criteria:	The diagnosis of NAME syndrome is made on the basis of finding two or more characteristic lesions in the proband or finding one characteristic lesion in the proband and a first-degree relative.
Cancer monitoring:	Cancer screening for at-risk individuals includes an echocardiogram every 3–5 years, careful skin examinations, checking serum cortisol levels, checking serum levels of insulin-like growth factor I and prolactin, testicular exam, thyroid exams, and careful endocrine review of systems.
Molecular findings:	Some families with Carney complex have been found to have germline mutations in the *PRKAR1A* gene. A few families have been found to have mutations in the *CNC2* gene. Little is currently known about either of these genes and researchers anticipate that additional genes will be identified to explain other families with NAME syndrome.
Genetic testing:	Not currently available

20. NEUROFIBROMATOSIS, TYPE 1

Incidence:	1 in 3,000 individuals
Penetrance:	100%
Inheritance:	Autosomal dominant (30–50% are *de novo*)
Gene:	*NF1* at 17q11.2
Cancer risks:	2–5%
Clinical features:	Neurofibromatosis, type 1 (NF 1) is one of the most common genetic disorders. There is widely variable expressivity to this syndrome, with some individuals severely affected and others only mildly affected. The hallmark features of NF 1 are the multiple café au lait spots and neurofibromas. Many affected individuals will develop Lisch nodules (hamartomas of the iris).

TABLE 4-4. DIAGNOSTIC CRITERIA FOR NEUROFIBROMATOSIS

Neurofibromatosis, type 1	Proband meets at least two criteria	1st-degree relative with NF1 6 or more café au lait spots 2 or more neurofibromas of any type or one plexiform neurofibroma Freckling of armpits or groin Optic glioma 2 or more Lisch nodules A distinctive bony lesion Dysplasia of sphenoid bone Dysplasia or thinning of long bone cortex
Neurofibromatosis, type 2	Proband meets at least one criteria	Bilateral eighth-nerve masses Unilateral eighth nerve mass plus 1st-degree relative with NF 2 Two of the following: Neurofibroma Meningioma Glioma Schwannoma Juvenile posterior subcapsular lenticular opacity

Source: Gutmann and Collins, 1998; MacCollin and Gusella, 1998.

Other features can include short stature, macrocephaly, learning disabilities, and seizures.

Although individuals with NF 1 almost always develop several benign tumors, few will go on to develop cancer. The risk of malignancy is about 2–5%; with malignant optic gliomas and neurofibrosarcomas occurring most frequently. Astrocytomas, meningiomas, epdendymomas, and pheochromocytomas have also been reported.

Diagnostic criteria: See Table 4-4 for the NF 1 diagnostic criteria. To distinguish from NF2, note that café-au-lait spots are present in virtually all individuals with NF1, but are present in only 50% of individuals with NF2.

Cancer monitoring: The clinical care of individuals with NF 1 typically involves the management of clinical symptoms as they occur. Cranial imaging can be performed as a screening measure, but early detection of brain lesions has not been found to significantly change outcome.

Molecular findings: Clinical criteria has been more useful in identify-
                       ing individuals with NF 1 than molecular studies.
                       Although linkage analysis is informative in some
                       families, direct DNA testing has been less successful at
                       identifying specific mutations in the lengthy (59 exons)
                       NF1 gene. The protein product of *NF1* is neuro-
                       fibromin that downregulates the proto-oncogene
                       p21-RAS. The loss of NF 1 leads to the activation of
                       the *p21-RAS* oncogene, resulting in uncontrolled cell
                       growth.
Genetic testing: Clinically available

21. NEUROFIBROMATOSIS, TYPE 2

Incidence: 1 in 40,000
Penetrance: 100% by age 60
Inheritance: Autosomal dominant
Gene: *NF2* at 22q12
Cancer risks: May not be increased
Clinical features: Neurofibromatosis, type 2 (NF 2) is characterized by
                       multiple spine and skin tumors. Most affected indi-
                       viduals become hearing impaired due to the pre-
                       sence of vestibular schwannomas (also called acoustic
                       neuromas) and the risk of cataracts is also increased.
                            Meningiomas are the most frequent tumors to
                       occur. Other benign tumors in the NF 2 spectrum
                       include astrocytomas, neurofibromas, spinal schwan-
                       nomas, and ependymomas. About 50% of individuals
                       with NF 2 develop café au lait spots. These tumors can
                       be difficult to manage clinically yet rarely become
                       malignant. In fact, rates of malignancy in people with
                       NF 2 may be similar to general population rates. Malig-
                       nant gliomas have been reported in people with NF 2.
Diagnostic criteria: Table 4.4 shows the diagnostic criteria for NF 2. To dis-
                       tinguish from NF 1, note that individuals with NF 2
                       do not have Lisch nodules and do not have associated
                       learning disabilities.
Cancer monitoring: Because it is not clear whether individuals with NF 2
                       are at increased risk for developing malignant tumors,
                       no routine cancer monitoring is recommended. The
                       clinical care of individuals with NF 2 typically
                       involves the management of clinical symptoms as they
                       occur. Clinical management often involves the surgi-
                       cal removal of tumors.

Molecular findings: Genetic testing is performed by linkage analysis or by direct DNA testing. Many protein-truncating mutations have been reported throughout the gene. Certain genotype-phenotype correlations have been reported, with frameshift mutations leading to more severe phenotypes than missense mutations. The *NF2* gene is 17 exons in length and its protein product is one of the cytoskeleton-associated proteins. This protein helps maintain the shape and membrane stability of the cell.

Genetic testing: Clinically available

22. NEVOID BASAL CELL CARCINOMA SYNDROME
(also Gorlin syndrome)

Incidence: 1 in 56,000 in the United Kingdom (new mutation rate is 40%)

Penetrance: 97%

Inheritance: Autosomal dominant

Gene: *PTC* at 9q22.3

Cancer risks: 90%

Clinical features: With the rates of skin cancer skyrocketing in the general population, it may be difficult to identify familial cases. Age of onset may be a useful feature as is the occurrence of multiple skin cancer diagnoses in the same person. Individuals with nevoid basal cell carcinoma syndrome (NBCCS), also called Gorlin syndrome, have a 75% risk of developing basal cell carcinoma by age 20 and a 90% risk by age 40. Carcinoma of the pancreas is also a feature of NBCCS. Other associated cancers include ovarian sarcomas and childhood medulloblastomas (5% risk). Fibrosarcomas have occurred secondary to radiation treatments.

   The main features of the syndrome are the multiple basal cell carcinomas (90%), jaw cysts (90% by age 40), and palmar and plantar pits (65%). Other features include cardiac fibromas, ovarian fibromas, meningiomas, cutaneous keratocysts and milia, and hamartous polyps of the stomach. Affected individuals may have characteristic physical features including tall stature, large head with frontal bossing, ocular hypertelorism, broad nasal root, enlarged mandible, ocular abnormalities, shortened fourth metacarpals, skeletal malformation of the spine and ribs, sellar bridging, and/or hydrocephalus. About 25% have

TABLE 4-5. Diagnostic Criteria for Nevoid Basal Cell Carcinoma Syndrome

Major Criteria	Minor Criteria
Proband meets either of the following: *2 major criteria, or 1 major criteria and 2 minor criteria*	
3+ Basal cell carcinomas < age 30 or >10 basal cell nevi	Congenital skeletal anomaly
Any odontogenic keratocyst or polyostotic bone cyst	Head circumference >97th percentile
3+ Palmar or plantar pits	Cardiac or ovarian fibroma
Ectopic calcification, lamellar or early (<20 yr) falx calcification	Medulloblastoma
At least 1 relative with basal cell nevus syndrome	Lymphomesenteric cysts
	Congenital malformation

Source: Lindor et al., 1998, p. 1045.

	ophthalmic abnormalities, and up to 10% have lowered intelligence.
Diagnostic criteria:	Criteria for NBCCS are listed in Table 4-5.
Cancer monitoring:	Individuals at increased risk for NBCCS are suggested to have annual examinations by a dermatologist beginning in early puberty and examinations every 6 months for the jaw cysts. They are advised to use sunscreen on a daily basis. Conservative early excision of basal cell tumors is recommended. Pediatricians should be aware of possible increased risk of medulloblastoma, although no screening is suggested. Adult women at risk for NBCCS should have careful gynecological examinations. The benefits of cancer screening in people with NBCCS have not yet been established. Affected individuals have increased sensitivity to radiation and should minimize their exposure to radiation.
Molecular findings:	The *PTC* (so-called "patched") gene encodes a transmembrane protein that, in *Drosophila*, represses hedgehog-mediated induction of several genes involved in cell-to-cell communication.
	Disruption of this signaling pathway may cause increased activity of hedgehog targets, leading to changed cell patterning and increased growth in numerous tissues. Perhaps 40% of cases represent *de novo* mutations.
Genetic testing:	Available on a research basis only

TABLE 4-6. DIAGNOSTIC CRITERIA FOR PEUTZ-JEGHENS SYNDROME

Proband meets both criteria

Histopathological confirmation of hamartomatous gastrointestinal polyp(s)

At least 2 of the following:
  Small bowel polyposis
  >1 relative with Peutz-Jeghers syndrome
  Pigmented macules of buccal mucosa, lips, fingers or toes

Source: Lindor et al,, 1998 p 1062

23. PEUTZ-JEGHERS SYNDROME

Incidence:	1 in 120,000
Penetrance:	Nearly 100%
Inheritance:	Autosomal dominant
Gene:	*STK11* at 19p13.3
Cancer risks:	50%
Clinical features:	Individuals with Peutz-Jeghers syndrome (PJS) have multiple hamartomatous polyps that can occur throughout the gastrointestinal tract (most commonly in the small intestine) and multiple pigmented spots on the lips and buccal mucosa. The pigmented spots typically present in infancy or childhood and occur in over 95% of cases. Complications from the gastrointestinal polyps include anemia and hemorrhaging; the pigmented skin lesions rarely cause medical problems.
	Individuals with PJS are at increased risk for developing colon cancer. Women with PJS are also at risk for developing cancers of the breast, pancreas, uterus, and ovary. Almost all affected women develop benign sex cord tumors of the ovary. Men with PJS appear to have lower risks of cancer than affected women but can develop cancer of the colon, pancreas, lung, or testes.
Diagnostic criteria:	Table 4-6 details the criteria for PJS.
Cancer monitoring:	Screening recommendations include upper endoscopies and colonoscopies. Men should also have regular testicular exams. Women should have regular mammograms, pelvic exams and PAP smears, and abdominal and pelvic ultrasound exams.
Molecular findings:	Little is known about the *STK11* gene other than it appears to be a tumor suppressor gene and is one of the serine threonine kinase genes.
Genetic testing:	Clinically available

24. RETINOBLASTOMA, FAMILIAL

Incidence:	1 in 3,500 to 1 in 25,000 births
	60% of cases are unilateral, sporadic
	15% of cases are unilateral, familial
	25% of cases are bilateral, familial
Penetrance:	90%
Inheritance:	Autosomal dominant (40% of familial cases are *de novo*)
Gene:	*RB1* at 13q14.1
Cancer risks:	90%
Clinical features:	About 90% of children with familial retinoblastoma (RB) will develop either unilateral or bilateral tumors in the retina. Children may first present with strabismus or leukoria (a white spot in the eye). The average age of onset for familial cases is 12 months, which is earlier than sporadic cases are diagnosed (average age is 3 years). It is rare for a child to be diagnosed with retinoblastoma after the age of five. Affected children who also develop a tumor in the pineal gland behind the eye are said to have "trilateral retinoblastoma."

Children with familial RB are also at increased risk for developing cancer in other organ systems, often within the field of radiation. The most frequently occurring second primary is osteosarcoma. Other tumors have also been reported including Ewing sarcoma, leukemia, lymphoma, melanoma, lung cancer and bladder cancer. The overall risk of second tumors may be as high as 26%.

A small number of children with RB will have 13q deletion syndrome. In addition to developing retinoblastoma tumors, affected children tend to also have moderately short stature, microcephaly, mental retardation, genital malformations, and ear abnormalities.

Diagnostic criteria:	Familial RB is diagnosed if at least one criterion is met:

    1. Bilateral retinoblastoma
    2. Unilateral retinoblastoma plus a positive family history
    3. Retinoblastoma (unilateral or bilateral) plus a second primary

Cancer monitoring:	At-risk children receive frequent careful ophthalmologic evaluations. These evaluations can include imaging the eye with CT scans or MRIs.

Molecular findings: Dr A G. Knudson used the two forms of RB (familial and sporadic) to demonstrate the important two-hit model (see Figure 3-3). *RB1* is a transcriptional regulator gene that binds with *TP53*. Clinical testing for germline mutations in the lengthy (27 exons) *RB1* gene has been challenging, but laboratories that perform a combination of tumor studies, linkage analysis, and DNA sequencing quote a detection rate of 80%. Because the vast majority of unilateral RB cases are not familial, it is not surprising that so few are found to have germline mutations.

Genetic testing: Clinically available

25. ROTHMUND-THOMSON SYNDROME

Incidence: Rare, about 200 cases reported worldwide

Penetrance: Nearly 100%

Inheritance: Autosomal recessive

Gene: *RECQL4* at 8q24.3

Cancer risks: Increased, but not quantified

Clinical features: The main features of Rothmund-Thomson syndrome (RTS) are skin atrophy marbleized pigmentation, telangiectasia (3-6 months of age), and cataracts. Many of the diagnoses occur in childhood. Other features are short stature, hypogonadism, congenital bone defects, soft tissue contractures, anemia, and poikilodermas. Osteosarcoma is the most frequently reported malignancy in RTS.

Diagnostic criteria: The diagnosis of RTS should be considered in anyone with osteogenic sarcoma and unusual skin findings.

Cancer monitoring: There is no established screening protocol for affected individuals. Individuals with RTS should have frequent dermatological examinations beginning in early childhood. At this time, there is no effective screening modality to look for bone cancers.

Molecular findings: A few families with RTS have been found to have germline mutations in the *RECQL4* gene. However, mutations in this gene do not appear to account for all families. The *RECQL4* gene is one of 5 known human *RECQL* helicase genes. Some families with Bloom syndrome and Werner syndrome have been found to have mutations in different *RECQL* genes.

Genetic testing: No testing currently available

TABLE 4-7. DIAGNOSTIC CRITERIA FOR TUBEROUS SCLEROSIS

Major Criteria	Minor Criteria
Definite TSC: Proband meets 2 major criteria or 1 major and 2 minor criteria *Probable TSC: Proband meets 1 major criteria and 1 minor criteria* *Possible TSC: Proband meets 1 major criteria or 2 or more minor criteria*	
Facial angiofibromas or forehead plaque	Multiple pits in dental enamel
Nontraumatic ungual or periungual fibroma	Hamartomatous rectal polyps
Hypomelanotic macules (4 or more)	Bone cysts
Shagreen patch	Cerebral white matter migration lines
Multiple retinal nodular hamartomas	Gingival fibromas
Corical tuber	Nonrenal hamartomas
Subependymal nodule	Retinal achromic patch
Subependymal giant cell astrocytoma	"Confetti" skin lesions
Cardiac rhabdomyoma	Multiple renal cysts
Lymphangiomyomatosis	
Renal angiomyolipoma	

Source: Hyman and Whittemore, 2000, p. 663.

TSC, tuberous sclerosis.

26. TUBEROUS SCLEROSIS

Incidence:	1 in 30,000
Penetrance:	Close to 100%
Inheritance:	Autosomal dominant (up to 60% are *de novo*)
Genes:	*TSC1* at 9q34
	TSC2 at 16p13.3
Cancer risks:	Increased but not quantified
Clinical features:	Individuals with tuberous sclerosis (TSC) have as high as 14% risks of developing childhood brain tumors. Almost all of the brain tumors are subependymal giant-cell astrocytomas. There may also be an increased risk of Wilms' tumor and renal cell carcinoma. Many benign tumors are associated with tuberous sclerosis, including renal lipomas, cardiac rhabdomyomas, retinal phakomas, and adenomas in the endocrine system. Also common are dental enamel pits and a skin abnormality termed the Shagreen patch.
Diagnostic criteria:	The diagnostic criteria for TSC is shown in Table 4-7.
Cancer monitoring:	There is no established monitoring regimen for individuals with TSC. Careful physical examinations are important to manage symptoms as they occur. Scans of the head and abdomen may also be helpful.

Molecular findings: Deleterious mutations in the *TSC1* or *TSC2* gene appear to confer similar phenotypes, with the exception that affected individuals with severe renal cystic disease are more likely to have deletions of both the *TSC2* and neighboring *AAPKD1* genes. *TSC1* and *TSC2* are both tumor suppressor genes. The *TSC1* gene encodes a protein called hamartin and the *TSC2* gene encodes tuberin.

Genetic testing: Clinically available

27. VON HIPPEL-LINDAU SYNDROME

Incidence: 1 in 36,000
Penetrance: 90%
Inheritance: Autosomal dominant
Gene: *VHL* at 3p25
Cancer risks: As high as 45%
Clinical features: von Hippel-Lindau syndrome (VHL) is characterized by a variety of tumors, most of which are benign. VHL is often diagnosed in the twenties or thirties, although childhood symptoms, usually retinal angiomas, can occur. VHL has wide expressivity with some people severely affected and others with only mild symptoms of the disorder.

VHL is characterized by clear cell renal carcinomas, pheochromocytomas, retinal angiomas (which can result in loss of vision), hemangioblastomas of the cerebellum, hemangiomas of the spine, and cysts and adenomas of the kidney and pancreas. Hemangiomas and cysts can occur in other tissues as well. The renal cell carcinomas occur in approximately one-third of cases and tend to be of clear cell histology rather than papillary. Islet cell tumors of the pancreas, paragangliomas, and adrenal hemangiomas have also been reported. A somewhat recent finding is that affected individuals may also develop progressive hearing loss as a result of tumors in the endolymphatic sac of the inner ear.

VHL is sometimes subdivided into two types:

1. VHL, type 1: affected individuals are at risk for developing the above features but do not develop pheochromocytomas (pheos), which are benign but potentially serious tumors of the adrenal gland.

2. VHL, type 2: affected individuals are at risk for developing pheos, in addition to the other VHL-

TABLE 4-8. DIAGNOSTIC CRITERIA FOR VON HIPPEL-LINDAU SYNDROME

Proband meets at least one criteria

Central nervous system (CNS) and retinal hemangioblastomas

CNS or retinal hemangioblastoma and at least 1 of the following:
  Multiple renal, pancreatic or hepatic cysts
  Pheochromocytomas
  Renal cell carcinoma

One or more relatives with confirmed VHL plus proband has at least 1 of the following:
  CNS or retinal hemangioblastoma
  Multiple renal, pancreatic or hepatic cysts
  Pheochromocytoma
  Renal cell carcinoma

Source: Lindor et al., 1998, p. 1062.
VHL, von Hippel-Lindau syndrome.

	associated symptoms. The pheos can occur in childhood or adulthood. Untreated pheos represent a high stroke risk.
Diagnostic criteria:	Diagnostic criteria for VHL are listed in Table 4.8. VHL is almost certainly underreported because of its wide spectrum of tumors and cysts and the great variability of symptoms even within a family.
Cancer monitoring:	Individuals with VHL should have annual physical examinations, ophthalmologic exams, red blood cell count, urinalysis, MRI of the central nervous system and spinal cord, and annual imaging for the kidneys and pancreas.
Molecular findings:	The *VHL* gene has three exons, and germ line mutations can be identified in more than 90% of families when PCR-based mutation detection and Southern blotting techniques are used. Large deletions and protein-truncating mutations are generally associated with lower risks of pheochromocytomas. *VHL* is a tumor suppressor gene that codes for a protein called elongin.
Genetic testing:	Clinically available

28. WERNER SYNDROME

Incidence:	1 in 50,000 to 1 in 1,000,000 (perhaps a higher incidence in Japan)
Penetrance:	Presumed 100%

Inheritance:	Autosomal recessive
Gene:	WRN (RECQL2) at 8p12
Cancer risks:	10%
Clinical features:	Werner syndrome (WS) is also termed adult progeria. Individuals with WS typically develop multiple "old age" complaints in their twenties or thirties. The average lifespan is age 47. Associated features include cataracts, graying hair and/or balding, decreased muscle mass, arteriosclerosis, scleroderma, endocrine failure, and adult-onset diabetes. An individual with WS may also have a thin face, beaked nose, high pitched and hoarse voice, stocky trunk, and slender limbs. The earliest sign of WS can be the lack of a puberty-related growth spurt.
	Associated cancers include soft tissue sarcomas, osteosarcomas, melanoma, thyroid cancer, and hematological malignancies. Cancers of the stomach and breast and benign meningiomas also appear to be part of the WS spectrum. Despite the rarity of this condition, it is the focus of much research because it may help further our understanding of the aging process.
Diagnostic criteria:	The clinical diagnosis of WS is made on the basis of premature aging, short stature, and loss of subcutaneous fat and muscle.
Molecular findings:	Mutations in the large WRN gene (35 exons) cause cells to undergo programmed cell death prematurely, which accelerates the aging process. The WRN (or RECQL2) gene is not involved in DNA repair, although it does appear to have an important role in maintaining genomic stability. The RECQL2 gene is one of 5 known human RECQL helicase genes. Some families with Bloom syndrome and Werner syndrome have been found to have mutations in different RECQL genes.
Genetic testing:	Available on a research basis only

29. WILMS' TUMOR (includes Drash syndrome, WAGR syndrome)

Incidence:	1 in 10,000
Penetrance:	Presumed 100%
Inheritance:	Autosomal dominant (only 1% are familial)
Genes:	WT1 at 11p13
	WT2 at 11p15.5
	FWT1 localized to 17q12-21

Cancer risks:	Close to 100% (WAGR syndrome has lower risks)
Clinical features:	Wilms' tumor (WT) arises from an embryonal stem cell in the kidney and is sometimes referred to as nephroblastoma. WT is usually diagnosed by age 5 and is the most common solid tumor in childhood. It is estimated that only 1% of WT cases are due to an underlying hereditary factor.

In familial WT, 10% of tumors are bilateral. Second primary tumors are rare, but soft tissue sarcomas and acute leukemias have been reported. It is assumed that these tumors are due to the effects of chemotherapy and radiation as much as the underlying genotype.

Diagnostic criteria:	Bilateral cases of WT are assumed to represent familial cases. Unilateral cases of WT are diagnosed as familial if there is a positive family history of the disorder or if the child has other associated features of Drash syndrome or WAGR syndrome (see below).
Drash syndrome:	Drash syndrome is characterized by WT and urogenital abnormalities, including male pseudohermaphroditism. The kidney tumor is usually diagnosed by 18 months of age and children typically present with bilateral disease. Affected children may also develop gonadoblastoma.
WAGR syndrome:	The following features are associated with WAGR syndrome: Wilms' tumor, aniridia (absence of the iris), genitourinary abnormalities, and mental retardation. Less than 50% of children with WAGR syndrome develop Wilms' tumor.
Cancer monitoring:	Children at increased risk for developing Wilms' tumor should be regularly evaluated with clinical examination and abdominal CT scan and/or ultrasound until age 5 years. Alpha-fetoprotein blood tests may also be helpful as a screening tool.
Molecular findings:	The *WT1* gene, composed of 10 exons, is a tumor suppressor gene. It codes for a transcription factor that appears to be regulated only in the normal kidney. The *WT2* gene can lead to the formation of a kidney tumor if both copies of the gene are maternal or paternal in origin (homozygous) rather than heterozygous. This type of genetic error can occur at either the germline or somatic level. Little is known about the *WT2* gene except that it is presumed to be a tumor suppressor gene.

The *WT2* gene comprises a small part of the *BWS*

region, which causes Beckwith-Wiedemann syndrome (BWS). Not surprisingly, children with BWS are at increased risk for developing Wilms' tumor.

Drash syndrome is associated with germline mutations at specific points in the *WT1* gene located on 11p13. WAGR syndrome, an example of a contiguous gene syndrome, is caused by a large 11p deletion (that includes the 11p13 region).

Genetic testing: Available on a research basis only

30. XERODERMA PIGMENTOSUM

Incidence: 1 in 250,000 (United States)
                    1 in 40,000 (Japan)
Penetrance: Close to 100%
Inheritance: Autosomal recessive
Genes: *XPA* at 9q34.1
                    XPB at 2q21
                    XPC at 3p25.1
                    XPD at 19q13.2
                    XPE at 11p12-p11
                    XPF at 16p13.2-p13.1
                    XPG at 13q32-q33
Cancer risks: May be greater than 90%
Clinical features: The primary problem in xeroderma pigmentosum (XP) is an inability to repair genetic damage caused by exposure to ultraviolet (UV) radiation. Individuals with XP typically have dry skin and chronic dermatological problems. About half of the individuals with this disorder have some clinical symptoms by 18 months. Symptoms, such as severe freckling, blistering, and irregular pigmentation, indicate an abnormal sensitivity to ultraviolet radiation. About 20% of affected children also demonstrate some neurological abnormalities, including mental retardation, microcephaly, and spasticity.

Individuals with XP have an astonishingly high risk for malignancy. The risk for basal and squamous cell carcinomas is thought to be 2,000-fold above the normal population risks. The average age for developing skin cancer is 8 years (compared with age 60 in the general population). Cutaneous angiosarcomas have also been reported. Benign skin abnormalities are common and include poikilodermas, epitheliomas, angiomas, fibromas, keratoses, and keratoacanthomas.

Also frequent are lesions of the eye such as telangiectasias and papillomas.

The risk of squamous cell carcinoma of the tongue, mucous membranes, eyes, and oropharynx is greatly increased. The risk of malignant melanoma is about 5%. There is as much as a 20-fold increased risk of other malignancies, including leukemias and solid tumors of the brain, lung, stomach, breast, uterus, and testes. The occurrence and progression of tumors associated with the syndrome result in lowered survival rates, with only 70% living to age 40.

Diagnostic criteria: Diagnosis is usually made on the basis of clinical features during childhood. By age 15, the characteristic skin findings are present in 95% of affected individuals. There are a few specialized laboratories that can confirm the defective DNA excision repair mechanism.

Cancer monitoring: Individuals with XP require frequent eye and skin examinations.

Cancer prevention: The primary prevention strategy is avoidance of UV radiation exposure by shielding the skin and eyes from sunlight. Affected individuals are also suggested to avoid cigarettes and charbroiled foods because they contain specific DNA-binding carcinogens.

Molecular findings: The underlying genetics of XP is complex. Six *XP* complementation groups have been identified. The underlying genetic defects are usually point mutations. Defects in complementation groups B, D, and G are rare; individuals with these defective genes are more likely to have the associated neurological problems. Otherwise, there seems to be little genotype-phenotype correlation.

Genetic testing: Available on a research basis only

4.2. CHROMOSOMAL ANEUPLODIES

All genetic counselors are familiar with the clinical features of Down syndrome, Klinefelter syndrome, and Turner syndrome. This section briefly describes these three syndromes and discusses the associated cancer risks.

1. DOWN SYNDROME

Incidence: 1 in 650 to 1 in 1,000 live births (risk increases with maternal age)

Genetic basis: Trisomy 21 or unbalanced translocation involving chromosome 21

Clinical features: Down syndrome is characterized by mild to moderate mental retardation and characteristic facial features, including epicanthal folds, broad nasal bridge, and macroglossia. Some children with Down syndrome require surgery to repair a cardiac or esophageal defect. In adulthood, individuals with Down syndrome frequently develop significant hearing loss and early-onset Alzheimer disease.

                        Children with Down syndrome have a 10- to 20-fold increased risk for developing acute lymphoblastic leukemia (ALL) and also have an increased risk of developing acute myeloid leukemia (AML). A rare type of leukemia termed acute megakaryocytic leukemia is increased by 200- to 400-fold among children with Down syndrome.

Genetics: Most cases of Down syndrome are caused by the presence of an extra number 21 chromosome (trisomy 21). There does not appear to be one specific region on the 21st chromosome that causes the Down syndrome phenotype; for this reason, Down syndrome can be considered a contiguous gene syndrome. Trisomy 21 usually occurs sporadically and is the result of a nondisjunction event during meiosis. The chances of having a child with trisomy 21 increase with advanced maternal age. In 10% or less of cases, Down syndrome has been caused by an unbalanced translocation. A parent with a balanced translocation involving chromosome 21 has a greatly increased risk of having an affected child.

                        The underlying genetic cause of Down syndrome is well established. However, the link between trisomy 21 and childhood leukemia remains a puzzle.

2. KLINEFELTER SYNDROME

Incidence   1 in 500 to 1 in 1,000 live births

Genetic basis: 47XXY

Clinical features: Klinefelter syndrome is associated with enlarged breasts, sparse facial and body hair, and small testes. Men with Klinefelter syndrome can exhibit significant behavioral and learning disabilities. However, features may be quite subtle and go undetected until the man and his partner present at an infertility clinic.

The most common types of cancer seen in men with Klinefelter syndrome are extragonadal germ cell tumors. The risk of testicular cancer is also increased. Men with Klinefelter syndrome have an estimated 7% lifetime risk for developing breast cancer. This risk represents a 66-fold increased risk over men in the general population (whose lifetime risk of breast cancer is well below 1%). Men with breast cancer who have a history of infertility should be worked up for Klinefelter syndrome.

Genetics: The genetic basis of Klinefelter syndrome is an extra X chromosome, which has occurred as a result of non-disjunction. Cases are generally sporadic.

3. TURNER SYNDROME

Incidence 1 in 2,000 to 1 in 2,500 live births

Genetic basis: 45X or abnormalities in the structure of the X chromosome

Clinical features: Turner syndrome is associated with short stature, webbed neck, broad-shield chest, and learning disabilities. Some women with Turner syndrome have malformations of the kidney or reproductive organs. Infertility is common and may be the presenting symptom that leads to the identification of the chromosomal anomaly.

Women with Turner syndrome are at increased risk for developing Wilms' tumor, neurogenic tumors, postestrogen endometrial tumors, leukemia, and gonadal tumors.

Genetics: Turner syndrome is typically caused by the loss of one X chromosome due to a nondisjunction event. Cases are generally sporadic. Some cases of Turner syndrome are mosaic meaning that only a portion of cells are missing one copy of the X chromosome.

4.3. REFERENCES

Birch, J, Hartley, A, Tricker K et al. 1994. Prevalence and diversity of constitutional mutations in the p53 gene among 21 Li-Fraumeni families Cancer Res 54: 1298–1304.

Burke, W, Petersen, G, Lynch, P et al. 1997. Recommendations for follow-up care of individuals with an inherited predisposition to cancer. I. Hereditary non-polyposis colon cancer. JAMA 277:915–919.

Easton, D, Ford, D, Bishop, D et al. 1995. Breast and ovarian cancer incidence in BRCA1-mutation carriers. Am J Hum Genet. 56:265–271.

Eng, C. 2000. Will the real Cowden syndrome please stand up: revised diagnostic criteria. J Med Genet 37:838–830.

Foulkes, W and Hodgson, S. 1998. Inherited Susceptibility to Cancer: Clinical, Predictive and Ethical Perspectives. Cambridge University Press, New York, NY.

Khoo, S Bradley, M, Wong, F et al. 2001. Birt-Hogg-Dube syndrome: mapping of a novel hereditary neoplasia gene to chromosome 17p12-q11.2. Oncogene, *in press.*

GeneTests. Children's Health Care System, Seattle, WA. World Wide Web URL: http://www.genetests@genetests.org.

Hodgson, S and Maher, E. 1999. A Practical Guide to Human Cancer Genetics, second edition. Cambridge University Press, Cambridge, UK.

Hyman, M and Whittemore, V. 2000. National Institutes of Health Consensus Conference: Tuberous sclerosis complex. Arch Neurol. 57:662–665.

Jackson, C and Puck, J. 1999. Autoimmune lymphoproliferative syndrome, a disorder of apoptosis. Curr Opin Pediatr 11:521–527.

Kim, S. 2000. Blue rubber bleb nevus syndrome with central nervous system involvement. Pediatr Neurol 22:410–412.

Li, F and Fraumeni, J. 1969. Soft-tissue sarcomas, breast cancer, and other neoplasms. A familial syndrome? Ann Intern Med 71:747–752.

Lindor, N, Greene, M, and the Mayo Familial Cancer Program. 1998. The concise handbook of family cancer syndromes. J Natl Cancer Inst 90:1039–1071.

Lynch, H. 1998. Introduction. In Offit, K (ed) Clinical Cancer Genetics. John Wiley & Sons, New York, NY, vx.

Offit K. 1998. Clinical Cancer Genetics: Risk Counseling and Management. John Wiley & Sons, New York, NY.

Online Mendelian Inheritance in Man, OMIM (TM). 2000. McKusick-Nathans Institute for Genetic Medicine, Johns Hopkins University (Baltimore, MD) and National Center for Biotechnology Information, National Library of Medicine (Bethesda, MD). World Wide Web URL: http://www.ncbi.nlm.nih.gov/omim/.

Rodriguez-Bigas, M, Boland, C, Hamilton, S et al. A National Cancer Institute Workshop on hereditary nonpolyposis colorectal cancer syndrome: meeting highlights and Bethesda guidelines. J Natl Cancer Inst 89:1758–1762.

Struewing, J, Hartge, P, Wacholder, S et al. 1997. The risk of cancer associated with specific mutations of BRCA1 and BRCA2 among Ashkenazi Jews. NEJM. 336:1401–1408.

Toro, J, Glenn G, Duray P et al. 1999. Birt-Hogg-Dube syndrome: a novel marker of kidney neoplasia. Arch Dermatology 135:1195–1202.

Vasen, H, Mecklin J, Khan P et al. 1991. The International Collaborative Group on hereditary non-polyposis colorectal cancer. Dis Colon Rect. 34:424–425.

Vasen, H, Watson, P, Mecklin, J et al. 1999. New clinical criteria for hereditary nonpolyposis colorectal cancer (HNPCC, Lynch syndrome) proposed by the International Collaborative Group on HNPCC. Gastroenterology 116: 1453–1456.

Vogelstein, B and Kinzler, K (eds). 1998. The Genetic Basis of Human Cancer. McGraw-Hill, New York, NY.

Whitelaw, S, Murday, V, Tomlinson, I et al. 1997. Clinical and molecular features of the hereditary mixed polyposis syndrome. Gastroenterology 112:327–334.

CANCER SITES AND ASSOCIATED SYNDROMES

> . . . uncertainty does not mean that we should do nothing: In the long tradition
> of the art of medicine, it behooves the clinician to practice and advise to the best
> of his/her ability given the knowledge of the day—and the knowledge grows
> day by day.
>
> *(Eng, 1997, p. 671)*

There are many readable chapters in this book—but this is not one of them. This chapter has been designed as a quick reference for genetic counselors and other clinicians who are interested in determining the possible hereditary cancer syndromes associated with a specific tumor type.

5.1. CANCER SITES AND ASSOCIATED SYNDROMES

The 10 tables in this Chapter list various cancer syndromes associated with specific sites of malignant and benign tumors. This includes tumors of the cardiovascular and respiratory systems, central nervous system, circulatory and lymphatic systems, connective tissue, endocrine system, gastrointestinal system, head and neck, reproductive system, skin, and urinary tract. The references used to compile these tables are listed at the end of the chapter. Refer to Section 5.2 for the full syndrome names abbreviated in these tables.

And now for the disclaimers . . . Diagnosis of a hereditary cancer syndrome requires a careful review of the client's personal and family history of cancer; in other words, the tables in this Chapter should be used to help consider the possibilities, not to make a diagnosis.

Also, in an effort to be inclusive, cancer syndromes have been listed with a cancer site even if the tumor type is a minor or uncommon feature of the syndrome. And even with the best intentions, it is quite possible that there are additional syndromes that could have been listed with certain tumor types.

Lastly, keep in mind that the identification of a particular cancer syndrome almost always involves more than a single tumor diagnosis. Please refer to Chapter 4 for the diagnostic criteria of 30 major hereditary cancer syndromes.

TABLE 5-1. CARDIOVASCULAR AND RESPIRATORY SYSTEMS—BENIGN AND MALIGNANT TUMORS

Tumor Site	Type	Cancer Syndrome
Heart	Cardiac fibroma	NBCCS
	Myocardial rhabdomyoma	TS
	Myxoid neurofibroma	NAME
	Myxoma (atrium)	NAME
Larynx	Carcinoma	BS, HNPCC
Lung	Carcinoma	BS, LFS, PJS, RB, XP
Pharynx	Hemangioma	BRBNS
	Squamous cell carcinoma	XP

TABLE 5-2. CENTRAL NERVOUS SYSTEM—BENIGN AND MALIGNANT TUMORS

Tumor Site	Type	Cancer Syndrome
Brain	Unspecified type	FA, LFS, XP
	Astrocytoma	FAMM, NF 1, NF 2, TS
	Ependymoma	NF 1, NF 2
	Gangliocytoma (dysplastic)	CS
	Glioblastoma	CS, TURCOT
	Glioma	AT, NF 2
	Hemangioblastoma	VHL
	Medulloblastoma	AT, ?BRBNS, FAP, NBCCS
	Meningioma	NBCCS, NF 1, NF 2, WS
Nervous system	Hemangioma (spinal cord)	VHL
	Neuroblastoma	BWS, LFS
	Neurofibroma (spinal cord)	NF 1, NF 2
	Paraganglioma	VHL
	Schwannoma (spinal cord)	NF 2

TABLE 5-3. CIRCULATORY AND LYMPHATIC SYSTEMS—BENIGN AND MALIGNANT CONDITIONS

Tumor Site	Type	Cancer Syndrome
Leukemia	Acute, unspecified	RB, WS, XP
	Acute lymphoblastic	BS, LFS
	Acute lymphocytic	BS, LFS
	Acute myelocytic	FA
	Acute nonlymphocytic	BDS
	Acute promyelocytic	AT
	Chronic lymphocytic	AT
Lymphoma	Non-Hodgkin, unspecified	BS, RB
	Non-Hodgkin, B cell	ALPS, AT
	Non-Hodgkin, T cell	AT
Anemia	Unspecified	PJS, RTS
	Aplastic	FA
	Hemolytic	ALPS
	Hypoplastic (congenital)	BDS
	Thrombocytopenia	ALPS

TABLE 5-4. CONNECTIVE TISSUE—BENIGN AND MALIGNANT TUMORS

Tumor Site	Type	Cancer Syndrome
Bone	Ewing sarcoma	RB
	Osteomas(jaw)	FAP
	Osteosarcoma	LFS, RB, RTS, WS
Soft tissue	Collagenoma	MEN 1
	Desmoid	FAP
	Fibroma	CS
	Leiomyosarcoma	AT, LFS
	Lipoma	BHD, CS, FAP, MEN 1
	Liposarcoma	LFS, NAME
	Neurofibroma	NF 1, NF 2
	Neurofibrosarcoma	NF 1
	Rhabdomyosarcoma	BWS, LFS, XP
	Soft tissue sarcoma, unspecified	LFS, WS

TABLE 5-5. ENDOCRINE SYSTEM—BENIGN AND MALIGNANT TUMORS

Tumor Site	Type	Cancer Syndrome
Adrenal gland	Adenoma	MEN 1
	Adrenal hemangioma	VHL
	Adrenocortical carcinoma	BWS, LFS, CARNEY
	Pheochromocytoma	MEN 2, NF 1, VHL
Parathyroid	Adenoma	BHD, MEN 1, MEN 2
	Carcinoma	MEN 1
Pituitary gland	Adenoma	CARNEY, MEN 1
Thyroid	Unspecified carcinoma	NAME, WS
	Adenoma	NAME, TS
	Follicular carcinoma	CS, FAP
	Medullary carcinoma	MEN 2
	Papillary carcinoma	CS, FAP

TABLE 5-6. GASTROINTESTINAL SYSTEM—BENIGN AND MALIGNANT TUMORS

Tumor Site	Type	Cancer Syndrome
Ampulla of vater	Periampullary carcinoma	FAP
Bile duct	Carcinoma	BOCS, FAP, HNPCC
Colon/rectum	Adenocarcinoma	BOCS, BS, FAP, HMPS, HNPCC, JP, LFS, MTS, NAME, PJS, TURCOT
Colon polyps	Adenomas	FAP, HNPCC
	Adenomatous polyposis	FAP
	Atypical juvenile	HMPS
	Hamartomas	CS, PJS
	Hemangiomas	BRBNS
	Juvenile hamartomas	JP
Esophagus	Carcinoma	BS
Gallbladder	Carcinoma	BOCS
Liver	Hepatoblastoma	BWS, FAP
	Hepatocellular carcinoma	ALPS, BWS, FA
Pancreas	Adenoma	VHL
	Carcinoma	AT, BOCS, BS, DNS, FAMM, JP, NAME, PJS, VHL
	Cysts	VHL
	Islet cell tumor (gastrioma)	MEN 1, VHL

Continued

TABLE 5-6. Gastrointestinal System—CONTINUED

Tumor Site	Type	Cancer Syndrome
Small intestine	Adenocarcinoma	FAP, HNPCC, JP, PJS
	Juvenile hamartoma	JP
Stomach	Adenocarcinoma	AT, BOCS, BS, FAP, HNPCC, JP, LFS, WS, XP
	Carcinoid	MEN 1
	Desmoid	FAP
	Gastric Teratoma (congenital)	BWS
	Hamartomas	JP, NBCCS, PJS
	Hemangiomas	BRBNS

TABLE 5-7. Head and Neck—Tumors and Other Associated Findings

Tumor Site	Type	Cancer Syndrome
Eye	Aniridia	WAGR
	Cataracts	NF 2, RTS, WS
	CHRPE	FAP
	Hemangiomas	BRBNS
	Iris hamartomas (Lisch nodules)	NF 1
	Leukoria (white spot)	RB
	Ocular melanoma	BOCS
	Optic glioma	NF 1
	Papillomas	XP
	Pinealoma	RB
	Retinal phakoma	TS
	Retinal angioma	VHL
	Retinoblastoma	RB
	Squamous cell carcinoma	XP
	Telangiectasia	AT, XP
Ear	Endolymphatic sac	VHL
	Vestibular schwannomas	NF 1
Mouth	Carcinoma	BS
	Dental enamel pits	TS
	Jaw cysts	NBCCS
	Mucosal papillomatosis	CS
	Mucosal neuromas	MEN 2
	Pigmented spots (lip, buccal mucosa)	PJS
	Squamous cell carcinoma	XP
	Trichilimmomas	CS

TABLE 5-8. REPRODUCTIVE SYSTEM—BENIGN AND MALIGNANT TUMORS

Tumor Site	Type	Cancer Syndrome
Breast	Adenocarcinoma (females)	AT, BS, BOCS, CS, ?HNPCC, LFS, PJS, WS, XP
	Adenocarcinoma (males)	BOCS, KS
	Sarcoma	LFS
Cervix	Unspecified type	BS
Germ cell tumor	Extragonadal	KS
	Gonadoblastoma	DRASH
	Sertoli-Leydig cell tumor	NAME
Fallopial tube		BOCS
Ovary	Adenocarcinoma	AT, BOCS, CS, HNPCC, PJS
	Benign sex cord tumor	PJS
	Fibroma	NBCCS
	Sarcoma	NBCCS
Peritoneum	Papillary serous carcinoma	BOCS
Prostate	Carcinoma	BOCS
Testes	Germ cell tumor	KS, NAME, PJS, XP
Uterus	Endometrial carcinoma	CS, HNPCC, PJS, XP
	Hemangiomas	BRBNS
	Myxoid uterine leiomyomas	NAME
	Uterine sarcoma	LFS

TABLE 5-9. SKIN—BENIGN AND MALIGNANT TUMORS AND ASSOCIATED
SKIN FINDINGS

Tumor Site	Type	Cancer Syndrome
Skin	Angiomas	XP
	Basal cell carcinoma	BS, FAP, NBCCS, RTS, XP
	Café au lait spots	AT, NAME, NF 1, NF 2
	Collagenomas	MEN 1
	Cutaneous angiosarcoma	XP
	Cutaneous keratocysts	NBCCS
	Cutaneous myxomas	CARNEY
	Dermal fibroma	NAME, XP
	Ephelides (freckles)	NAME, XP
	Epidermoid cyst	FAP
	Epitheliomas	XP
	Fibroangiomas (facial)	MEN 1
	Fibrofolliculomas	BHD

Continued

TABLE 5-9. SKIN—*CONTINUED*

Tumor Site	Type	Cancer Syndrome
	Hamartomas	CS
	Keratocanthomas	CS, MTS, XP
	Keratoses	XP
	Lentigines	LAMB
	Macules (black-brown)	NAME
	Melanoma	AT, CS, DNS, FAMM, LFS, RB,WS, XP
	Nevi/hemangioma (blue)	BRBNS, LAMB
	Nevi (dysplastic)	DNS, FAMM, NAME
	Pigmented spots	CARNEY, PJS, RTS, XP
	Poikilodermas	RTS, XP
	Scleroderma	WS
	Sebaceous cyst	FAP
	Sebaceous gland toumor	MTS
	Shagreen patch	TS
	Squamous cell carcinoma	FA, RTS, XP
	Telangiectasia	AT, RTS
	Trichilimmomas	BHD, CS
	Trichodiscomas	BHD

TABLE 5-10. URINARY TRACT—BENIGN AND MALIGNANT TUMORS

Tumor Site	Type	Cancer Syndrome
Bladder	Carcinoma	RB
Kidney	Adenoma	VHL
	Cyst	VHL
	Lipoma	TS
	Renal cell carcinoma	BHD, CS, HNPCC, TS, VHL
	Wilms' tumor	BS, BWS, TS, WT
Renal pelvis	Transitional cell	HNPCC
Urogenital	Malformations	DRASH, WAGR
Ureter	Carcinoma	HNPCC

5.2. A LISTING OF THE CANCER SYNDROME ABBREVIATIONS

ABBREVIATION	*SYNDROME*
ALPS	Autoimmune lymphoproliferative syndrome
AT	Ataxia-telangiectasia
BDS	Blackfan-Diamond syndrome
BHD	Birt-Hogg-Dube syndrome

ABBREVIATION	SYNDROME
BOCS	Breast-ovarian cancer syndrome
BRBNS	Blue rubber bleb nevus syndrome
BS	Bloom syndrome
BWS	Beckwith-Wiedemann syndrome
CARNEY	Carney complex
CS	Cowden syndrome
DNS	Dysplastic nevus syndrome
DRASH	DRASH syndrome
FA	Fanconi anemia
FAMM	Familial astrocytoma—malignant mole syndrome
FAP	Familial adenomatous polyposis
HMPS	Hereditary mixed polyposis syndrome
HNPCC	Hereditary nonpolyposis colon cancer
JP	Juvenile polyposis
KS	Klinefelter syndrome
LAMB	LAMB syndrome
LFS	Li-Fraumeni syndrome
MEN 1	Multiple endocrine neoplasia, 1
MEN 2	Multiple endocrine neoplasia, 2
MTS	Muir-Torre syndrome
NAME	NAME syndrome
NBCCS	Nevoid basal cell carcinoma syndrome
NF 1	Neurofibromatosis, 1
NF 2	Neurofibromatosis, 2
PJS	Peutz-Jeghers syndrome
RB	Retinoblastoma, familial
RTS	Rothmund-Thomson syndrome
TSC	Tuberous sclerosis
TURCOT	Turcot syndrome
VHL	von Hippel-Lindau syndrome
WAGR	WAGR syndrome
WER	Werner syndrome
WT	Wilms' tumor
XP	Xeroderma pigmentosum

5.3. REFERENCES

Easton, D, Ford, D, Bishop, D et al. 1995. Breast and ovarian cancer incidence in BRCA1-mutation carriers. Am J Hum Genet. 56:265–271.

Eng, C. 1997. From Bench to Bedside . . . but when? Genome Research 7:669–672.

Eng, C. 2000. Will the real Cowden syndrome please stand up: revised diagnostic criteria. J Med Genet 37:838–830.

Foulkes, W and Hodgson, S. 1998. Inherited Susceptibility to Cancer: Clinical, Predictive and Ethical Perspectives. Cambridge University Press, New York, NY.

GeneTests. Children's Health Care System, Seattle, WA. World Wide Web URL: http://www.genetests@genetests.org

Hodgson, S and Maher, E. 1999. A Practical Guide to Human Cancer Genetics, second edition. Cambridge University Press, Cambridge, UK.

Hyman, M and Whittemore, V. 2000. National Institutes of Health Consensus Conference: Tuberous sclerosis complex. Arch Neurol. 57:662–665.

Jackson, C and Puck, J. 1999. Autoimmune lymphoproliferative syndrome, a disorder of apoptosis. Curr Opin Pediatr 11:521–527.

Kim, S. 2000. Blue rubber bleb nevus syndrome with central nervous system involvement. Pediatr Neurol 22:410–412.

Lindor, N, Greene, M, and the Mayo Familial Cancer Program. 1998. The concise handbook of family cancer syndromes. J Natl Cancer Inst 90:1039–1071.

Lynch, H and de la Chapelle, A. 1997. Genetic susceptibility to non-polyposis colorectal cancer. J Med Genet 36:801–818.

Offit, K. 1998. Clinical Cancer Genetics: Risk Counseling and Management. John Wiley & Sons, New York, NY.

Online Mendelian Inheritance in Man, OMIM (TM). 2000. McKusick-Nathans Institute for Genetic Medicine, Johns Hopkins University (Baltimore, MD) and National Center for Biotechnology Information, National Library of Medicine (Bethesda, MD). World Wide Web URL: http://www.ncbi.nlm.nih.gov/omim/

Rodriguez-Bigas, M, Boland, C, Hamilton, S et al. . . . A National Cancer Institute Workshop on hereditary nonpolyposis colorectal cancer syndrome: meeting highlights and Bethesda guidelines. J Natl Cancer Inst 89:1758–1762.

Toro, J, Glenn, G, Duray, P et al. 1999. Birt-Hogg-Dube syndrome: a novel marker of kidney neoplasia. Arch Dermatology 135:1195–1202.

Varley, J, Evans, D, and Birch, J. 1997. Li-Fraumeni syndrome—a molecular and clinical review. Br J Cancer 71:1–14.

Vasen, H, Watson, P, Mecklin, J et al. 1999. New clinical criteria for hereditary nonpolyposis colorectal cancer (HNPCC, Lynch syndrome) proposed by the International Collaborative Group on HNPCC. Gatroenterology 116:1453–1456.

Vogelstein, B and Kinzler, K (eds). 1998. The Genetic Basis of Human Cancer. McGraw-Hill, New York, NY.

Whitelaw, S, Murday, V, Tomlinson, I et al. 1997. Clinical and molecular features of the hereditary mixed polyposis syndrome. Gastroenterology 112:327–334.

6

COLLECTION AND INTERPRETATION OF CANCER HISTORIES

> I view a pedigree like a quilt, stitching together the intimate and colorful scraps
> of medical and family information from a person's life.
>
> *(Bennett, 1999, p. 8)*

Cancer risk assessment relies on the careful collection and interpretation of the client's personal and family histories of cancer. The first section of this chapter focuses on how to collect a comprehensive cancer history and discusses difficult issues that can arise. The latter section describes the important elements to consider when assessing and classifying cancer histories. The chapter ends with three case examples.

6.1. COLLECTING A CANCER HISTORY

The purpose of gathering family history information is to determine the likelihood that a client has a hereditary cancer syndrome. This section discusses strategies for collecting a cancer history, including examples of questions to ask and methods of confirming histories. Please see Appendix B for a review of basic pedigree symbols.

6.1.1. GENERAL STRATEGIES

As with other aspects of the genetic counseling session, there is an art to taking a comprehensive cancer history. Although the pattern of cancer among first- and second-degree relatives is the most relevant information in terms of the client's risks, cancer histories typically extend three or more generations and often include third-degree relatives (first cousins, great aunts, and great uncles).

Here are some general strategies for collecting a cancer history:

1. *Obtain confirmation on tumor diagnoses*—Even clients who are good historians can provide inaccurate or misleading information. This is why obtaining confirmation of the diagnosis, in the form of a pathology report or physician's note, remains the gold standard. Unfortunately, the process of obtaining the necessary documentation can be incredibly time consuming and frustrating for both client and counselor. And sometimes, even with the best of efforts, it is not possible to obtain the needed records. Thus, it may be better to ask clients to focus their efforts on obtaining records on diagnoses that are key to interpreting the cancer history rather than attempting to confirm each diagnosis.

2. *Include nonmalignant findings*—Certain cancer syndromes have well-recognized nonmalignant features. These include associated benign lesions (sebaceous cysts with Gardner syndrome), physical features (macrocephaly with Cowden syndrome), and even birth defects (aniridia with familial Wilms' tumor). Thus, it is important to record nonmalignant tumors and diseases when collecting the family history, especially if the feature seems to track with the cancer occurrences in the family.

3. *Extend pedigree around each cancer diagnosis*—The purpose of taking the history is to determine whether the various cases of cancer in the family could be due to the same underlying genetic factor. One way to help answer this question is to extend the pedigree further in branches of the family that contain cases of cancer. In other words, counselors should obtain information about first- and second-degree relatives for each family member who has had cancer. In some cases, the client might need to contact certain distant relatives to obtain this information.

4. *Do not neglect the unaffected relatives*—Identifying a family with two siblings who have had similar cancers may seem significant until learning that they are part of a sibling set of 12. Looking for evidence of a dominant cancer syndrome relies on assessing the proportion of at-risk relatives who have gone on to develop cancer. Of course, smaller families may be more difficult to assess. In addition, it is important to gather information about both sides of the family

even if it seems obvious which side of the family has the cancer predisposition. Sometimes, it turns out that the less interesting side of the family is actually the one that has the hereditary cancer syndrome.

5. *Consider the accuracy of the historian*—Clients are more likely to accurately report a cancer diagnosis in first-degree relatives than in more distant relatives. This is hardly surprising since clients are more apt to be directly involved in the care of a close family member. The site of cancer may also influence accuracy rates. Although reports of breast cancer, prostate cancer, and melanoma are usually quite accurate, reports of other forms of cancer have much lower rates of accuracy. This includes cancers of internal organs (such as pancreas or small intestine), cancers that are often sites of metastasis (including bone, lung, and colon cancers), and tumors that are rare or have lengthy names (such as hamartomas or leiomyosarcomas).

6. *Help clients identify strategies for expanding history*—The counselor depends on the client's ability and willingness to obtain a comprehensive family history. However, counselors should recognize that obtaining this information can be tedious, time consuming, and, in some cases, an emotional landmine. It may be helpful for counselors to suggest ways to obtain information with a minimum of effort or involvement by other relatives. For example, a client may not feel comfortable contacting a distant cousin about his newly diagnosed cancer, but perhaps an aunt would either know the information or could find out.

7. *Use history as a psychosocial tool*—It is almost impossible to gather a family history without hearing about the stories behind the cancer diagnoses. In addition to eliciting the pattern of cancer in the family, the family history discussion can also provide information about relationships with other family members, the clients' perceptions of risk, and even attitudes toward cancer monitoring or genetic testing. In addition, it might be important to note the points at which the client becomes emotional or quiet; these "triggers" might be a clue as to how clients might react to the news that they are at increased risk for cancer.

8. *Standardize pedigree nomenclature*—Constructing a cancer pedigree is like cursive handwriting; there is a correct form to follow, but everyone has their own style. Some cancer risk programs use a quadrant system or different types of shading to denote different types of cancer. It might also be useful to distinguish between cancers that have been fully documented and those that have not. Programs may also want to standardize the abbreviations used for specific types of tumors and the symbols used to denote whether the individual has had a premalignant tumor or has undergone genetic testing.

9. *Decide on confidentiality practices*—Cancer risk programs also need to decide on the information that will not be included on the pedigree. This might include full names of relatives, genetic test results, and other potentially sensitive information (such as adoption status, mental illness, alcoholism, or HIV status). If in doubt, ask clients whether certain ancillary information should be included on the finalized form of the pedigree. Pedigrees forwarded to other institutions should not include names or other identifying information unless the relative has given permission for this information to be released.

10. *Review completed pedigrees with clients*—It is a good policy to confirm the completed pedigree with each client. Errors can occur while initially taking down the information or when transposing the pedigree to a computerized form. After reflection, clients may also have additional or revised information to include in the pedigree.

6.1.2. KEY QUESTIONS TO ASK ABOUT THE CLIENT'S MEDICAL HISTORY

Questions about cancer histories typically begin with the clients themselves. This section suggests the types of questions to ask clients presenting in a high-risk clinic. These questions will obviously differ depending on whether the client has had cancer.

The client's date of birth will be recorded in his or her medical chart, but it is worth rechecking this information at the time of the visit. The client's age is an important factor in determining appropriate medical management once the risk assessment has been completed and may also raise or lower the risk of having an inherited predisposition.

Clients who have never had cancer should be questioned about the following.

1. *Presence of syndromic features*—Some hereditary cancer syndromes are associated with observable physical features. Examples include congenital defects (like hemihypertrophy associated with familial Wilms' tumor) and premalignant conditions (such as dysplastic nevi associated with familial melanoma). The features will sometimes be obvious to the genetic counselor, but, in general, clients should be referred to a physician to perform a careful physical examination and order appropriate diagnostic tests.

2. *Current surveillance practices*—Many clients will already be undergoing surveillance for cancer. For clients being monitored, it is useful to obtain the following information: types of screening tests performed, frequency of screening, and results and dates of any abnormal screening tests. Whenever possible, obtain a copy of the

surveillance reports. If the family turns out to have a hereditary cancer syndrome, this information may be useful in determining the client's risk status.

3. *Other cancer risk factors*—There are several established environmental factors that can increase the risks of specific forms of malignancy. In addition, certain medical conditions such as diabetes or ulcerative colitis can greatly increase cancer risks. Counselors may want to ask a few questions about the client's occupational exposures, medical conditions or problems, dietary habits, and use of tobacco and alcohol.

Clients who have had cancer should be questioned about the following:

1. *Cancer diagnosis*—Clients are usually, but not always, able to provide their exact cancer diagnosis. Regardless, clients should be asked to bring in written confirmation of their diagnosis including the client's age at diagnosis and the date of the diagnosis. If the counselor is planning to assist the client in obtaining medical records documentation, also obtain the names of the hospitals where the client has been treated. It is also useful to learn specifics about how the cancer was first detected. This allows clients to share their personal cancer experiences which can provide insights beyond the specifics of the cancer diagnosis.

2. *Cancer treatment and follow-up*—Standard methods to treat cancer include surgery, chemotherapy, and radiation. Counselors may want to ask a few questions about the treatment they underwent (or are still going through) and what recommendations have been made regarding follow-up.

3. *Current status and prognosis*—In discussing plans for obtaining additional family history information or blood specimens for genetic testing, it is important to be aware of the client's current cancer status and short-term prognosis. It is also useful to know where clients are in their treatment because clients in active treatment are likely to have different concerns than those who are long-term survivors. Also, making arrangements for genetic testing might differ depending on the client's current status (e.g. terminally ill) or treatment history (e.g. underwent donor bone marrow transplant).

6.1.3. KEY QUESTIONS ABOUT THE CLIENT'S RELATIVES

Accurate interpretation of the client's cancer history hinges on collecting detailed information about relatives who have developed cancer. It is important to obtain the following information about family members who have had cancer (see Table 6-1).

TABLE 6-1. SAMPLE FAMILY HISTORY QUESTIONS TO ASK

What type of cancer was diagnosed?
Do you know the exact diagnosis?
Where was your relative diagnosed and/or treated?
Did the relative develop any other types of cancer?
Do you know whether the second cancer spread from the original tumor?
How old was your relative at diagnosis?
What year was the cancer diagnosed?
Is your relative still living?
  If yes, how old is your relative now?
  If no, what year and at what age did your relative die?
What was your relative's occupation?
Did your relative smoke cigarettes?
Was your relative exposed to any other harmful agents that might have caused
cancer?

1. *Exact diagnosis for each cancer*—Attempts should be made to obtain
   precise information for each cancer diagnosis in the family. This information will be crucial in determining whether the family could have
   a hereditary cancer syndrome. Certain features of the diagnosis
   (unusual histology, bilaterality) may also be important in the
   assessment.

   In an ideal situation, a client would state with conviction, "My
   mother had invasive ductal carcinoma of the breast." Realistically,
   however, a client is more likely to know only the site of cancer in the
   body, "My mother had breast cancer." Sometimes even the site of
   cancer is unknown, and the client will relate, "My mother had some
   type of cancer; it could have been breast cancer." Thus, confirmation
   of the cancer diagnoses in a family with medical records becomes
   extremely important. (Section 6.1.4 discusses strategies for confirming pedigree information.) Clients will sometimes report that a relative has had two separate cancer diagnoses and counselors will need
   to sort out whether these two cancers represent separate primaries or
   metastatic disease.

2. *Ages and dates*—Because age of onset is an important variable of inherited cancers, genetic counselors need to ascertain the age at which
   family members were diagnosed. The age at diagnosis is what is most
   important, not the age at which they began noticing symptoms. Other
   useful information includes the approximate date (year) cancer was
   diagnosed, current ages of relatives, or, if they are deceased, the age
   and year of death. Clients may be more likely to remember the relative's death than when they were diagnosed with cancer. If this is
   the case, it may be helpful to ask whether the relative was diagnosed

within a few years of death or was diagnosed many years earlier. Obtaining the dates of when cancer was diagnosed or when death occurred will make it easier to request written confirmation of the cancer diagnosis. In addition, it may be possible to obtain tumor specimen blocks for individuals who died within the past 10–20 years, which could be utilized in certain DNA studies.

3. *Environmental exposures*—Certain cancers are known or suspected to be associated with specific environmental agents. In these cases, it is useful to determine whether exposure to a particular carcinogen could have contributed to the development of cancer. Such clustering of exposures is rare and would not be expected to lead to multiple cases of cancer within the family (although this is possible if several family members smoke cigarettes or all have the same occupational exposures). The most important carcinogens to ask about are cigarettes, alcohol, radiation, asbestos, and DES *in utero* (females).

4. *Questions regarding unaffected relatives*—Counselors should also ask a few questions about the relatives who have not developed cancer. Useful information includes determining relatives' current ages and whether they are routinely screened for cancer. Also, whether they have undergone any prophylactic surgeries. If family members are deceased, document the age when they died and the cause of death. Counselors should specifically ask about any non-malignant features of the syndrome in question. For example, Cowden syndrome is associated with benign skin lesions and fatty tumors (lipomas). If there is any possibility that a relative had a syndromic related feature, request medical records documentation. It is important to find out how old the relatives were when they died because family members who were cancer-free in their eighties can provide more information than living unaffected relatives who are in their twenties.

6.1.4. Obtaining Confirmation

Because inherited forms of cancer are recognized almost solely on the pattern of cancer in the family, it is crucial for pedigrees to reflect accurate information. However, family histories are notoriously inaccurate, especially regarding relatives who live far away or who have died a long time ago.

The confirmation process involves obtaining prior permission from the relative in question (or if deceased, the designated next of kin). The following information is usually needed: the relative's full name (including maiden name), the relative's date of birth, the approximate date of diagnosis (or death), and the name of the hospital where the cancer was diagnosed. If the individual is deceased, it may be necessary to include the actual or approximate date of death. Lack of precise information can make the task of confirming information even more tedious—and much less likely to be successful. Unfortunately, the process of obtaining confirmation of cancer diagnoses can be quite laborious, often taking months to complete.

Sometimes, clients are stymied about how to go about obtaining documentation. The red tape involved in obtaining copies of a medical record can be daunting to individuals who are unfamiliar with hospital procedures, and they may be intimidated by the thought of contacting an unfamiliar physician's office or hospital. Medical records departments often require that requests be made in writing. It may be useful to provide clients with sample release forms and instructions for how to obtain the relevant records. Counselors should provide clients with general instructions as to how to obtain documentation; counselors may even want to assist families with these efforts.

There are several levels of confirmation, which are discussed below (see Table 6-2).

1. *Verbal confirmation*—Collecting a comprehensive cancer history may require conversations with more than one family member. Reviewing the pedigree with multiple family members allows counselors to confirm the information already obtained and also to learn additional information. Ask clients for permission to speak to their relatives. Speaking directly with the relatives who have had cancer tends to be most useful. If this is not possible, the person's spouse or another close relative is the next best option.

2. *Pathology report*—Obtaining the pathology report is the best method of confirmation. Pathology reports are issued for almost every type of malignancy. The diagnosis of cancer almost always involves an analysis of the malignant cells. The pathology report will include the full name and age of the patient, date of analysis, the name of the tumor, site of origin, and grade. Reviewing pathology reports should be done in conjunction with a physician (preferably an oncologist or pathologist). Pathology reports are typically part of the individual's medical record; however; it may be easier to obtain a copy directly through the hospital's pathology department.

TABLE 6-2. SOURCES FOR CONFIRMING CANCER HISTORY

Client's relatives
Pathology report(s)
Physician clinic notes
Hospital discharge summaries
Autopsy report
Death certificate

3. *Hospital summary notes*—If the pathology report is not accessible, another option is to review other entries in the medical record, such as surgical records, hospitalization discharge notes, or summaries of outpatient visits. Counselors should look for information recorded close to the time of diagnosis.

4. *Autopsy report*—A number of deceased individuals undergo autopsy examinations. This information might be useful to look for evidence of a malignancy or other syndromic features. This report is typically included in the individual's medical record.

5. *Death certificate*—Another possible source of confirmation is the death certificate. The death certificate will list the individual's cancer diagnosis if it is considered the primary cause of death and sometimes includes the cancer diagnosis if it is considered a secondary cause of death. However, family members who were long-term cancer survivors and died of natural causes are less likely to have the diagnosis listed on the death certificate. The death certificate usually indicates whether an autopsy has been performed (which is more likely to mention the prior cancer diagnosis). Death certificates are a matter of public record and should be obtainable, provided the client has enough information to locate it. Required information typically includes where the person died (city and state) and date of death. It may also be helpful to have date of birth, name of parents and spouse, and place of birth. Clients should be warned that there is usually a fee associated with obtaining copies of death certificates.

6.2. Challenges to Collecting an Accurate History

Counselors depend on clients to provide accurate and complete family histories. Yet cancer histories can be notoriously inaccurate. This can occur because clients have lost touch with some of their relatives or because they never paid attention to their relatives' medical histories. Perhaps most challenging are the clients who report their family histories with conviction, which turn out to be false. This section discusses reasons why the cancer history might be inaccurate or incomplete and strategies that counselors can use to elicit better histories.

6.2.1. Family History Information is Incomplete

It can be difficult to obtain a comprehensive cancer history. In some cases, the problem lies in the client's skill as a historian. Some clients are much better at recounting their family histories than others. Clients may be poor historians for the following reasons:

1. *Family members live far away*—It is rare these days to find an extended family that has remained in the same city or region. Members of a family have frequently scattered to different parts of the country and may only get together on special family occasions, if at all. As a result, some clients may be unaware of the medical histories of entire branches of the family. Alternatively, they may have heard about the diagnosis from an indirect (and potentially unreliable) source. Also, clients may feel awkward about asking for more detailed family history information from relatives whom they barely know. Even among family members with solid relationships, clients may hesitate to ask too many questions. They may not want the person to worry or may be afraid of making them sad.

2. *Clients are not prepared to answer questions*—Clients may not be good at remembering dates and may be hazy about who died from what. For this reason, it is helpful to have informed clients beforehand about the types of questions they will be asked during the genetic counseling visit. It may also be the counseling session itself that has hampered the client's ability to remember detailed information. Questions about family history may cause some clients to feel "put on the spot" or swamped with emotional memories; neither is conducive to providing accurate information.

3. *Cancer is not discussed in the family*—A generation ago it was not unusual to call cancer "The big C," as though uttering the word itself was too frightening. Although it is now more common for people to talk about their cancer diagnoses, some individuals remain fiercely private about their medical histories. Sometimes relatives hide their cancer diagnoses out of misguided attempts to "protect" other relatives from knowing what they are going through. Counselors need to be sensitive to the fact that clients may have been rebuffed in their efforts to obtain family history information, or they may want to honor their relatives' wishes about "not wanting to talk about it." Clients may also hesitate to ask too many questions, because they do not want their relatives to become worried or distressed. The inability to obtain cancer information may also reflect a lack of opportunity to discuss the subject. If clients only see their relatives on festive occasions, it may be awkward to discuss details about their cancer diagnoses.

In the above scenarios, clients may not be aware of their family histories but probably do have access to the information. In collecting a cancer history, counselors may want to utilize the following strategies:

- ask specific questions about each family member to help jog the client's memory,

- link ages or dates with other family events or special occasions,
- help the client identify relatives who might have answers to specific questions,
- compile a list of questions that would help in the assessment of the family history,
- consider who in the family might have the needed information and create a strategy for obtaining this information, and
- because completing the history is a process, reassure clients that it is okay for them not to have all needed information at the first visit (otherwise, they may not return).

6.2.2. FAMILY HISTORY INFORMATION IS NOT AVAILABLE

In certain situations, clients may have difficulty accessing family history information. This can occur because of the following reasons.

1. *Lost contact with relatives*—Family members who live far apart may, over time, lose contact with one another. Clients may have little awareness of the current health status of certain relatives and may not even have current contact information for them. There may be one or two relatives, such as a parent or grandparent, who act as the glue that keeps everyone together. Upon their death, family members may have much less contact with each other. The death of key relatives also causes clients to have less information about certain individuals in the family. This is also true if a parent has died young and the other parent remarried. Clients may have little information about that side of the family and have no way to learn more about it.

2. *Estrangement from family*—Relationships may be full of conflict or practically nonexistent; in either case, clients may have less than complete information about their relatives' cancer history. Sometimes even families in the same city have not spoken to each other in years. There may be complicated reasons for the estrangement, such as drugs or abuse. Individuals who are estranged from family members will have no way of obtaining confirmation of their family history and may in fact have less than complete information about their relatives. Sometimes, in the tradition of Hatfield and McCoy, who made family feuding an art form, it is not the client who has broken off contact with others but someone from a previous generation.

3. *Adoption*—The amount of information an adopted individual has about his or her biological family can vary. Usually, the following information is provided about the biological parents: age at the time of the birth, medical information, and race, ethnicity, and religion. Clients can sometimes obtain additional information by contacting

the agency that arranged the adoption, and some adult clients have eventually tracked down their biological parents. However, most of the time, clients will have limited facts about their family histories and no access to obtaining this information.

In the above-listed situations in which access to information may be limited, counselors can consider utilizing the following strategies:

- focus on obtaining information on key relatives or diagnoses,
- gain an understanding of the barriers to obtaining this information,
- discuss alternative ways of obtaining this information, such as contacting other relatives or friends of the family, and
- accept that it may not be possible for clients to provide more additional information and reassure clients that this is okay.

6.2.3. REPORTED HISTORY IS FALSE

The most challenging counseling situations can occur when clients provide information about their family histories that turns out to be inaccurate. These types of situations can occur when clients are

1. *Mistaken about the cancer diagnosis*—Cancer diagnoses among relatives may turn out to be benign lesions that have been biopsied or removed. The relative may have undergone surgery for reasons that were unrelated to a cancer diagnosis. For example, the client's aunt had a hysterectomy because of a benign uterine fibroid not uterine cancer. Relatives may also be assumed to have cancer if they have medical conditions that lead to invasive procedures or treatments. Examples include gastric ulcers and inflammatory bowel disease.

2. *Confused about the diagnosis*—Clients may make assumptions about the site or type of cancer among relatives or may be confused about which relatives had what cancers. They may know, for example, that the relative had colon polyps but not that the polyps were hamartomas. In addition, clients frequently do not distinguish between the primary site of cancer and sites of metastatic disease. In fact, it may be the metastatic cancer that is more likely to be remembered, as it is probably what led to the relative's death. Clients may also have little knowledge of anatomy or medical terminology. Thus, "stomach cancer" may mean any malignancy in the abdomen and "uterine cancer" may mean any female reproductive cancer. Vague reports of a "brain tumor" can also be problematic, as it can be used for anything from a benign cyst to a hemangioblastoma or malignant astrocytoma.

3. *Deliberately fabricating history*—It is rare that clients deliberately falsify their family histories of cancer, but, when it occurs, it creates a diffi-

cult and awkward counseling dilemma. Clients might provide fabricated histories because they want to ensure that they will be monitored closely or have access to prevention options, such as prophylactic surgery. In addition to providing fabricated cancer histories, clients may also falsely claim that there is a deleterious gene mutation in the family. Sometimes, it is not the client who has fabricated the history but, rather, another relative. Clients or relatives may fabricate their cancer histories because they are seeking sympathy or attention. This type of behavior can also indicate the presence of an emotional disorder termed Munchausen syndrome. Individuals with Munchausen syndrome, which has been observed more frequently among women, are hypochondriacal and may actually seek out painful, invasive procedures.

Falsely provided information, whether deliberate or not, can wreak havoc on the interpretation of the family history. Counselors can employ the following strategies to help ensure that the recounted history is correct:

- encourage clients to confirm the history with other family members rather than making assumptions about the diagnoses,
- obtain documentation of cancer diagnoses, especially if key to the interpretation of the family history,
- diagnoses that appear questionable should be explored further, but in a respectful and gentle manner, and
- if there is evidence that the history has been fabricated, carefully consider the potential ramifications if this information is shared with the client. Unless the corrected information is germane to the risk assessment, it might be best not to challenge the claims of the relative or client.

6.3. INTERPRETING A CANCER HISTORY

Ancient mapmakers marked rough water, "Here there be serpents." as a warning by which to navigate. In exploring our medical family trees we become the cartographers of our ancestry, mapping the very stuff from which we are made. We can use what we find to protect ourselves, our children, our children's children.

(Adato, 1995, p. 60)

As DNA testing becomes more widely available, demonstrating which families have inherited susceptibilities to cancer will become a more exact science. Until then, the identification of a hereditary cancer syndrome relies on the careful interpretation of a cancer history. This section describes general features of hereditary cancer syndromes and discusses possible ways to classify the patterns of cancer within families.

6.3.1. FEATURES OF INHERITED CANCERS

Taking a good cancer history is easier if counselors understand why the answers are being sought. This section describes eight general pedigree features that are indicative of hereditary forms of cancer. These features are also listed in Table 6-3. The presence of at least some of these features raises the likelihood that cancers in the family are due to an inherited factor.

1. *Several relatives with same or related cancers*—The first, and foremost, feature of a cancer history is obviously the presence of malignancy. In general, pedigrees should include at least two first-degree relatives (or one first-degree and two second-degree relatives) who have developed the same or related cancers. The more family members affected with cancer, the stronger the likelihood that there is a genetic predisposition. However, the presence of the same or related types of cancer in a few relatives is more striking than multiple family members with different cancers. This is because a cancer susceptibility gene is typically associated with specific forms of cancer. It is important to become familiar with the spectrum of cancers that could be linked to the same underlying genetic factor. For example, certain breast cancer syndromes are associated with cancers of the ovary, colon, thyroid, and/or bone.

2. *Younger age of onset than is typical*—Inherited forms of cancer typically have earlier ages of onset than sporadic tumors. This is true for pediatric as well as adult forms of cancer. The pediatric hereditary cancer syndromes (such as retinoblastoma) may occur several months earlier, whereas some of the adult-onset syndromes (such as hereditary colon cancer) may occur several decades earlier. The presence of one or more family members who have developed malignancies at unusually young ages is strongly suggestive of an inherited form of cancer. However, malignancies occurring at later ages may also be due, in part, to inherited factors.

3. *Autosomal dominant pattern of cancer*—The majority of hereditary cancer syndromes identified to date follow autosomal dominant

TABLE 6-3. PEDIGREE FEATURES SUGGESTIVE OF A HEREDITARY CANCER SYNDROME

Three or more relatives with similar or related cancers
At least 1 relative diagnosed at a younger than usual age
At least 1 relative with more than one primary
At least 1 relative with bilateral, multisynchronous tumor
At least 1 relative with a common tumor at an unusual age
At least 1 relative with a rare tumor
Absence of environmental risk factors

inheritance patterns. Thus, the pattern of cancer should occur in more than one generation and exhibit a vertical pattern of transmission (i.e., grandparent, parent, child). In other words, the presence of cancer in a parent-child pair tends to be more compelling than in a sibling pair. However, the dominant pattern of inheritance can be subtle due to incomplete penetrance, small family size, young ages of the majority of family members, or, in a syndrome with predominantly female cancers, few at-risk women.

4. *Presence of rare tumors*—Cancer can cluster in families due to a variety of factors including inherited factors, shared exposures to carcinogens, or simply random chance ("bad luck"). However, the clustering of tumors, which occurs rarely in the general population, is more difficult to explain by chance alone, providing evidence for an inherited basis. Examples include sebaceous gland tumors associated with Muir-Torre syndrome and childhood adrenal gland tumors associated with Li-Fraumeni syndrome. Pedigrees suggestive of inherited forms of cancer may also include malignancies that have developed in an unusual subgroup. This includes children who develop typically adult-onset cancers, men who develop breast cancer, and nonsmokers who develop early-onset lung cancer.

5. *Excess of multifocal or bilateral cancers*—Most tumors are monoclonal, meaning that the population of malignant cells has arisen from a single cancer cell. Individuals with inherited forms of cancer more frequently present with malignancies that are multifocal (more than one tumor within the same organ) or bilateral (tumors that have occurred in both paired organs).

6. *Excess of multiple primary cancers*—Cancer survivors who have an inherited susceptibility to cancer are at substantially increased risks for developing subsequent malignancies. Individuals with a hereditary colon cancer syndrome, for example, are also at increased risk for developing extracolonic tumors.

7. *Presence of other nonmalignant features*—Certain hereditary cancer syndromes are also associated with benign tumors or other physical characteristics. Examples include multiple nevi in individuals with dysplastic nevus syndrome and multiple benign tumors and cysts in von Hippel-Lindau syndrome. There are also a few syndromes that are associated with congenital defects including CHRPE, a distinctive eye finding associated with familial adenomatous polyposis.

8. *Absence of environmental risk factors*—It is also important to consider potential environmental causes of tumors. This is especially true for cancers commonly associated with nongenetic risk factors, such as lung cancer. In addition, certain forms of cancer are associated with

preexisting medical conditions. Examples include lymphoma and Kaposi sarcoma in HIV-positive individuals, colon cancer in those with ulcerative colitis, and testicular cancer in men born with undescended testes. There are also certain malignancies with well-established risk factors such as lung cancer (tobacco) and stomach cancer (*H. pylori* infection). Some cancer survivors have increased risks of subsequent malignancies, because of the cancer treatments they have undergone. For example, women who had thyroid cancer treated with irradiation are at greater risk to develop breast cancer.

6.3.2. CLASSIFYING CANCER HISTORIES

Once the family history has been assessed, genetic counselors will determine whether the family is likely to have a hereditary form of cancer. There are various ways of classifying familial patterns of cancer; as described in this section.

The pattern of cancer in a family can be classified as one of the following:

1. *Hereditary form of cancer*—Families with a hereditary form of cancer typically have several of the features listed in Table 6-3 . This makes it more likely that the family has an underlying hereditary predisposition to cancer. Clients may be at risk for one or more types of cancer, which should be dictated by the parameters of the syndrome rather than the pattern of cancer in the client's family.

2. *Familial cluster of cancer*—Families with a few relatives who have developed similar or related forms of cancer may be designated as having a familial cluster of cancer. Specific cancers may appear to cluster in a family and may confer somewhat increased risks to close relatives. However, a cluster of cancer does not establish the presence of a known hereditary cancer syndrome or predictable inheritance pattern. Familial clustering of cancer is more likely caused by a combination of genetic and environmental effects.

3. *Cancers induced by carcinogen*—The pattern of cancer in the family is thought to be environmentally linked. Examples include occupational exposures or broad exposures to carcinogens, such as toxic well water or extensive nuclear radiation. Certain carcinogens are linked with specific forms of cancer. If several members of a family have similar exposures, then the cancers that occur may resemble a familial pattern. For example, multiple cases of liver cancer in a family might be due to hepatitis B exposures rather than an inherited predisposition.

4. *Sporadic form of cancer*—It is important to keep in mind that most cases of cancer do not have an obvious hereditary basis or link with carcinogens. Thus the cancer in the family may very well represent

sporadic cases, even if more than one family member has developed cancer. This is especially true if family members have developed commonly occurring cancers at standard ages.

6.3.3. CLASSIFYING FAMILIES AT LOW, MODERATE, HIGH, OR UNCERTAIN RISK

As cancer risk counselors, it may be most helpful to assess histories in terms of the likelihood that the family has a hereditary predisposition to cancer. Distinguishing between families that are at low, moderate, or high risk for having a hereditary cancer syndrome will be helpful in the subsequent risk assessment and follow-up recommendations (see Chapter 7, Section 7.3). Of course, in some cases, it will not be possible to interpret the history of cancer as presented. This section discusses four categories of risk: low, moderate, high, and uncertain. Please keep in mind that the definitions of risk listed in this section are provided as a general guide only and may differ from how others use these terms.

Based on the collection and interpretation of the cancer history information, the family can be categorized as one of the following:

1. *Family at low risk*—A family at low risk for having a hereditary cancer syndrome has a negative or noncontributory history of cancer. Figure 6-1 shows an example of a low-risk pedigree. Although there are several cases of cancer in the family, the cancer types are ones that frequently occur among older individuals. This pattern of cancer is therefore unlikely to be due to a common inherited factor.

   Features of low-risk families typically include the following:

   - few, if any, first- or second-degree relatives with cancer,
   - cancers that are not usually associated with a hereditary syndrome,
   - cancers that have occurred at typical ages,
   - cancers that occur commonly in the general population,
   - cancer that has occurred in only one generation, and
   - no unusual tumor characteristics or other physical findings.

2. *Family at moderate risk*—A family at moderate risk for having a hereditary predisposition has some features suggestive of a cancer syndrome. However, the family may not quite meet criteria for the syndrome or the family may have certain features that are inconsistent with the syndrome. As an example, see Figure 6-2. In this pedigree, the client has one feature (two small renal cysts) that could be associated with von Hippel-Lindau syndrome (VHL). Further tests revealed no other manifestations of VHL. Although the client's

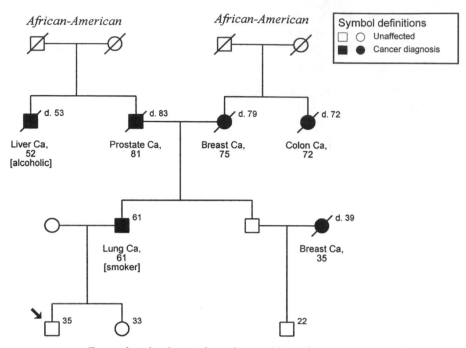

FIGURE 6-1. Example of a low-risk pedigree. Note the occurrences of common cancers at typical ages. Most affected individuals are over age 60. The one early-onset breast cancer case is not in a blood relative! See text for further explanation.

first-degree relatives demonstrate no signs of VHL, she does have a second-degree relative with renal cell carcinoma; a cardinal feature of VHL. This constellation of features does not meet diagnostic criteria for VHL (see Table 4-8). However, there is a small possibility that the family has VHL and thus, the client may wish to consider genetic testing for *VHL* mutations.

In the initial assessment of this family, the genetic counselor might compare the pedigree features that are suggestive of VHL with the features that are not.

Features in pedigree suggestive of VHL:

• client's two renal cysts
• uncle with renal cell carcinoma

Features not suggestive of VHL:

• client does not have other, more common, manifestations of VHL
• father (presumed obligate carrier) had no signs of VHL

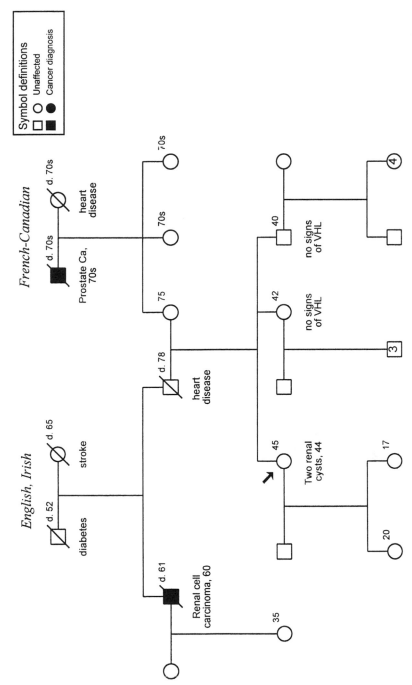

FIGURE 6-2. Example of a moderate-risk pedigree. Client's personal and family history have some features that are suggestive of von Hippel-Lindau syndrome (VHL) and others that are not. See text for explanation.

3. *Family at high risk*—The pedigree of a family at high risk shows strong evidence for having an inherited predisposition. The pattern of cancer in the family is consistent or highly suggestive of a specific hereditary cancer syndrome. See Figure 6-3 for a "textbook" example of a family with familial adenomatous polyposis (FAP). In this family, close family members should be counseled about their 50% risk of inheriting the predisposition to developing polyposis. Clients at high risk should be counseled that they meet criteria for a particular syndrome, even if genetic testing is not informative. In other words, regardless of the outcome of genetic testing, the client and/or family has the syndrome by clinical criteria.

4. *Family at uncertain risk*—Even the most skilled genetic counselor will not be able to provide a risk assessment for every client. As discussed previously in Section 6.2, some clients are better historians than others. There may be key information that is missing or there may be doubts about the accuracy of the verbal history given. In these cases, counselors should delay the assessment and interpretation of the family history until additional information and/or documentation has been obtained. If it is not possible to obtain further information, counselors can either say to clients that the pedigree is not interpretable or can offer the range of possible interpretations.

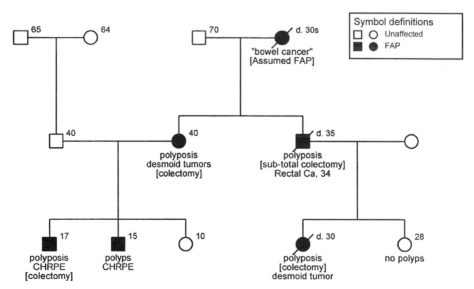

FIGURE 6-3. Example of a high-risk pedigree. This pattern of cancer is consistent with familial adenomatosis polyposis (FAP).

6.4. CASE EXAMPLES

Collecting and interpreting cancer histories present many challenges. The three case examples in this section illustrate some of these challenges.

6.4.1. CASE 1: HAVING A SYNDROME SEEMS A LOT WORSE

"I just want them off," stated Kelly emphatically, pointing to her breasts. Her recent needle biopsy, the third one in 5 years, had revealed benign changes but not cancer; however, 30 year old Kelly said she was tired of panicking every time she felt a lump. Her worries about breast cancer began in her teens, when she first learned about her significant family history of breast cancer. She had appointments with both the breast surgeon and program psychologist to discuss this option further.

The counselor briefly discussed the option of prophylactic mastectomy, then suggested they take a more comprehensive look at her family history of cancer. They began with Kelly's own medical history. Other than fibrocystic breast disease, Kelly said that she was in good health; her only vice was drinking one glass of red wine each evening. Kelly's mother and maternal aunt had been diagnosed with perimenopausal breast cancer. In addition, the aunt's daughter had developed ovarian cancer at the unusually young age of 29. To seemingly clinch the diagnosis of hereditary breast-ovarian cancer syndrome (BOCS), a maternal uncle had recently had a tumor removed from his breast. To be complete, the counselor also asked Kelly about the paternal side of her family, which was negative for cancer. The family was of French-Canadian descent.

The counselor pondered the initial pedigree (shown in Fig. 6-4) as she considered Kelly's risks of having an inherited susceptibility to breast cancer. The counselor considered the diagnoses of ovarian cancer and male breast cancer to be key features of the pedigree, since perimenopausal breast cancer among a pair of sisters was more likely to be sporadic rather than due to a germline *BRCA1* or *BRCA2* mutation. Because Kelly had not brought in any medical records, the counselor considered whether these two reported diagnoses were likely to be true. She started with the uncle's possible diagnosis of breast cancer.

"It would be helpful to find out whether your uncle really did have breast cancer or if he had some other type of tumor."

"I'm pretty sure it was breast cancer. I remember hearing about it from my mother. You know, I almost brought her with me today, because she keeps track of all this stuff. She was a nurse for 30 years so everyone tells her everything. Hey, I could call her." She pulled out a cell phone from her purse. "Would that be okay?"

At the counselor's assent, Kelly placed her call. "Hi, Ma. Look I'm at my appointment and I need to know if Uncle Billy had breast cancer. Oh, he

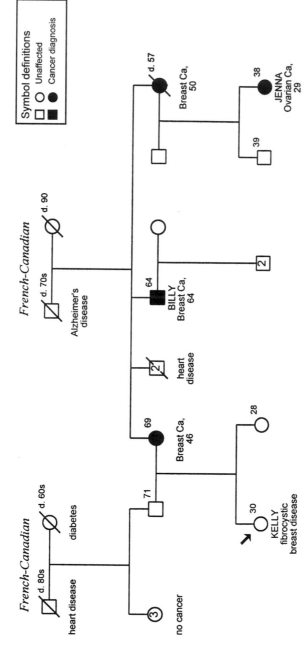

FIGURE 6-4. Kelly's initial pedigree. The undocumented pattern of cancer in this family is highly suggestive of hereditary breast and ovarian cancer.

didn't, then what did he have? Okay, thanks." Kelly hung up the phone and said somewhat sheepishly, "Well, I guess I was wrong about that. He had something removed from under his arm, but it was not cancer. My mother said it was a fatty tumor."

The counselor changed the information on the pedigree and asked whether her uncle had had other benign tumors.

"I don't think so." Kelly replied, but without conviction. "But I've had a few; do you need to know that? Right now I have one on my thigh and one on the back of my neck. My doctor says they aren't going to cause me any problems, so I don't need to have them taken out. I also had two small ones removed from my shoulder about 10 years ago. Oh and my mother has had a few removed as well—I remember one on her arm—but nothing that was cancer." From this information, the counselor began to consider the possibility that this family could have Cowden syndrome but decided to continue ruling out hereditary breast-ovarian cancer syndrome before mentioning it.

"It is also important to find out what type of ovarian cancer your cousin had. Some types of ovarian cancer are linked to breast cancer and are likely to be caused by an underlying inherited factor and other types are not."

Kelly said that she had no idea what type of ovarian cancer her cousin had, then pulled out her cell phone again. "Ma, do you know what type of cancer Jenna had? Yeah, I know it was ovarian, but what type? Okay, call me when you find out." Kelly turned back to the counselor, "She's going to call my cousin to find out. She should be able to get the answer. My mother is really good at tracking down this type of information."

The counselor then said she had a few more questions to ask Kelly about her own medical history. She began with, "Have you ever had thyroid cancer?"

"No, but did I mention that my mother did?" This time Kelly didn't even wait for the counselor's follow-up question; she immediately called her mother to find out what type of thyroid cancer she had. After hanging up, Kelly announced, "She said it was the follicular type. Does that make sense? She had radiation treatments for it. And she says to tell you that her grandmother (my great-grandmother) also had thyroid cancer. Oh, and she says that my Uncle Billy had a goiter about 10 years ago, I don't know if that's important or not."

The counselor added all of this information to the pedigree and continued, "Have you ever had any lesions removed from your face?"

"Yeah, I've always had terrible skin. It's like I never outgrew acne! My internist scraped off a few things from my face last year. He didn't even send them to the lab to be analyzed; he knew they weren't going to be cancer."

While the counselor was silently wishing that the lesions had been analyzed by a pathologist, she continued questioning Kelly, "Why do you say your skin is terrible?"

"Well, I've always had really dry skin. And whenever I get a cut, it doesn't heal right." Kelly showed the counselor a scar on the back of her hand that was raised and coarse. "You should see the terrible breast scars I have from all those biopsy procedures."

"Do you have any unusual bumps on your tongue?" Kelly nodded and said that her tongue was sort of strange looking, it had always been like that. At the counselor's request, Kelly stuck out her tongue and the counselor noticed the multiple papules and furrowed appearance.

At this point, Kelly was looking curiously at her. The counselor smiled and said, "I bet you're wondering why I'm asking all these questions that don't seem to have anything to do with breast cancer." When Kelly smiled back and nodded, the counselor explained that she was exploring the possibility that Kelly's family could have a specific breast cancer syndrome. She explained that a syndrome was a group of physical or medical problems that clustered together because of a common underlying genetic risk factor. She said that breast cancer was part of several different cancer syndromes and that it was important to sort out which syndrome, if any, her family had. This would help determine Kelly's risks of developing breast cancer. The shrill ringing of Kelly's cell phone interrupted the conversation. She answered the call and reported to the counselor that her cousin had had a borderline tumor of the right ovary. The ovary was removed and no further treatment was required.

The counselor explained that this type of ovarian tumor was less likely to be caused by a hereditary factor. She went on to say, "But there is one cancer syndrome that is associated with breast cancer, thyroid cancer, and noncancerous tumors. It is called Cowden syndrome. Most people have never heard of Cowden syndrome because it is so rare."

"You think I have this syndrome?" Kelly asked in surprise.

"I think it is a possibility. We have a physician here who specializes in genetics. I would like to ask him to evaluate you for signs of Cowden syndrome; would that be alright?" Kelly agreed to this evaluation, and the counselor excused herself to page the genetics fellow and the breast surgeon. Both agreed with this plan, and the genetics fellow corroborated that Kelly and her family probably met criteria for Cowden syndrome. Kelly was given a follow-up appointment with a dermatologist to have two facial lesions removed and analyzed; the diagnosis hinged on the pathology of the lesions.

Later that morning, Kelly met with both the breast surgeon and the psychologist to discuss prophylactic surgery (which suddenly seemed to be a less urgent issue). She returned in 2 weeks to meet with the dermatologist. The two lesions were trichillemmomas. Kelly also obtained her mother's medical records, confirming her diagnoses of follicular thyroid carcinoma and invasive ductal carcinoma of the breast as well as the several lipomas and facial papules she has had removed over the years. Thus, Kelly and her family did meet diagnostic criteria for Cowden syndrome. (Figure 6-5 shows

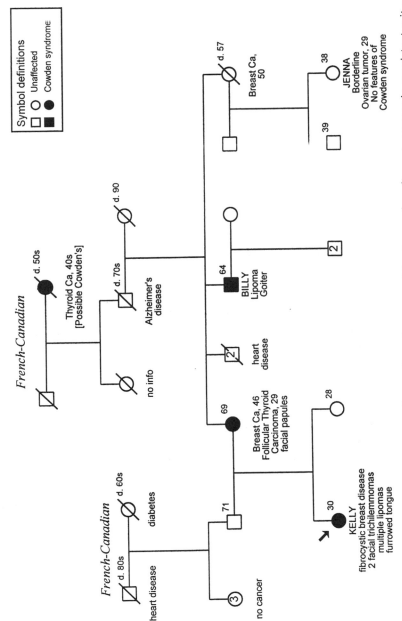

FIGURE 6-5. Kelly's final pedigree. The confirmed pattern of benign and malignant tumors is consistent with Cowden's syndrome.

the final pedigree). Kelly returned to meet with the genetic counselor and genetics fellow to discuss features of Cowden syndrome, the option of *PTEN* gene testing, and recommendations for medical monitoring, most importantly, thyroid function tests. In some ways, the issue of prophylactic surgery was less straightforward with the diagnosis of Cowden syndrome and Kelly is still considering whether to pursue surgery. It also took her a lot of time to adjust to the diagnosis. As Kelly explained it, "Somehow having a syndrome seems a lot worse than having a family history."

Key Points of Case:

1. Importance of asking about noncancerous features—see Section 6.1.1
2. Strategies for dealing with incomplete family history—see Section 6.2
3. Assessing features of pedigree suggestive of Cowden syndrome—see Section 6.3.1 and Chapter 4, entry 9

6.4.2. CASE 2: UNRAVELING FAMILY SECRETS

As the client and genetic counselor settled into chairs in the exam room, a loud pager went off. The counselor was relieved to realize that it was the client's pager, not his. As a first-year surgical resident, Gina Lu was undoubtedly overworked and sleep deprived but looked both alert and calm as she quickly dispatched the call. This was her first visit to the long-term survivor's clinic. She had been treated for a malignant liver tumor (hepatoblastoma) at the age of 2 and had completely recovered. In fact, she had not thought much about her cancer history until hearing a Grand Rounds presentation on the potential long-term effects of childhood cancer. The main purpose of her visit was to learn whether she was at increased risk for second malignancies or infertility, because of the treatments she had received.

Gina reported that two maternal relatives had been diagnosed with cancer as adults; one had lung cancer, the other had throat cancer. Both had been long-term smokers. Gina's mother was alive and well in her fifties, and Gina had one older brother and one younger half-brother, both of whom were fine. As far as she knew, there was no history of cancer on her father's side of the family. Gina's father had died from influenza complications at age 36, and her paternal grandmother had died in her fifties (see Fig. 6-6). Most of Gina's paternal relatives were still in Shanghai and she has had little contact with them since her mother's remarriage.

The counselor discussed the low likelihood that Gina could have a hereditary cancer syndrome based on this family history. There was certainly no reason to suspect that her childhood cancer was linked to the two adult-onset cancer diagnoses in the family. However, given the association of hepatoblastoma with familial adenomatous polyposis (FAP), the counselor felt that it was reasonable to ask Gina to obtain more information about her paternal relatives in order to rule out a possible inherited predisposition.

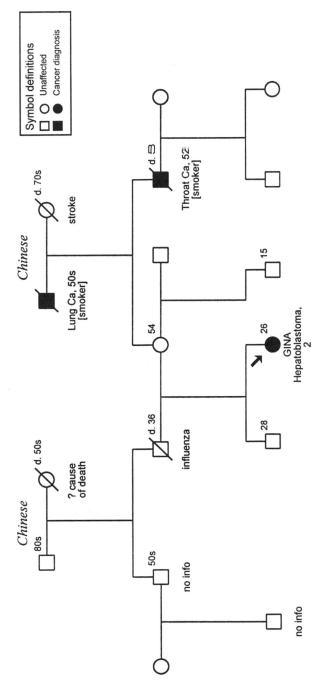

FIGURE 6-6. Gina's initial pedigree. Gina is a long-term survivor of childhood cancer who does not appear to have a contributing family history of cancer.

Therefore, the counselor explained the association between FAP and hepatoblastoma (while stressing that most cases of hepatoblastoma were sporadic) and requested that she obtain more information about her father's illness and the paternal side of her family.

They discussed ways of obtaining additional information about her paternal relatives. Gina said that her mother still became upset whenever her father's name was brought up and hesitated to ask her for more information. She did have contact information for her paternal uncle but felt awkward about contacting him out of the blue and asking potentially sensitive questions about his medical history. The counselor asked whether her older brother might have any additional information. Gina did not think so but thought she could enlist his help in gathering the information. He had spent a few years in Shanghai as an exchange student and had kept in closer contact with their uncle. The counselor also suggested that she try to obtain the medical records or death certificate for her father to confirm his cause of death. Gina agreed to do this and made a list of the requested information.

Gina went on to meet with the program nurse practitioner, radiation oncologist, and reproductive endocrinologist. She was given information about potential long-term problems from her radiation exposure. Gina denied any symptoms that could be indicative of colon cancer or other digestive tract problems. She underwent standard blood screening, thyroid function tests, and scheduled a one-time cardiac echocardiogram. She was reassured that, because she was having regular menses, she was likely fertile; a further fertility workup was discussed but not performed. Gina made plans to return annually to the long-term survivor's clinic.

The following year, Gina was scheduled to meet only with the nurse practitioner. During the appointment, the counselor was paged to join them. Gina explained that her older brother had recently visited their paternal uncle and had uncovered two additional diagnoses of cancer in her family— their paternal grandmother had died from stomach cancer and her grandmother's brother had died at age 30 from colon cancer. This history coupled with Gina's own cancer diagnosis created a pattern that was more worrisome. Rather than ruling out FAP, this new information (if true) actually strengthened the possibility.

The genetic counselor and nurse practitioner presented to Gina two possible strategies for resolving whether she had FAP. One strategy was to continue pursuing documentation of the family history. The other strategy was for her to undergo two screening tests: a sigmoidoscopy and a slit-lamp eye exam to look for signs of CHRPE, an eye finding associated with FAP. As a second-year surgical resident, Gina had even less free time than last year, but her brother promised to continue efforts to track down the information about their paternal relatives. The counselor stressed the importance of learning whether anyone (including her father) had ever been diagnosed with polyposis. Gina was less than enthusiastic about the prospect of undergoing a total colectomy but also expressed concerns about her physically demanding career path. Thankfully, the pathology from the polyps revealed no overt malignancy, and the procedure and reconstruction of an ileal pouch went smoothly. An upper endoscopy exam was negative. Gina took a short leave of absence from her residency program and moved back home so that her mother could care for her during her recovery period.

The genetic counselor revised the family pedigree (see Fig. 6-7) and continued to stay in touch with Gina at her follow-up appointments. Both Gina and her older brother, who had no signs of polyposis, eventually underwent *APC* gene testing. Interestingly, in follow-up conversations, Gina denied any anger toward her mother for keeping her father's diagnosis a secret, claiming that this course of action was understandable given the circumstances. The counselor was surprised by this shift in attitude but realized that Gina's need for her mother's help and support outweighed possible feelings of anger and betrayal—at least for the present.

Key Points of Case:

1. Importance of documentation—see Section 6.1.4

2. Strategies for dealing with incomplete family history—see Section 6.2.1 and 6.2.2

3. Assessing features of pedigree suggestive of familial adenomatous polyposis—see Section 6.3.1 and Chapter 4, entry 10

6.4.3. CASE 3: TRUTH IS STRANGER THAN FICTION

Leann arrived an hour late to her genetic counseling appointment, blaming it on the fierce rainstorm and heavy traffic. She removed her dripping wet coat and gratefully accepted a cup of coffee from the hospital volunteer. Although the counselor was less than pleased about the late clinic arrival, she could not help but like Leann, who turned out to be a very pleasant, albeit anxious, client. And given the history of breast cancer in her family, she had every right to be concerned!

As shown in Figure 6-8, four of Leann's maternal relatives had been diagnosed with breast cancer; two women had bilateral disease. The most recent diagnosis was in Leann's cousin who was only 30 years old. Leann and her sister, Marte, were both cancer free, but Marte had recently undergone a prophylactic mastectomy after receiving a positive *BRCA2* genetic test result. Leann said that Marte has been encouraging her to undergo surgery as well. Leann was still uncertain whether she would ever do this but thought it made sense to learn her genetic test results.

Leann and the counselor talked about the option of genetic testing. At that time, there were two options at the hospital—a research testing program and a clinical testing program. After listening to both options, Leann decided to enroll in the research testing program. The counselor explained that she

going a sigmoidoscopy but agreed to set up appointments with an
mologist and a gastroenterologist. She also agreed to recontact the c(
if her brother learned any additional information.

About a month later, Gina dropped by to report that her CHRF
had been negative and that her grandmother had not had cancer a
The tumor in her stomach had been a large, unresectable benign tum(
had scheduled a sigmoidoscopy exam but was hoping that with th
information she no longer needed it.

Although the negative eye exam was reassuring, the counsel
nurse practitioner explained that this finding did not reduce the pos
that her grandmother could have had FAP; benign tumors (desmoids
cardinal features of the variant form of FAP called Gardner syndrome
who had obviously read up on FAP, countered that, since FAP had vir
100% penetrance, her father's unaffected status reduced the likelihoo
this was the case even though he died at age 36. The counselor agree
tactfully reminded her that young children were not always told the d
about a parent's illness. As they began to discuss her father's illness,
to broke down into tears as she recalled how her father was sud(
whisked away to the hospital and died several days later. She said tha
had tried to remain detached and objective as she pursued obtainin;
death certificate (which had finally been requested) but confessed tha
was almost afraid to read it. She also seemed to feel that her actions
disrespectful to her mother, as though she were admitting that she did
trust what her mother had told her.

They discussed this issue in more depth and explored ways to help C
get through this process of discovery. They also talked about her moth
possible reaction if she learned that her children were seeking this infor
tion and what it would be like for Gina to learn that her mother had kno
about information but had not shared it. Gina, a medical professional hers
had a difficult time justifying why her mother would have hidden t
information from them and felt that this was unlikely to be the case. T
counselor also suggested that Gina might want to speak to the program ps
chologist about these issues. Gina seemed somewhat resistant to this id
until the counselor had the inspired idea of suggesting that her older broth
be included in these discussions. Gina agreed that it might be beneficial f(
the two of them to strategize about how best to approach their mother an
an appointment was set up.

Gina received her father's death certificate 2 days before her sigmoi
doscopy. The document listed "pneumonia" as the primary cause of deatl
and "colon polyposis" as the underlying cause. The only benefit to the timin;
of this report was that it prepared Gina—a little—for her sigmoidoscopy
exam, which revealed extensive polyposis. Gina's grief and anger regarding
her father's diagnosis were quickly overwhelmed by her feelings of fear and
shock regarding her own diagnosis. Not only was she fearful about under-

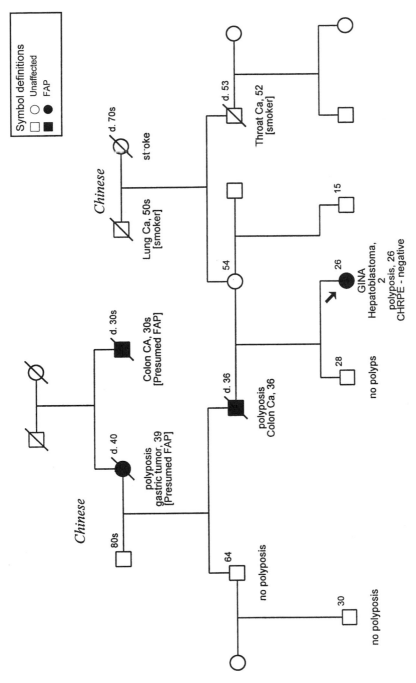

FIGURE 6-7. Gina's final pedigree. The confirmed pattern of benign and malignant tumors is consistent with familial adenomatous polyposis (FAP).

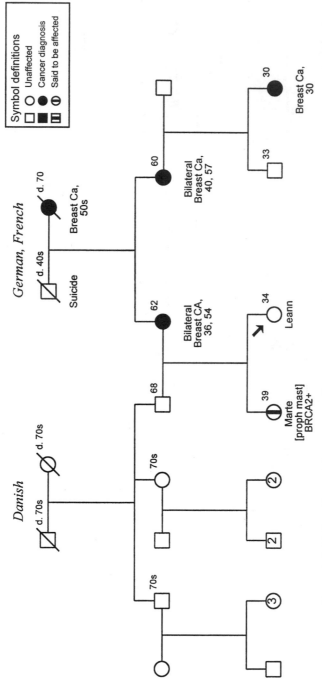

FIGURE 6-8. Leann's initial pedigree. The pattern of breast cancer in this family and positive *BRCA2* result are consistent with hereditary breast and ovarian cancer.

would need to obtain two pieces of documentation in order to be tested: a copy of the genetic test result and a pathology report of her mother's breast cancer diagnoses.

Leann hesitated, then said, "Getting the test result will be easy, I'll get that from my sister. But the pathology report might be a problem. My mother is really secretive about her breast cancer diagnosis. She doesn't like to talk about it, so I'm not sure I can get this from her."

The counselor assured her that, if it were easier, she could obtain the pathology report on another relative who has had breast cancer. She handed Leann her business card, which listed her phone number and her fax number.

A faxed copy of the aunt's breast cancer diagnosis arrived a few days later. The pathology report revealed ductal carcinoma in situ (DCIS) at age 57. There was no mention of an earlier breast cancer diagnosis. The counselor called Leann and got permission to speak to the aunt directly. The counselor called the aunt and began by thanking her for releasing the pathology report. The aunt confirmed that she was undergoing treatment for DCIS. When the counselor asked her whether she also had breast cancer many years ago, the aunt confided, "To tell you the truth, I didn't have breast cancer before. My breasts were always uncomfortably large, so I finally went in and had them reduced. But I was sort of embarrassed to tell anyone. It happened around the time my sister was diagnosed with breast cancer, so I guess everyone in the family thought I had it too." The counselor asked whether it would be okay to tell Leann that her aunt had not had bilateral breast cancer, but the aunt was reluctant to change her story at this date.

After discussing the situation with the other members of the testing team, the counselor called Leann and said that they would need a pathology report from one additional family member. Leann did not question why, and the counselor did not offer a further explanation. Leann felt that her cousin would be willing to release documentation of her breast cancer diagnosis and agreed to contact her. Leann called back the next day and asked if a breast cyst was the same thing as breast cancer, because that was what her cousin had been found to have. The counselor said the two were very different and that a cyst was not even considered precancerous.

Leann sighed as she realized she would need to try and obtain her mother's pathology report after all. Because Leann sounded so reluctant to approach her mother, the counselor told her that the program could waive this requirement if she truly felt that she could not obtain these records. But Leann said that she was willing to try and decided to ask her sister for some advice about how best to do this. The counselor also reminded her about the need for her sister's genetic test result.

Leann called back the following week and asked if her grandmother's pathology report would be acceptable. The counselor said this would be fine and agreed to send Leann a release form that she could send to her grandmother. The counselor subsequently received a call from the grandmother, who was puzzled about why the counselor thought she had had breast cancer. Leann's grandmother then recalled that she had had a "breast cancer scare" years earlier. In great detail, she described finding a lump and having it evaluated. Luckily, the breast biopsy had been negative. She then told several rambling stories about her other on-going health problems. After a fairly lengthy story about breast cancer—in a friend of hers—the counselor finally managed to redirect the conversation back to the purpose of the phone call. When the counselor asked if it was alright to tell her grand-daughter that she had not had breast cancer, she indignantly replied, "Certainly not. It isn't any of her business. If my family doesn't care enough to call me or come visit, why should I care about them?" She then slammed the phone down.

A week later, the counselor received a handwritten note from Marte stating that she had been found to have a *BRCA2* mutation. The counselor called Leann and told her that she appreciated receiving this note, but she really needed the actual laboratory DNA report in order to proceed. She reiterated that Leann could not undergo single-site analysis unless the laboratory knew the exact site of her sister's mutation. Leann promised to call her sister again.

The counselor then received a faxed note from Marte granting permission to obtain her result from her doctor's office. The counselor spoke with Marte's physician, who verbally confirmed the *BRCA2* result; however, he didn't have a copy of the test result on file. The physician said that Marte had been tested elsewhere and that, because of confidentiality concerns, she had preferred not to give him a copy of her results. He did confirm that she had undergone prophylactic mastectomies and faxed the normal pathology findings from the breast tissue.

As the counselor was pondering what to do next, her phone rang. It was Leann who stated that she had finally approached her mother about documenting her breast cancer and her mother had agreed to think about it. Leann was relieved that the conversation had gone smoothly and then added, "Marte says that you should have her test results already because she was tested through your program."

"Marte was tested through our program?" the counselor asked in surprise. As the only genetic counselor on staff, she usually recognized the names of the people who had undergone testing.

"She says that she participated in a research project about 3 years ago and provided all the records." There was a separate research project going on at the time, so the counselor concluded that was why her name did not sound familiar. The counselor promised to look up the test result but indicated that she would need Marte's consent to release the information. As the counselor hung up the phone, she was relieved at the thought that this case might actually be wrapped up soon. She then considered what she would do if she did not receive permission from Marte to release the test result. But, as it turns out, this was not a problem; she received a faxed permission statement from Marte late that afternoon. However, there was an even bigger problem—there was no evidence that Marte had ever been enrolled in this study let alone tested through it.

At the weekly meeting of the testing team, the counselor summarized her attempts to obtain documentation of the test result and cancer history so that Leann could be tested. The testing team discussed possible strategies if it turned out that Marte had never been tested. The team also agreed that the counselor needed to honor the requests from relatives that their medical history information remain private.

The counselor called Leann the next day and told her that she could not find any records that Marte was tested through their center. Leann was puzzled by this and said that she would ask her sister to call. She also said that her mother had agreed to release her medical records (which were at the hospital), as long as she didn't need to speak to anyone directly. The counselor agreed that she would not call her.

Upon receiving the mother's release form, the counselor ordered her medical record. According to the records, Leann's mother was diagnosed with lobular carcinoma at age 57, but there was no mention of the earlier diagnosis. However, there were several references to a previous diagnosis of lobular carcinoma in situ (LCIS). As the counselor leafed through the medical record, she also found mention that the woman's mother (Leann's grandmother) was an alcoholic, which suddenly put their somewhat erratic phone conversation into perspective. At least she now had confirmation of a breast cancer, although it looked as though it was the only breast cancer in the family! (See Figure 6-9 for the revised pedigree.)

When the counselor took Marte's phone call later that afternoon, she braced herself for a hostile or erratic encounter. However, Marte had a friendly manner and chuckled when told that the counselor could not identify her records. "I'm so sorry, I completely forgot that I was tested under a different name. At the time I came in, I was up for a promotion at work and was absolutely paranoid about confidentiality. So I used a fake name—try looking up the information under "Mary,"—that is the name I used. And I'd appreciate it if you didn't tell my sister about this—she already thinks I'm crazy!" The counselor agreed to keep this information private, although she felt like she was holding way too many secrets for this family already.

"Mary" had been evaluated by their cancer risk program about 4 years earlier. After reviewing her clinic file, the counselor did remember her as a very anxious client who became furious when told about the standard waiting period between when a prophylactic mastectomy was requested and when the procedure was actually performed. There was no mention that BRCA1 or BRCA2 testing had ever been performed.

After further discussions with the testing team, the counselor told Leann

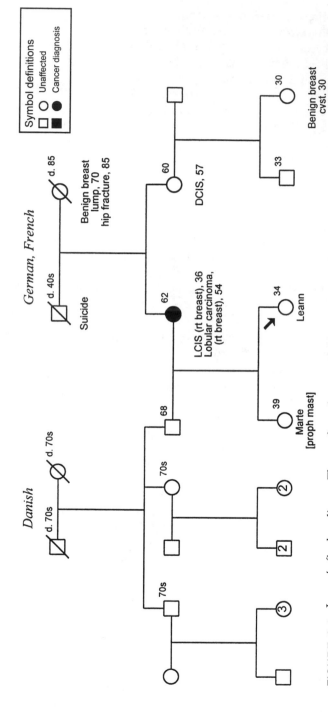

FIGURE 6-9. Leann's final pedigree. The confirmed pattern of breast cancer in this family is unlikely to represent an inherited form. Note that the positive *BRCA2* result turned out to be fabricated. LCIS = lobular carcinoma in situ; DCIS = ductal carcinoma in situ.

that it would not be possible to use Marte's prior research test result, there-fore, Leann would need to undergo full gene analysis if she wanted to pursue testing. She also explained that Leann was no longer eligible for the research program but could be tested clinically. Without disclosing specific informa-tion about her relatives' altered diagnoses, the counselor did explain that her likelihood of having a *BRCA1* or *BRCA2* mutation was much lower than initially estimated. Despite this, Leann elected to undergo full *BRCA1* and *BRCA2* gene analysis, and was relieved to learn that the test did not iden-tify a mutation. When Leann later confided that she did not plan to share this result with any of her relatives, the counselor was not surprised—the legacy of secrets in the family was continuing.

Key Points of Case:

1. Importance of confirming history—see Section 6.1.4

2. Strategies for dealing with incorrect family histories—see Sections 6.2.2 and 6.2.3

3. Revised history is less suggestive of breast-ovarian cancer syn-drome—see Sections 6.3.3 and Chapter 4, entry 8

6.5. REFERENCES

Adato, A. 1995. Living Legacy: knowing your medical family tree can save your life. LIFE magazine, April Issue, 60.

Bennett, R. 1999. The Practical Guide to the Genetic Family History. Wiley-Liss, New York, NY.

Bennett, R, Steinhaus, K, Uhrich, S et al. 1995. Recommendations for standardized human pedigree nomenclature. Am J Hum Genetics 56:745–752.

Claus, E, Risch, N, and Thompson, W. 1994. Autosomal dominant inheritance of early-onset breast cancer. Implications for risk prediction. Cancer 73:643–651.

Cummings, S and Olopade, O. 1998. Predisposition testing for inherited breast cancer. Oncology 12:1227–1242.

Eccles, D, Evans, D, and Mackay J. 2000. Guidelines for a genetic risk based approach to advising women with a family history of breast cancer. UK Cancer Family Study Group (UKCFSG). J Med Genet 37:203–209.

Foulkes, W and Hodgson S, (Eds.). 1998. Inherited Susceptibility to Cancer: Clinical, Predictive and Ethical Perspectives. Cambridge Univ. Press, Cambridge, UK.

Gray, J, Brain, K, Norman, P et al. 1999. A model protocol evaluating the introduc-tion of genetic assessment for women with a family history of cancer. J Med Genet 37:192–196.

Kelly, P. 2000. Just the facts, ma'am. In Assess Your True Risk of Breast Cancer. Owl Books, New York, NY.

Kerr, B, Foulkes, W, Cade, D et al. 1998. False family history in the family cancer clinic. Eur J Surg Oncol 24:275–279.

Offit, K and Brown, K. 1994. Quantitating familial cancer risk: a resource for clinical oncologist. J Clin Oncol 12:1724–1736.

Parent, M, Ghadirian, P, Lacroix, A et al. 1997. The reliability of recollections of family history: implications for the medical provider. J Cancer Education 12:114–120.

Peters, J and Stopfer, J. 1996. Role of the genetic counselor in familial cancer. Oncology 10:159–66, 175.

Schmidt, S, Becher, H, and Chang-Claude, J. 1998. Breast cancer risk assessment: use of complete pedigree information and the effect of misspecified ages at diagnosis of affected relatives. Hum Genet 102:348–356.

Schuette, J and Bennett, R. 1998. Lessons in history: obtaining the family history and constructing a pedigree. In A Guide to Genetic Counseling. Eds.: Baker DL, Schuette JL, and Uhlmann WR. Wiley-Liss, New York, NY, 27–54.

Sijmons, R, Boonstra, A, Reefhuis, J et al. 2000. Accuracy of family history of cancer: clinical genetic implications? Eur J Hum Genet 8:181–186.

Weil, J. 2000. The pedigree as a psychosocial instrument. In Psychosocial Genetic Counseling. Oxford Univ. Press, Oxford, UK, 102–105.

Westman, J, Hampel, H, and Bradley, T. 2000. Efficacy of a touchscreen computer based family cancer history questionnaire and subsequent cancer risk assessment. J Med Genet 37:354–360.

THE CANCER GENETIC COUNSELING SESSION

With cancer risk-assessment services, coupled with innovative cancer diagnostic and preventive services and research, we have the potential to make great strides in cancer prevention and control.

(Weitzel, 1999, pgs. 2491-2492)

Chapter 7 outlines the components of a cancer genetic counseling session, starting with the logistics of setting up a high-risk clinic. Also included in this chapter are risk assessment discussions for clients at high, moderate, low, or uncertain risk; descriptions of various client populations; and three case examples.

7.1. LOGISTICS

Setting-up a high-risk cancer program requires a team of providers and the resolution of many logistical issues, including time and space allotments, billing policies, scheduling protocols, and case review procedures.

7.1.1. THE TEAM OF PROVIDERS

High-risk cancer programs typically involve a multidisciplinary team of providers. These providers have different roles in the care of clients at high risk for cancer but also need to work closely together. It is also important to develop a referral network for clients who need to meet with additional specialists. These specialists may be located at the same medical center or based elsewhere in the community.

Personnel in a high-risk cancer program include the following:

1. *Genetic counselor*—Most genetic counselors have masters degrees in genetic counseling and are certified by the American Board of Genetic Counseling. The educational training of genetic counselors encompasses a strong foundation in molecular and clinical genetics as well as counseling skills, a necessary cadre of knowledge for providing cancer counseling. Genetic counselors will collect a comprehensive family history, conduct the risk assessment, and arrange genetic testing. In some programs, the genetic counselor will be the primary genetics specialist and will thus be responsible for researching and describing the features of hereditary cancer syndromes. Because counselors typically have the most contact with clients, another important role will be to act as a liaison between the client, DNA laboratories, and other health care providers.

2. *Oncologist*—Oncologists are the primary caregivers for individuals with cancer and will often provide care to at-risk relatives as well. The role of the oncologist in a high-risk cancer program is to offer medical management recommendations tailored to the client's situation. For example, a woman with a *BRCA1* mutation is usually not a candidate to take hormone replacement therapy, but, if she has a strong family history of heart disease, this recommendation might be tailored to her particular situation.

3. *Geneticist*—In some programs, the director of the high-risk clinical program is a geneticist rather than an oncologist. In other programs, geneticists are called upon as needed, such as when the diagnosis of a cancer syndrome requires a specialized physical examination or review of tests. If there is no appropriate geneticist on staff, counselors should establish a way to refer patients to a geneticist at another local hospital.

4. *Advanced practice nurse*— Nurses have long had an important educational role in caring for patients and can either work side-by-side with genetic counselors or in other, related roles in the high-risk clinical program. A nurse with advanced genetics training may collect family history information and provide risk assessments in a role similar to that of genetic counselors. Alternatively, the nurse may focus on the medical responsibilities, such as taking personal medical histories or conducting physical examinations.

5. *Mental health provider*—Mental health providers include psychologists, social workers, family therapists, and psychiatrists. Mental health providers are valuable members of a high-risk clinic or predisposition testing program and can help in the management of difficult cases. Most medical centers have psychologists or social workers on staff who can be asked to participate in the care of high-

risk families. If there is no one appropriate on staff, another option is to connect with someone in private practice or at another local medial center.

6. *Other physician specialist(s)*—Some high-risk programs have additional medical specialists as part of the team of providers. In a high-risk program, this can include a breast surgeon, gynecological oncologist, radiologist, gastroenterologist, or dermatologist. In a long-term survivor's clinic, the team of providers can include an endocrinologist, radiation oncologist, fertility specialist, neurologist, and cardiologist.

7. *Administrative support staff*—In any clinical endeavor, there needs to be at least one person dedicated to scheduling appointments and making arrangements for the impending visit (registration, parking, and so forth). This individual can also remind clients about the importance of obtaining medical records documentation and bringing in certain tests or slides for review. Although in some centers this may be the genetic counselor's role, larger centers usually have one or two administrative personnel to handle scheduling issues.

7.1.2. TIME AND SPACE

Having sufficient time and space to provide quality cancer genetic counseling can be among the two greatest challenges facing providers.

1. *Time involvement*—Initial cancer counseling sessions can take 1–3 hours, which may greatly exceed the amount of time usually allotted for oncology appointments or general genetic counseling sessions. Having this block of time is important to review the pattern of cancer in the family and accurately identify a hereditary cancer syndrome and provide cancer risk assessment and follow-up. Strategies to help shorten the appointment time include collecting the pedigree and medical records documentation before the visit.

    Follow-up appointments are the rule rather than the exception and can serve several purposes: to clarify and review information given in the initial session, update new family history information, discuss new or changed screening recommendations, and arrange for genetic testing. With the exception of genetic testing visits (discussed at length in Chapter 9), follow-up meetings are typically shorter, from 30 to 60 minutes.

2. *Space allotment*—Although clients can be counseled in an exam room, a consult room that looks less "medical" is preferable. Ideally, the available clinic space will include both consult and exam rooms as well as a private workspace to discuss cases and perform dictations. In reality, clinical programs must make do with the space they are

given—as long as it consists of an office or room in which the client can be given full attention and privacy. Hallways, patient waiting rooms, or even modules are not appropriate settings for genetic counseling encounters.

7.1.3. BILLING ISSUES

Methods of billing vary from program to program. Some high-risk programs bundle the clinical charges so that clients are charged one flat fee rather than charged separately for each provider seen. In other programs, the genetic counselor will bill separately, often under the physician's name. Unfortunately, genetic counseling services are reimbursed less consistently than other medical interventions. For this reason, some high-risk programs have elected not to charge for genetic counseling services, relying instead on departmental or grant support.

In the United States, standardized codes are used for billing. Because there is currently no specific billing code for genetic counseling, programs must rely on codes that come closest to fitting the intervention. For more specific information about reimbursement of genetic services, an excellent resource is available through the American College of Medical Genetics (Greenstein, 2000).

Billing codes are based on three variables:

1. *Type of visit*—The encounter will be categorized as either an initial visit or a follow-up visit.
2. *Complexity*—Visits are further categorized by their complexity, ranging from low to high complexity.
3. *Time*—This refers to the time spent providing in-person counseling, excluding the time spent collecting the personal or family history. Because the majority of genetic counselors do not have the opportunity to be licensed, it may be possible to bill only for the time the physician was physically present for the counseling session.

7.1.4. SCHEDULING AN APPOINTMENT

Once the program begins to grow, it is important to develop a standardized method for scheduling appointments. In doing this, the following questions should be answered:

1. *Who makes the appointments?*—It is useful to have one central phone number that clients can use to make appointments. Clients will also feel more comfortable calling the clinic if they know with whom they will be speaking. Having multiple ways to make an appointment may

be appreciated by potential clients, but this can lead to client and/or staff confusion.

2. *What is the referral process?*—Some programs accept self-referrals, whereas others prefer to have a referral from a physician. In some cases, the client's insurance plan will require a referral by the primary care provider.

3. *Who is eligible to attend the clinic?*—The clinic may agree to see anyone who is interested in making an appointment or may require that clients have significant family histories of cancer. When the program is initially set up, it may be wise to make appointments with the majority of people who call as a way of encouraging referrals. However, as time passes and clinic appointments become more in demand, it will probably become necessary to set some minimum criteria.

4. *What medical records documentation is required?*—Ideally, clients will provide complete medical records documentation on each of their relatives who has had cancer. Of course, in the real world, this rarely happens. Clients may bring documentation of a single affected relative, if they bring in any. Clients who have had cancer themselves may not even bring in documentation of their own cancer diagnosis. Programs should decide as a matter of policy what documentation will be required for the visit. For example, it seems reasonable to require that clients minimally bring documentation of their own cancer diagnoses and/or documentation of all affected first-degree relatives. The documentation requirements may differ, depending on which cancer syndrome is being considered. Clients with family histories of breast cancer probably require less documentation than clients with histories of colon polyps or other abdominal malignancies. If the requested documentation is not available, programs can either delay the initial visit or require a second visit when the documentation is available. Clients should also be made aware that the accurate interpretation of the family history may require documentation beyond first-degree relatives. In the absence of medical records documentation, counselors should include the caveat that the subsequent risk assessment is based on verbal information only.

5. *What should be sent to clients before their appointments?*—Clients should routinely be sent letters with details about the appointment, including the appointment time, clinic location, approximate length of session, and instructions for registration and parking. It may also be helpful to remind clients to bring documentation of the cancer history and to provide a brief description of the genetic counseling session to give prospective clients a clearer idea of what to expect from the encounter. Reminder phone calls to clients 1 or 2 days before their

appointments helps reduce the number of "no shows" to the clinic but is a time-consuming practice.

7.1.5. CASE REVIEW

To ensure quality care, counselors should routinely review cases with others. Case review can take different forms as outlined below.

1. *Case review conference*—High-risk clinic programs often hold a pre-clinic case conference to consider the client's risk calculations based on the preliminary pedigree and to formulate an outline of topics that should be discussed during the session. Programs also typically hold a conference to review cases seen that day or week. The post-clinic case review conference is an opportunity to discuss the complexities of each case and decide on appropriate follow-up. It also provides an opportunity to educate team members about each other's areas of expertise and allows team members the opportunity to discuss and formulate program policies.

2. *Genetic counseling colleagues*—Working with clients who may be at risk for a hereditary cancer syndrome can cause challenging diagnostic or counseling dilemmas. Counselors who work in isolation or with a small group of providers may find it useful to gather feedback from cancer genetic counselors in the broader genetic counseling community. One useful resource for members of the National Society of Genetic Counselors (NSGC) is the Cancer Risk Counseling Special Interest Group, which has an active e-mail list serve.

3. *Medical and mental health providers*—Some challenging cases may require input from colleagues in related fields, such as medical specialists, laboratory researchers, or mental health providers. Members of your clinical team may be able to help identify such resources. Another option is to contact other cancer genetic counselors who may have suggestions or links with needed specialists.

4. *Formal consult*—Hospitals often have forums for formal or informal consults. This type of consult may involve making a presentation to a panel of experts or may simply provide an opportunity for a round-table discussion. Tumor conferences can provide a way to discuss and resolve dilemmas about diagnosis or treatment. The genetics information may be an important factor in this discussion. Other conferences are set-up to discuss ethical or mental health issues raised by the case. Most of these conferences do not result in binding recommendations, although some do provide a written summary of comments.

TABLE 7-1. MAJOR COMPONENTS OF A CANCER GENETIC COUNSELING SESSION

Contracting
Collecting personal and family medical history
Interpreting pattern of cancer in family
Describing features of cancer syndrome
Providing cancer risk assessment
Suggesting early detection and prevention strategies
Discussing genetic testing options

7.2. ELEMENTS OF THE COUNSELING SESSION

Education is mainly a process of providing information in a manner which is accessible to the counselee. Counseling is an interactive process which incorporates past and immediate psychosocial issues into the process of information transfer. . . . We feel that it is important to distinguish the need for genetic education from the need for counseling and to provide for both needs.

(Baty B al., 1997)

The major components of a cancer genetic counseling session consists of the following: contracting; collecting and interpreting the family history; describing features of a cancer syndrome; providing a risk assessment, discussing cancer monitoring, and describing genetic testing options (see Table 7-1). This section details each of these cancer genetic counseling topics. As you read through this section, consider the words of two experienced cancer genetic counselors, which are provided in Table 7-2. Refer also to Section 8.2.2 for suggestions of counseling techniques to use during the session.

7.2.1. CONTRACTING

The first few minutes of a cancer genetic counseling session set the stage for the ensuing discussion. Contracting is the merging of counselor and client expectations of the session. Counselors will need to do the following:

1. *Listen to the client's goals*—Client goals can include learning their risks of cancer based on family history, starting the genetic testing process, maximizing prevention strategies, and gaining answers about specific medical issues (for example, hormone replacement therapy). Client and counselor goals should match, but this does not always occur. Counselors should be careful not to assume that they know what the client most hopes to gain from the session. While some clients are interested in finding out whether their family could have an inherited predisposition to cancer, others will be more interested in learning about appropriate monitoring or possible prevention strategies.

TABLE 7-2. HELPFUL SUGGESTIONS FROM TWO CANCER COUNSELORS

Suggestions from June Peters, MS[1]	Suggestions from Beth Peshkin, MS[2]
To triage the patient appropriately, learn whether the issues are genetic, medical, psychosocial, educational, or epidemiological. Often multiple referrals are required.	Recognize factors that may influence a patient's perception of risk, such as cause of cancer, life experiences with cancer, level of optimism and control, and educational level.
The prudent counselor should be reluctant to provide risk estimates without first obtaining confirmation of diagnoses.	Compare risk with baseline risk of getting the disease and with actuarial risk of other events; mention limitations/exceptions to data presented.
Clustering of sporadic and environmentally induced cases can mimic genetic inheritance patterns.	Usually, patients' precounseling perception of risk is higher than the realistic risk, so patients are often reasured especially when we say risk rarely exceeds 50%.
Empirical risk estimates are only available for certain [hereditary] cancer families.	Flip risks around to emphasize risks that patient won't develop cancer.
	Age-specific or lifetime cumulative risks are more helpful than relative risks.

Source: [1] Peters, 1992. [2] Peshkin, Personal Communication, 1993.

Sometimes, clients have agendas that differ from their stated goals. A skilled genetic counselor should be able to elicit these underlying goals during the ensuing discussion.

2. *Communicate the counselor's goals*—This is generally an educational or information-oriented goal, such as "we will review your family history to determine whether there could be a hereditary component to the cancer in your family" or "I will describe the pros and cons of genetic testing so you can decide whether this is something you would like to do." The counselor can also indicate whether these goals are likely to be reached during the session or whether additional sessions might be needed. For example, some centers allow clients to proceed with genetic testing on the day of their initial visit, whereas other centers require one or more separate visits.

3. *Outline the clinic visit*—It is helpful for clients to know what to expect during the entire high-risk clinic visit. Outlining the clinic visit can include reminding clients of the providers with whom they will be meeting and mentioning the general topics that each provider will discuss. This sets the boundaries for what will be covered by the

genetic counselor and gives clients an opportunity to mention additional topics they would like covered in the visit.

4. *Assess the underlying motivators*—It is also useful to determine the motivation for the client's visit. It may be that the client's physician made the referral or that the client has decided it is time to gather more information. Other motivators include a new cancer diagnosis or death in the family. A few clients may be experiencing worrisome symptoms and find it less frightening to meet with a genetic counselor than their physician. (Obviously, such patients need to be told that this appointment does not negate the need to be seen by their physician!)

5. *Set the tone*—A final purpose of contracting is to help put the client at ease. Helpful ways to do this include making sure the client is comfortably seated, opening the session with a few minutes of small talk, and using a soothing voice. Clients need to feel that it is safe to discuss their personal and family histories and that the counselor will carefully listen to them.

7.2.2. COLLECTING AND INTERPRETING THE FAMILY HISTORY

Risk assessment and follow-up recommendations will depend on the pattern of cancer in the client's family. This section provides a brief description of collecting and interpreting family history information (refer to Chapter 6 for more specific information).

1. *Collection of the family history*—Some high-risk programs request the family history information before the counseling session. This can be accomplished with a mailed questionnaire or an intake telephone call. Having the information before the visit can help with case preparation. However, it is important to review the family history during the session as additional information might be revealed that will lead to altered histories (and greatly altered discussions!).

2. *Interpretation of the family history*—Diagnosis of certain rare cancer syndromes may require specialized examinations or diagnostic tests. In these cases, the genetic counselor can discuss the possible diagnoses and the importance of these tests. Sometimes, the diagnosis of a hereditary cancer syndrome is based solely on the pattern of cancer in the family. In these cases, the counselor may feel comfortable sharing the interpretation of the family history directly with the client. If the client is not expecting such a diagnosis, it may be better to gently suggest the possibility and then resume the discussion with the physician present or at a later visit.

7.2.3. DESCRIBING SPECIFIC INHERITED DISORDERS

This section concentrates on how to best present information about inherited cancer disorders. These strategies are particularly important in discussing cancer disorders but may also be useful in other genetic counseling situations. When describing specific inherited forms of cancer, it is helpful to

1. *Start with what the client knows*—Clients will vary in terms of familiarity with cancer terminology and details about specific cancer syndromes. Some have long been aware that the cancers in their families are hereditary, whereas others may be shocked to learn this news. In addition to assessing the extent of the client's knowledge about the cancer syndrome, it is also useful to determine the reliability of their information.

2. *Pay attention to family folklore*—For every case of cancer within a family, there may be a story that attempts to explain why the tumor developed. These explanations can range from exposure to chemicals to eating the wrong types of food. By addressing these stories (rather than simply dismissing them), clients are more likely to listen to the counselor's "story" that the malignancies may be due to an underlying inherited component.

3. *Describe the name and features of the cancer syndrome*—The discussion about the syndrome should begin with naming it. This includes providing correct pronunciation and spelling of the syndrome, as well as its standard abbreviation (for example, MEN 2B for multiple endocrine neoplasia syndrome, type 2B). Explaining how the syndrome was given its name may make the term seem less intimidating. Descriptions of the cancer syndrome should include specific tumors associated with the syndrome, typical ages of onset, mode of inheritance, and other features (such as bilaterality) particular to the syndrome. All medical terminology needs to be simplified and defined, and the discussion needs to be adapted to each client's educational level and amount of detail he or she is ready to hear. In some hereditary cancer syndromes, like von Hippel-Lindau syndrome, benign tumors are the most common feature, which may make it important to describe the differences between benign and malignant tumors. Exploring reactions to the words "cancer" and "syndrome" may also be appropriate.

4. *Discuss certainty of diagnosis*—In certain cases, the diagnosis of an inherited cancer syndrome is unequivocal. However, more typically, there will be a certain level of uncertainty that needs to be addressed. Counselors should describe those features that are consistent and inconsistent with the syndrome. If the family history raises the possibility of more than one cancer syndrome, each should be described.

It is optimal to wait until the family history has been completely documented before providing a risk assessment and follow-up recommendations, however, this is not always feasible.

5. *Consider emotional impact of discussion*—Clients may come to the genetic counseling session fully prepared to hear about a particular cancer syndrome. Others may be surprised and even shocked to learn about a possible hereditary link. Clients may be alarmed that their cancer history is being taken so seriously or annoyed that they are considered "low risk" despite the history of cancer. Any of these emotions can influence how the client reacts to the discussion.

7.2.4. RISK ASSESSMENT

Two patient perspectives on the use of numerical risks:
  Well, I have an analytical mind and I like to know [my numerical risks] so that I can go and think about it and decide what I am going to do based on it."
  ...I am not sure that percentages are the best way really. I mean its perhaps too black and white.... I'm not that keen on figures. I think words are kinder.

(Hallowell, et al., 1997, p. 279)

In general, people have a difficult time comprehending risk estimates. This makes the discussion about cancer risks, with its inherent uncertainties, especially challenging.

Before sharing risk estimates with clients, it is important to ascertain the accuracy and source of the available risk information. Risk estimates associated with cancer syndromes that are rare or newly described may be greatly overinflated (because it is the most striking families that are written up in case reports) and/or based on a very small series of cases. Over time, the cancer risks associated with a particular cancer syndrome may change. The wise counselor, therefore, always qualifies any risk figures given.

Provided that numerical risk estimates do exist for the syndrome under discussion, counselors then have to decide how best to describe these figures. Concepts of probability are a source of confusion to many clients. Certain statistics like 50/50, zero, and 100% are easy to convey because people tend to understand "all or nothing" situations. Unfortunately, the statistics used in clinical cancer genetics are rarely this straightforward—hence the need for so many different ways to describe risk. Counselors can present risk statistics in a variety of ways, including percentages, odds, and ranges (see Table 7-3). Keep in mind that a single approach will not work with every client and some clients will benefit from having the information presented in more than one format.

General strategies for presenting risk estimates include the following:

TABLE 7-3. DIFFERENT WAYS IN WHICH TO DESCRIBE CANCER RISK
ESTIMATES

Category	Name	Description
Numerical descriptions	Gambling odds	The odds are 12 to 1 that you will not develop colon cancer.
	Percentage	You have a 30% chance of developing colon cancer.
	Proportion	You have a 1 in 10 chance of developing colon cancer.
	Range	You have a 10–20% chance of developing colon cancer.
Word descriptions	Relative risk	Your risk of colon cancer is 3 times higher than the average person.
	Analogy	To understand your risk of colon cancer, think about flipping a coin 10 times—9 times it will come up heads (no cancer) and once it will come up tails (cancer).
	Comparison	Your risk of developing colon cancer is higher than the average person.
	General description	You are at high risk of developing colon cancer.

Source: Hallowell et al., 1997, p. 280.

1. *Ask clients what they perceive their risks to be*—This will let counselors know whether clients are gauging the risks correctly or whether they are vastly overestimating or underestimating the risks. Counselors can also explore why clients feel they are at such increased or decreased risk.

2. *Provide absolute risks rather than relative risks*—Although textbooks are fond of using relative risks, these can provide the wrong impression. To state that one has a 200-fold increased relative risk of a certain cancer might translate into an absolute risk below 10%. The former statistic is certainly more dramatic, which is why it shows up in media reports, but may be alarming and misleading to use with clients.

3. *Utilize a range of risks*—Sometimes using a single number makes it appear as though this is the absolute truth, when in fact this is seldom the case. Using a range of risks may be the safer approach, especially if published statistics are not firm.

4. *Use of numerical risks*—Most genetic counselors would agree that clients should at least be given the option of hearing published numerical risk estimates. Keep in mind that some clients will not intuitively know that 1 in 50 and 2% are the same figure. And keep in mind that continued questions about statistical minutia might be masking the client's underlying feelings of fear or helplessness. Exploring these underlying feelings may be the better counseling strategy.

5. *Describe risks in two or three different ways*—Describing the risk figures in a few different ways increases the likelihood that the client will understand the risks in a meaningful way. Sometimes it is useful to compare the risks of developing cancer with other risks that are familiar. It may be tempting to rattle off the statistics in multiple different ways, but this may be even more confusing to clients. Better to state the risk estimate in a certain way and ascertain if the client comprehends it. If in doubt, try stating the risk in a different way.

6. *Find ways to illustrate concepts of risk*—The use of visual aids to illustrate probability concepts is helpful. Suggestions include the use of drawings or even different colored marbles in a jar. Analogies can also be useful. These can include stories about flipping a coin or pulling a green sock out of a drawer full of white socks.

7. *Pay attention to how the client perceives the risks*—One problem with providing numerical risks is that different clients will interpret the same numbers differently. This phenomenon is termed risk perception. For example, some clients given a 10% risk of cancer will feel optimistic about this low risk, whereas others will consider a 10% risk to be alarmingly high. The factors that influence clients' risk perception include their previous life experiences, their coping styles, and the nature of the perceived threat. A client's perception of risk represents a subjective and personal viewpoint, not a wrong answer that needs correction.

8. *Learn how the client wants the information presented*—Matching client preferences is what is most important. Clients who are not mathematically savvy may become overwhelmed or confused if presented an array of numbers. Conversely, clients who are seeking such figures will become increasingly frustrated with and even suspicious of counselors who avoid the use of hard data. However, it is not always easy to discern what the client prefers. Even asking clients for their preferences is not a guarantee; clients may not know or they may give you the answer they think you want to hear. (The public is well aware of the medical profession's eagerness to quote numerical statistics!)

7.2.5. CANCER MONITORING

> For counselors the central issue in counseling is to provide the individual with
> an estimation of risk, while for the counselee it is what to do about a risk they
> already perceive to be high.
>
> (Kelly, 2000, p. 173)

The purpose of early detection strategies is to find signs of cancer at earlier
and potentially more curable stages. Many, but not all, clients in high-risk
cancer families are familiar with the recommended early detection strategies.
Early detection strategies include educating people about appropriate
medical screening procedures and educating them about possible warning
signs of cancer. (Refer to Chapter 2 for more information about monitoring
for breast, colon, or ovarian cancer.)

Early detection procedures include standard screening tests (like mammograms), which may be initiated at earlier ages and more frequent intervals, as well as unusual screening procedures (like MRIs) targeted at those
considered to be high risk. Clients need to be informed that none of the
screening tests is 100% effective in detecting tumors at early stages.

Before meeting with clients, genetic counselors will want to become
familiar with standard monitoring recommendations. This can be done by
checking with the oncologists within their hospital and reading published
studies on particular cancer syndromes. To obtain general information about
cancer surveillance, counselors may want to contact the American Cancer
Society or National Cancer Institute. Counselors may also prefer to keep discussions general and tell clients to check with their personal physicians for
specific recommendations.

Some clients are extremely conscientious about following guidelines;
others seem to decline or delay initial or important follow-up screening tests.
In addition to discussing screening options, counselors may wish to explore
what might be keeping an individual from following a particular recommendation. Some of the common reasons why people may not follow
through with screening recommendations are described below.

1. *Cost*—Specific monitoring tests can range from fairly inexpensive
   blood tests to costly sophisticated imaging techniques. Although
   certain monitoring tests are covered by insurance, this is not always
   the case, particularly if the test has not been proven to be beneficial.

2. *Fear*—Feelings of fear and anxiety play major roles in why people do
   not always follow recommended monitoring guidelines. These monitoring tests are looking for signs of cancer—something the average
   person would rather not find. Scheduling and undergoing monitoring tests forces people to face the possibility that cancer might be
   detected. In addition, clients may not be ready to admit to themselves
   that they are at risk for developing cancer. Clients may also avoid

scheduling such tests in order to keep other family members from worrying excessively.

3. *Lack of information*—High-risk individuals may not be aware of the appropriate monitoring tests; given how quickly the field changes, their physicians may not be aware of them either. Some individuals may be aware of the recommended screening but are not sure how to arrange the tests. For individuals with hereditary cancer syndromes that can affect multiple organ systems, such as von Hippel-Lindau syndrome or neurofibromatosis, it can be difficult to find one provider who feels comfortable managing all aspects of the disorder.

4. *Access*—Clients might have different degrees of access to monitoring programs. They may face vast geographic distances, transportation problems, insurance difficulties, and even language barriers. In addition to discussing recommended monitoring, counselors should also ascertain whether there are any potential problems with access. Hospitals often have social workers or patient advocates who can help resolve these types of problems.

7.2.6. OPTION OF GENETIC TESTING

Some clients will be given the option of genetic testing. Initial discussions about genetic testing can include

1. *Appropriateness of testing*—Counselors should describe the available genetic tests and indicate their appropriateness given the pattern of cancer in the family. If it is appropriate for the family to pursue genetic testing, then the next step is to determine whether the client is the best family member to initially test. If not, then it may be necessary to discuss the involvement of other relatives in the testing process.

2. *Determine client's interest in testing*—Some clients will express immediate interest in testing, whereas others will make it clear that this is not something they wish to pursue. All clients should be told of the availability of genetic testing, but the discussion can be brief if the client is not interested. Clients should never be made to feel they are being coerced into testing. However, counselors may wish to explore potential barriers to being tested. It may turn out that a high risk client does want to be tested, but is reluctant to involve his affected sister into the process. The counselor and client in this situation can consider testing strategies that would not necessitate his sister's involvement.

3. *Describe potential results*—As a way of helping clients decide whether they want to pursue genetic testing, counselors should describe the

possible results and the interpretation of these results. This often includes the limitations of the results and possibility of nondefinitive results.

4. *Provide information about testing process*—For clients interested in genetic testing, counselors should explain the testing protocol at their institution and clearly delineate the next steps of the testing process. This includes the informed consent procedures, fees, how much blood is needed for the test, which laboratory will perform the analysis, and the manner in which results are given. If this is a research testing program, clients need to be made aware of alternative ways in which they can be tested.

7.3. COUNSELING CLIENTS AT LOW, MODERATE, OR HIGH RISK

[My daughter's] odds are either fantastic, because they can't all have it, or they're terrible, because [her mother and grandmother] both had it.
>   *(Baker, 1991, p. 188, quote from man whose wife and mother-in-law*
>   *both died of breast cancer)*

On the basis of the patterns of cancer in their families, clients will be counseled about the likelihood of having a hereditary cancer syndrome. Clients can be broadly categorized as being at low risk, moderate risk, or high risk. In some cases, it is not possible to determine whether the family has an inherited predisposition to cancer so the level of risk remains uncertain (refer to Chapter 6 for a more detailed explanation of these risk categories). As this section demonstrates, discussions of risk and medical management vary for clients assessed to be at low, moderate, high, or uncertain risk. Please keep in mind that the definitions of risk listed in this section are provided as a general guide only and may differ from how others use these terms.

7.3.1. CANCER RISK ASSESSMENT—LOW RISK

Clients at low risk for having a hereditary cancer syndrome may be quite relieved to learn that, in fact, their risks of cancer are not as high as expected. Although the main focus of a clinical program is to identify clients at high risk, providing reassurance to individuals at low risk also serves an important purpose.

1. *Likelihood of cancer syndrome*—Clients at low risk can be told that there is no evidence that their family has a hereditary cancer syndrome. The counselor can explain how this conclusion was reached by pointing why the pattern of cancer in the family is not suggestive of a cancer

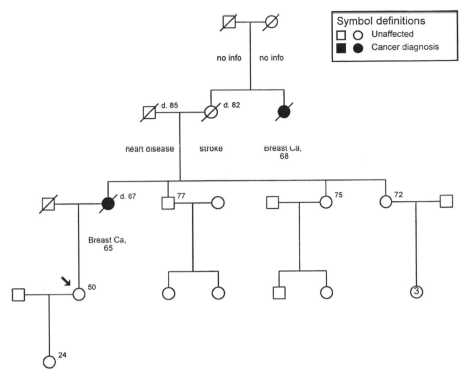

FIGURE 7-1. Example of a low-risk pedigree. This pedigree reveals a client at low risk for having a hereditary breast cancer syndrome.

syndrome. Figure 7-1 depicts a client assessed to be at low risk for a hereditary cancer syndrome. In this instance, the counselor could explain to the client, "Yes, it's true your mother and great-aunt had breast cancer but both were in their sixties when diagnosed, and, of your many relatives on that side of the family, no one else has ever developed cancer."

2. *Risk of developing cancer*—In most cases, clients at low risk can be quoted general population risks of cancer. This type of information is available through the American Cancer Society. Having a single first-degree relative with a certain form of cancer may increase the client's risks by two- to threefold; therefore, it might be appropriate to discuss possible increased risks of cancer based on a combination of genetic and environmental factors. For example, a woman in the United States has a 1–2% lifetime risk of developing ovarian cancer. If her mother has been diagnosed with ovarian cancer (and there is no other family history of cancer), then the woman's risks of ovarian cancer

might be increased to 2–6% over her lifetime. Empiric risk tables might also be useful in determining a client's risks for specific cancers. For example, when determining risk estimates for breast cancer, it may be helpful to utilize the Claus model (1994) or Gail model (1989).

3. *Risks for other family members*—Sometimes, clients have sought genetic counseling because of concerns about other family members, especially offspring or siblings. Clients at low risk can usually be reassured that other family members are also unlikely to be at increased risk. Referring again to Figure 7-1, the client's daughter is even less likely to have an inherited predisposition to breast cancer, especially if her mother remains cancer–free (and her father's family has no history of breast cancer).

4. *Monitoring suggestions*—It is generally appropriate for clients at low risk to follow standard guidelines for cancer screening. The American Cancer Society has excellent materials about cancer screening, including detailed information about appropriate breast, colon, cervical, and skin examinations. Although clients may be at low risk for developing an inherited form of cancer, they may have other significant cancer risk factors that need to be considered. Thus, clients should be encouraged to speak to their physicians before making any changes in their cancer-monitoring regimens.

5. *Option of genetic testing*—Genetic testing is not indicated for clients at low risk because of the extremely low likelihood of a meaningful positive result. Such testing is unlikely to be beneficial and, similar to other medical tests, contains the risk of identifying a false positive result (such as a variant of uncertain significance) that could lead to unnecessary medical screening and increased client anxiety. In most cases, clients at low risk will be relieved to learn that they do not meet criteria for genetic testing, as long as the rationale for the decision is explained. However, there will be certain clients (for example, physician clients) who insist on being tested regardless of their low *a priori* risks. Clinical programs may want to set a policy in advance about whether they will honor such requests.

7.3.2. Cancer Risk Assessment—Moderate Risk

Clients at moderate risk for having a hereditary cancer syndrome may be among the most challenging to counsel. Some families will turn out to have low penetrant cancer susceptibility genes (when such genes are identified), whereas, in other families, the pattern of cancer is most likely the result of random events.

1. *Likelihood of cancer syndrome*—Clients at moderate risk for having a cancer syndrome range from those whose histories come close to meeting diagnostic criteria to ones in which a cancer syndrome is unlikely but cannot be completely ruled out. See Figures 7-2 and 7-3 for two examples of moderate risk pedigrees. By comparing these pedigrees to clinical criteria for hereditary nonpolyposis cancer syndrome (HNPCC), note that the pedigree in Figure 7-2 almost meets Amsterdam II criteria. Although the client can be given information about HNPCC, , it would not be appropriate to diagnose the family as having HNPCC based on this pattern of cancer. The family depicted in the second pedigree (Fig. 7-3) is much less unlikely to have HNPCC, although this cannot be completely ruled out. Counselors should be cautious in ruling out cancer syndromes if there

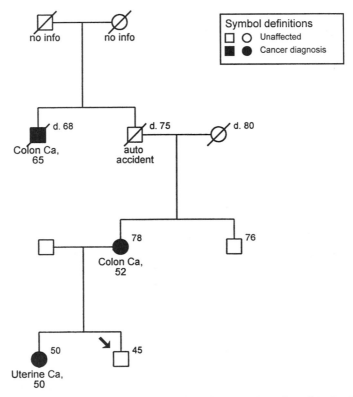

FIGURE 7-2. Example of a moderate-risk pedigree. Note that this family almost meets Amsterdam II criteria (refer to Table 4-3) for hereditary nonpolyposis colon cancer syndrome.

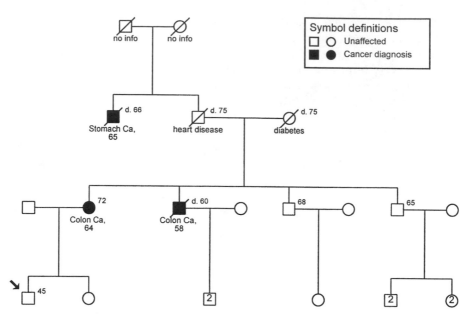

FIGURE 7-3. Example of a moderate-risk pedigree. Note that this family is less likely to have hereditary nonpolyposis colon cancer (HNPCC) than the family in Figure 7-2, but HNPCC cannot be completely ruled out.

are few at-risk relatives or if the family almost meets criteria for a syndrome.

Most counselors would agree that clients at moderate risk should be given at least general information about the possible cancer syndrome in the family. This discussion might elicit additional information from the client that helps confirm or rule out the cancer syndrome in question. Diagnoses should be confirmed with medical records whenever possible, and clients should be encouraged to stay in touch with the program. If the family does have a hereditary cancer syndrome, then additional cancer diagnoses will almost certainly occur over time. The family should adopt a "watchful waiting" attitude. If no new tumors have occurred over the next several years, then the family is less likely to have a strong inherited predisposition to cancer and the next generation may be considered at lower risk.

2. *Risk of developing cancer*—The level of increased risk will depend on the pattern of cancer in the family. Clients with pedigrees that come close to meeting criteria for a known hereditary cancer syndrome should be counseled about the syndrome-related cancer risks. Counselors should be clear that the client's cancer risks *may be* as high as the syndrome-related risks but that the risks might also be much

lower. Counselors can either provide a range of risks or quote two sets of risks given the two separate scenarios (for example, family has/does not have HNPCC). Clients with pedigrees that have only slight evidence of a hereditary cancer syndrome should also be counseled with a range of risks, although it may be appropriate to stress that the client is unlikely to have the maximum risks quoted. Counselors who tell clients that their family "probably" or "probably does not" have a cancer syndrome need to be certain that these conclusions are based on concrete evidence, that is, a documented pedigree, not because of pressure from clients to interpret their risks in a certain way. As a way of explaining the various interpretations of risk, it may be helpful to discuss with clients the concepts of reduced penetrance and variable expressivity, the potential combined influences of genetic and environmental modifiers, and the common incidence of sporadic cancers.

3. *Risks for other family members*—If clients are assessed to have moderately increased risks, then it is possible that risks are increased for other family members as well. Depending on the degree of relatedness, other family members may also be at potentially higher risk. When asked about risks for other relatives, counselors may want to provide general information rather than a numerical value.

4. *Monitoring suggestions*—Recommendations about monitoring will be based on the pattern of cancer in the family, taking into account the features associated with the syndrome in question. In most cases, it is suggested that clients at moderate risk undergo specialized and/or more frequent cancer monitoring. Over time, these monitoring efforts may shift the likelihood of a hereditary cancer syndrome if any additional cancers are identified.

5. *Option of genetic testing*—Genetic testing may be quite helpful to moderate-risk families.. A positive result will confirm the presence of a hereditary cancer syndrome, and a negative result will reduce, albeit not eliminate, the likelihood of an inherited cancer. As a rule, moderate-risk families should be offered genetic tests that are available clinically. If testing is only available on a research basis, counselors will need to determine whether the family meets eligibility criteria before raising it as an option with the client.

7.3.3. CANCER RISK ASSESSMENT—HIGH RISK

In many ways, counseling clients at high risk for cancer is the most straightforward. Counselors can use published data on the cancer syndrome regarding the associated types of cancer, estimates of risk, and appropriate monitoring.

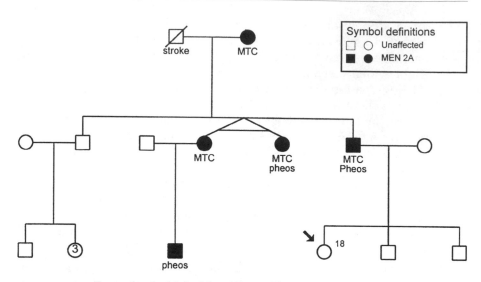

FIGURE 7-4. Example of a high-risk pedigree. The pattern of benign and malignant tumors in the family is consistent with multiple endocrine neoplasia, 2A (MEN 2A). [MTC = medullary thyroid carcinoma; Pheos = pheochromocytomas]

1. *Likelihood of cancer syndrome*—High-risk families are ones that are consistent with or highly suggestive of having a hereditary cancer syndrome (see an example of a pedigree consistent with multiple endocrine neoplasia, type 2 in Fig. 7-4). Counselors should describe the features of the specific hereditary cancer syndrome and compare it with the client's personal and family history. Clients may need time to adjust to the information. Some may want to know why such a diagnosis had never been made before; they may feel bitterness at past providers or hope that the counselor's assessment is wrong. It is important to provide written literature, including information about support groups, if available. Counselors should also offer to review the information at a later date through follow-up telephone calls or visits.

2. *Risk of developing cancer*— In most cases, there is nothing in physical appearance to distinguish carriers from noncarriers. Thus, a client's risks to develop cancer are based on the cancer risks associated with the syndrome as well as the client's position in the pedigree and inheritance pattern of the syndrome. There are a few cancer syndromes that have physical characteristics or features that make it obvious whether the client has the genetic predisposition and the associated risks of cancer. Examples include nevoid basal cell carcinoma syndrome, Cowden syndrome, and neurofibromatosis.

3. *Risks for other family members*—The likelihood that other relatives have the familial syndrome is based on their placement in the pedigree. Since most cancer syndromes have less than 100% penetrance, it is not possible to rule out risks to offspring of unaffected individuals. However, given the size of the family, it may be possible to identify the branches of the family at highest risk.

4. *Monitoring suggestions*—High-risk clients will typically be recommended to adhere to a monitoring schedule that is more frequent or involved than usual. For some of the hereditary cancer syndromes, there are published guidelines for monitoring, which should be utilized. Unfortunately, effective screening modalities do not exist for many types of cancer.

5. *Option of genetic testing*—Genetic testing is now clinically available for several of the major hereditary cancer syndromes. High-risk clients should be offered genetic testing in order to determine the underlying cause of the syndrome and to clarify which family members are truly at risk. Some clients will need time to consider whether to pursue genetic testing, and, of course, not everyone will be interested in being tested.

7.3.4. CANCER RISK ASSESSMENT—UNCERTAIN RISK

And then there are the reported family histories of cancer that are so vague or incomplete that it is not possible to accurately assign risk. In some cases, this is a temporary problem that will be resolved after the client speaks to other relatives or obtains needed medical records. However, sometimes it is just not possible to obtain any further information. Therefore, counselors may be faced with providing some type of risk assessment despite the incomplete history.

1. *Likelihood of cancer syndrome*—If it is not possible to determine the likelihood of a cancer syndrome with any degree of certainty, be honest with the client. Discuss the usual features of the syndrome in question and compare it with the client's family history. Sometimes it hinges on one key diagnosis—brainstorm about possible ways to obtain this information. Despite the incomplete or unconfirmed history, it may be appropriate to distinguish between clients who are unlikely to have a hereditary cancer syndrome and those for whom it is a distinct possibility. Counselors who do provide some level of assessment need to qualify their responses appropriately. For example, "Based on what you have told me, your family is unlikely to have a hereditary breast cancer syndrome—provided your grandmother really did have stomach cancer, not ovarian cancer."

2. *Risk of developing cancer*—Clients should be told that it is not possible to provide them with exact figures of risk. Counselors may want to provide a range of risks based on the different possibilities or provide clients with the best "guesstimate" based on the information at hand. In either case, it is important to qualify answers carefully and to emphasize that any additional family history information could dramatically alter the estimates of risk.

3. *Risks for other family members*—If it is difficult to sort out whether the client is at increased risk, then determining risks for other family members may be even more difficult. Counselors may want to limit their comments to generalities or to further emphasize that an accurate assessment is not possible given the limited information about family history.

4. *Monitoring suggestions*—Monitoring suggestions should be based on the pattern of cancer in the family rather than the possibility of a syndrome. If the family might have a syndrome for which monitoring is noninvasive and/or known to be effective, it may be appropriate to adjust recommendations accordingly. In these cases, counselors can say something like "to be safe, we will talk to you about screening *as if* you were at risk for an inherited form of colon cancer." Monitoring suggestions also need to take into account the client's current age, his or her position in the pedigree, and the presence of any other cancer risk factors.

5. *Option of genetic testing*—Genetic testing is not usually indicated unless the client is likely to be affected and the result will be straightforward to interpret.

7.4. THE CLIENTS

Without a doubt, this genetic journey has been not only one of the greatest challenges of my life, but also one of the loneliest.

I had to discover on my own the lessons that people with chronic diseases and women with breast cancer can learn from others in similar situations: We are now in a new, different and permanent place in our lives and only those who are there with us really understand what we are going through.

(Prouser, 2000)

No two genetic counseling sessions are alike. This is because clients come with widely different issues and concerns. This section describes the major counseling issues that can arise in the different groups of people presenting for cancer genetic counseling. Although each client needs to be treated on an individual basis, it may be helpful to read the general description of client issues within this section.

7.4.1. UNAFFECTED ADULTS AT HIGH RISK

High-risk adult clients are individuals who have never had cancer themselves but who have increased risks of developing specific adult-onset malignancies based on their family histories.

1. *Motivations*—Clients at high risk for cancer are usually highly motivated to learn how to minimize their chances of developing—or dying from—cancer. Thus, clients will be eager to hear about any and all early detection and prevention strategies, even those that are still in experimental phases. They may feel that meeting with a genetic counselor will help them gain a sense of control over their high-risk status. This may make them eager to learn the genetics information but can also lead to them holding unrealistic expectations of what genetic testing can tell them. Some clients may also want to establish relationships with appropriate caregivers (in case they ever do develop cancer).

2. *Risk perception and coping strategies*—Adults at high risk frequently overestimate their risks of developing cancer. This inflated perception of risk can lead to a variety of coping strategies, from an obsession with gathering medical facts to adopting a fatalistic attitude about developing cancer. The client's risk perception and coping strategies can affect his or her understanding of the cancer risk assessment and influence the discussion about genetic testing and preventive strategies.

3. *Family issues*—Common family issues include complicated communication patterns, lack of emotional support for at-risk relatives (compared with those with cancer), and varying attitudes about genetic testing or preventative measures. These family issues may complicate the logistics around genetic testing and may certainly play a role in the client's view of risk and his or her ability to cope with the risk. Some families will be very supportive of the decision to pursue testing whereas other families may find it difficult to even discuss the option of testing.

7.4.2. SURVIVORS OF ADULT-ONSET CANCERS

Many genetic counseling clients have had cancer themselves as adults. For this discussion, a survivor is defined as someone who has completed cancer treatment and whose cancer is in remission.

1. *Motivations*—Cancer survivors are often motivated to seek genetic counseling to obtain answers on behalf of their children or other family members. Some are seeking answers for why they developed

cancer, although this may be less of an issue for long-term survivors. They may also be concerned about the risks of developing a second cancer in addition to being concerned about recurrence.

2. *Potential impact of the session*—Cancer survivors may underestimate the emotional impact of the genetic counseling session. They may find that the discussion brings back unpleasant memories about their cancer experience and brings to the surface fears about themselves or other family members. They may also enter the genetic counseling session assuming they already have all the facts, only to be quite dismayed when new information is presented, such as the possibility that their offspring could also be at increased risk.

3. *Perception of medical providers*—Some cancer survivors have become strong advocates for their own medical care and believe that they have to argue for each service they feel they need. Thus, they can be demanding or argumentative about wanting to meet with a genetic counselor or about undergoing a genetic test. Many cancer survivors express gratitude for the care they received by their physicians and continue to hold special relationships with their oncologists or surgeons. These clients may not believe the risk assessment if it varies widely with what their physician has told them.

7.4.3. ADULT SURVIVORS OF CHILDHOOD CANCER

Although parents of a child with cancer may seek genetic counseling, this section focuses on the needs of the survivors themselves. Overall cure rates of pediatric-onset cancers is approaching 90%. Thus, there is an ever-growing number of adults who are also survivors of a childhood malignancy.

1. *Motivations*—Adult survivors of childhood cancer typically seek genetic counseling to learn about their risks of additional cancers and/or to determine the risks of cancer to offspring. As they enter adulthood, they may also need assistance transitioning their care from pediatric to adult specialties.

2. *The late-effects issues*—As more and more children survive their cancers, it has become clear that the current methods of cure can lead to a host of serious medical, emotional, and learning problems. The severity of these problems depends on many factors, including the site and type of cancer, methods of treatment, and the age at which treatment was initiated. Interest in long-term survivorship issues is quite recent; therefore, only a handful of long-term survivor clinics exist. Survivors may be unaware that they are now at increased risk for developing significant medical problems, such as cardiac or pulmonary disease. Some survivors have struggled for years with significant psychological and learning problems without recognizing the

connection to the brain irradiation they received at a young age, and, until recently, few were told of their potential infertility as a secondary effect of alkylating agents.

3. *Poor historians*—Survivors of adult-onset cancers are usually knowledgeable about their own cancer diagnoses; however, this is often not the case with survivors of childhood cancers. Survivors may have been shielded from detailed information about their treatment. A few survivors may not even be aware they had cancer; the euphemism "tumor" or "growth" could have been used.

7.4.4. THE RECENTLY DIAGNOSED CANCER PATIENT

Genetic counselors may also be called upon to see adult clients who have been recently diagnosed with cancer.

1. *Motivations*—Adult clients who have recently been diagnosed with cancer may want genetic information to assist them in making decisions about treatment. They may also be searching for an explanation as to why they developed cancer. They may be motivated to seek answers from genetic counselors but may also be afraid to hear what the counselor has to say.

2. *State of mind*—Newly diagnosed clients may be in a state of shock. In a short span of time, they need to come to terms with their cancer diagnosis—a life-altering event. They often need to make rapid decisions about treatment and make drastic adjustments to their lives. This series of events can cause clients to feel overwhelmed or vulnerable—even before the genetic counseling discussion begins. Their high levels of stress may make it difficult for clients to follow the conversation or to even provide accurate pedigree information.

3. *Timing issues*—Those with long-standing family histories of cancer may be more than ready to pursue genetic testing. Others may be surprised to learn about the possibility of a hereditary cancer syndrome and will need time to adjust to this information before proceeding with testing. Clients should dictate the timing of the genetic counseling and testing encounters, but counselors may want to remind them that there is seldom urgency in making decisions about genetic testing.

7.4.5. THE TERMINALLY ILL PATIENT

On occasion, genetic counselors will be asked to meet with patients who are terminally ill.

1. *Motivations*—Typically, terminally ill patients seek genetic counseling because they have decided to pursue genetic testing for the sake of

their families. They may have come to this decision on their own or at the urging of family members. They are usually aware that this information will not be helpful to them other than perhaps providing them with peace of mind that either the test result was negative or that they have potentially helped other family members avoid a similar fate (if the result is positive). Some are not interested in undergoing clinical testing but may be willing to donate and store a specimen to give their family the option of testing in the future.

2. *Counseling challenges*—Providing genetic counseling to terminally ill patients and their families presents special challenges. Patients may have some physical or intellectual limitations due to brain metastases or high dosages of pain medications. Traveling to the center for the genetic counseling appointment may be difficult. Most individuals are aware of their poor prognosis (although this is not always the case!) and will be in different phases of acceptance. In a few cases, it will be difficult to have any direct interaction (even over the telephone) with the client and counselors will find themselves dealing with the client's spouse or close relatives. Special issues can include discussions of banking a blood specimen or arranging for someone else to receive a pending genetic test result. These interactions can be further complicated by the family's grief and the counselor's potential discomfort or inexperience in dealing with terminally ill patients and their families.

3. *Family issues*—Patients who are imminently close to death may weave in and out of the conversation, in which case other family members may need to become the primary clients. Family members may display intense fear, anger, or grief, which may be directed at all health care providers, including genetic counselors. Even when family members are focused on learning the information, they may have a difficult time remembering any complicated instructions.

7.5. CASE EXAMPLES

The following three cases illustrate some of the issues that can arise during a cancer genetic counseling session.

7.5.1. CASE 1: IS IT A CLOCK OR A BOMB?

Ellen seemed tense as she greeted the genetic counselor and sat down in the consult room. She admitted that coming to a cancer hospital was difficult. "Guess that's why it has taken me so long to make the appointment to come in." The counselor assured her that this was not unusual and asked what she hoped to get out of the clinic visit. Ellen took a deep breath and said it was time to figure out why so many people in her family had developed breast cancer.

In a soft voice, she said, "Ever since my sister was diagnosed with breast cancer, my doctor has been urging me to have my breasts and ovaries removed. I know it's the smart thing to do, but I'm only 33. I haven't been married that long and we are still trying to get our business off the ground. It's not that I never want to have a baby, just not right now. I guess that's why I'm here, because I feel like I'm running out of time to make a decision. I'm so confused—I can't tell if this internal ticking I'm hearing is my biological clock or a cancer bomb!" They both laughed at this vivid description, and the counselor assured her that she had plenty of time in which to make a final decision about prophylactic surgery.

The counselor filed away this concern to bring up again later and then continued with contracting the session. "For today's visit, I'd like to gather more information about your family history, give you an estimate of your risks of developing cancer, and talk a little about genetic testing. How does that sound?"

"That would be fine. Are we also going to talk about what I can do about my risks?" The counselor assured her that the medical oncologist would be joining them to discuss appropriate monitoring and possible prevention strategies.

They then reviewed Ellen's family history. She had provided a cursory pedigree when making her appointment that provided the starting point of the discussion. Several members of Ellen's large Irish kindred over three generations had developed breast cancer, including one maternal uncle (see Fig. 7-5). Ellen's branch of the family had not been spared. Her mother and older sister had both been diagnosed with premenopausal breast cancer. Taking the family history took time because Ellen wove in anecdotes about her relatives. The counselor recognized how important it was for Ellen to describe her relatives as people rather than cases. When the pedigree was completed, the counselor paused and together they looked at the many darkly shaded pedigree symbols.

"Do you have any thoughts about what could be causing cancer in the family?"

"Well, if it's not the water, then I guess it's genetic."

"My guess is you are probably right." The counselor paused to assess Ellen's reaction to this statement, but Ellen just smiled and did not appear to be overly surprised or upset. So the counselor continued by discussing the features of breast-ovarian cancer syndrome, using the family history as her primary visual aid.

The counselor then turned the discussion to the next topic, "What do you think are your chances of getting cancer?"

"Oh, I think my chances are really high. My older sister and I look so much like our mother that I wasn't really surprised when she got breast

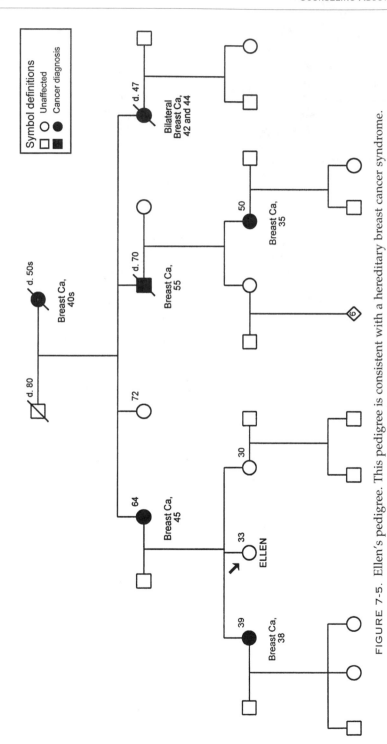

FIGURE 7-5. Ellen's pedigree. This pedigree is consistent with a hereditary breast cancer syndrome.

cancer. Frankly, I've always assumed I would get it In some strange way, I think that's why I went into nursing, to stay close to the medical profession."

The counselor went on to discuss the genetics and associated cancer risks of hereditary breast cancer syndrome. Mindful of Ellen's nursing background, the counselor was careful not to simplify the terminology too much but was aware that even medical professionals hear things differently when they themselves are the patients.

"Some people with a *BRCA1* or *BRCA2* mutation never develop cancer. But the risks of cancer—especially breast and ovarian—are higher. Are you a numbers person—would you like to hear what the risks are? Or are you already familiar with this information?" Ellen did want to know the statistics, which she carefully wrote down, explaining that she planned to share the information with her sisters and cousins.

They then talked about genetic testing. Ellen's older sister had already volunteered to be tested and several family members had expressed interest in having predictive testing once the genetic factor was identified. Ellen was certain that she herself would also be tested, some time in the future.

At this point, the counselor decided to reopen the issue of prophylactic surgery. Ellen reiterated that she could not decide whether to go ahead and have a baby, which her husband and family were urging her to do, or to make plans to undergo surgery, which seemed to her the more logical medical choice. Although the counselor reminded her that the decision to have prophylactic surgery could wait until after resolving whether to have a baby, Ellen clearly felt that this was an "either/or" situation.

The counselor considered mentioning the potential usefulness of genetic testing in making this decision but decided it would be more helpful to explore why Ellen was feeling so pressured and conflicted about this issue. When Ellen volunteered that her mother had been pregnant when diagnosed with breast cancer, the counselor felt this was likely to be an important contributing factor and was prepared to discuss the issue in more depth. When Ellen went on to say that she needed help making the "right decision" so that no one would be mad at her *and* said defensively that not every Irish-Catholic girl was cut out to be a good parent, the counselor realized this dilemma had actually triggered many different issues for her. She further realized that helping Ellen sort out these issues would take a much greater investment of time—and a different level of counseling skill—than she could provide.

The counselor acknowledged the many issues that Ellen raised and agreed with her that making this decision would not be easy. She suggested that Ellen consider meeting with someone to help her sort out these issues and come to the "right decision" for her. Ellen seemed amenable to the suggestion and wrote down the name and phone number of a local family therapist to whom the counselor had referred other high-risk clients.

The oncologist then joined the session and discussed the appropriate breast cancer screening regimen. She also suggested adding surveillance for ovarian cancer. Clearly focused on her risks of breast cancer, Ellen requested information about chemoprevention options, but realized this was another strategy that was on hold if she was considering a pregnancy. Because Ellen seemed reluctant to ask the physician about possible breast cancer risks during pregnancy, the counselor asked it on her behalf. The oncologist reassured Ellen that pregnancy itself does not seem to cause breast cancer, although it may hasten the growth of an existing tumor. Ellen looked thoughtful at this information but did not say anything.

The session ended with plans for Ellen to be seen in the high-risk clinic once a year and for her to contact the genetic counselor if and when her sister wanted to arrange *BRCA1* and *BRCA2* testing. The counselor made a note to herself to revisit the issue of prophylactic surgery if Ellen did eventually undergo genetic testing.

Key Points of Case:

1. Elements of counseling session—see Section 7.2, especially 7.2.1 and 7.2.6
2. Educational issues for client—see Section 7.3.3
3. Counseling issues for client—see Sections 7.4.1 and Chapter 8, Sections 8.1.3 and 8.3.2

7.5.2. CASE 2: THE STRONG SILENT TYPE

Each time the genetic counselor asked about the health status of a particular family member, Terry answered with "Dead." The counselor blinked the first time he heard the response and almost laughed. However, after glancing at Terry's face, he became less certain that the answer was meant to be funny; humor is tricky when you don't know the person. So the counselor continued to ask questions about the several relatives who had been diagnosed with gastric cancer. This became a somewhat frustrating ordeal, since Terry seemed reluctant to provide any detailed information, even about his own diagnosis of gastric cancer 6 weeks earlier. At first, the counselor thought he might be feeling uncomfortable in the major medical center but eventually decided that Terry was simply not much of a talker. When he did speak, it was a succinct response, with very little emotion.

Terry had agreed to meet with a genetic counselor at the dual requests of his wife and oncologist but kept glancing out the window and locking and unlocking his hands. To the query, "What do you hope to accomplish from our meeting today?" Terry answered "I dunno." After further encouragement, he shrugged his shoulders and said, "Get information I guess. Got two sons."

Excerpts from the genetic counseling session went something like this:

Counselor:	Do you worry about your boys developing stomach cancer?
Terry:	Yeah.
Counselor:	How are you doing with your diagnosis?
Terry:	Okay, I guess.
Counselor	What do you know about genetics?
Terry:	Not much.
Counselor:	Are you interested in genetic testing?
Terry:	I'm not sure.

After getting yet another curt response, the counselor inwardly sighed and decided to shift gears. In his most empathetic manner, he looked at Terry and said, "It must be difficult to talk about this after all you've been through." Terry just looked at him blankly and shrugged, "Not really." *Wrong gear*, the counselor thought to himself as he considered what next to try. As he watched Terry shift uncomfortably in anticipation of the next question, it struck him that the encounter had taken on the feel of an interrogation. As he mentally reviewed their conversation, the counselor was chagrined to realize that his focus on getting Terry to "open up" to him had had the opposite effect—and had pretty much derailed the session. Clearly, his usual conversational counseling technique was not going to be effective with this client.

So the genetic counselor decided to try something different and said briskly, "Okay, that should be all the information I need from you right now." He deliberately put aside his pen and paper as a way of underscoring that the "interrogation" was over. "Now it's my turn to talk. Let me tell you what we understand about familial stomach cancer. Of course, if you have any questions, feel free to interrupt me." He then launched into a mini-lecture about the inheritance pattern and underlying genetics of gastric cancer. He also discussed an ongoing research project and described what participation would entail.

Rather than being put off by this didactic approach, Terry seemed to become more attentive and relaxed. He even began asking a few questions, mainly about the logistics of the research study. The counselor deliberately kept his responses brief and curbed his natural inclination to ask follow-up questions.

They ended the session with the counselor agreeing to send Terry extra copies of the counseling session summary letter so that he could share them with other family members. He also agreed to discuss the project with Terry's primary oncologist. Terry said he would be willing to participate in the study if his doctor thought it was a good idea. Terry also said his wife would probably have lots of questions (which she did!).

About 2 months later, one of Terry's brothers called to make a genetic counseling appointment. He admitted to having some initial reluctance about coming in but said that his brother had convinced him. Curious, the counselor asked what his brother had said about the encounter. The counselor was pleased and somewhat amused when told, "My brother says you are really easy to talk to."

Key Points of Case:

1. Elements of counseling session—see Section 7.2, especially 7.2.1 and 7.2.6

2. Issues for client newly diagnosed with cancer—see Section 7.4.4

3. Counseling techniques - see Chapter 8, Section 8.2.2

7.5.3. CASE 3: A MILLION TO ONE ODDS

Jason was slouched in the waiting room chair wearing baggy pants, an oversized T-shirt, and a backward baseball cap. On the clinic form, it indicated that he was 22 years old and that this was his first visit to the long-term survivor's clinic. His thick medical chart revealed two primary cancer diagnoses: an osteosarcoma of the lower leg at age 3, at which time one leg was amputated below the knee, and a rhabdomyosarcoma of the upper arm at age 14, which was successfully excised, sparing the arm.

Jason's family was well known to the genetic counselor. As shown in Figure 7-6, Jason's brother had been diagnosed with an osteosarcoma at age 12 and his father was currently being treated for his third cancer. Jason was part of a classic Li-Fraumeni syndrome (LFS) family that had been participating in a genetic studies project for over 10 years. A deleterious $TP53$ mutation had been identified, and adult family members had been offered individual genetic counseling and testing appointments; few had elected to undergo predictive testing.

The counselor knew that Jason's main reason for coming to the long-term survivor's clinic was to coordinate his follow-up care. He had not seen a physician in over 3 years. At today's visit, he would undergo a thorough physical exam, blood and urine screening tests, and an endocrine check. He would also be meeting with a clinical psychologist. The counselor's "game plan" going into the session was to review general information about LFS and the familial $TP53$ result. Because Jason almost certainly carried the familial mutation, it did not seem necessary to discuss genetic testing. She tucked an LFS fact sheet into his clinic chart as well as the lab report documenting the familial mutation.

The counselor greeted Jason, and they walked together to the assigned exam room. Jason seemed to move comfortably with his prosthetic leg, limping only slightly. After they sat down, the counselor outlined the clinic

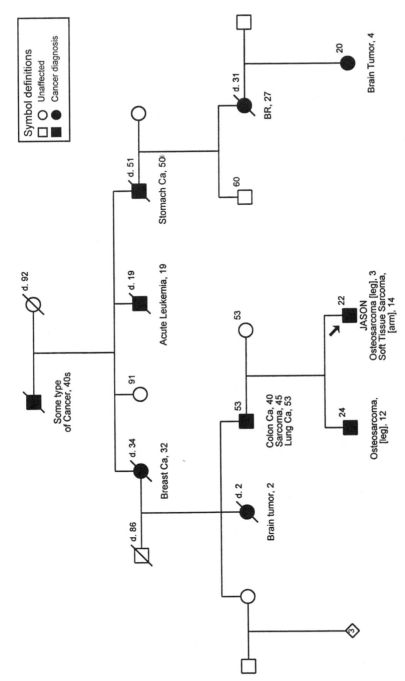

FIGURE 7-6. Jason's pedigree. This pedigree is consistent with Li-Fraumeni syndrome.

visit. She explained that he would be meeting with several providers with different areas of expertise. She indicated that her role was to discuss his personal and family history of cancer. Upon hearing this, Jason immediately launched into a 10-minute recital of the cancer diagnoses in his family. Because of his eagerness to provide the information, the counselor redrew the pedigree rather than pulling out the computerized version she already had on the family.

When they completed the family history, the counselor returned to contracting the session. She asked what questions he most wanted answered today. Jason leaned forward in his chair and said, "It seems so strange that my brother and I both developed bone cancers. I guess I'm curious about it. I remember one doctor telling us it was a million to one odds that we'd both come down with cancer. Think of that. A million to one. And then I got cancer in my arm. What are the odds of that happening?! My Dad says we deserve to win the lottery sweepstakes to balance out all the rotten luck we've had. We haven't won anything big, but I did win $20 last week."

"Do you have any ideas about why it might have happened—the cancers, not the lottery?" clarified the counselor, trying hard to stay focused and rein in this very engaging, talkative client.

Jason nodded eagerly, "Don't worry, I have lots of ideas about it. First, there's all the chemicals at my Dad's job. He works in a photoprocessing lab and is always getting stuff on his clothes. It drives my Mom crazy. She probably should have thrown the clothes away but didn't. Another possibility is all the power lines near our house. Personally, I think that's the problem. I know of two other people on our street who have gotten cancer—one guy has lung cancer and one guy has Hodgkin's disease. I can get you their phone numbers if you want to talk to them. I also read somewhere that eating food that's been microwaved can cause cancer. All the beams and stuff. Do you think that's true? Of course, my family didn't have a microwave when I was growing up, but I sure use it a lot now. But I try not to cook anything longer than 2 minutes. That's safer, don't you think?" Jason stopped talking as abruptly as he had started and looked expectantly at the counselor.

The counselor didn't say anything right away. She wasn't sure where to begin. She rapidly considered how best to acknowledge his concerns about the environment, gently suggest that none of these theories was likely to explain the cancer in his family, bridge to discussing genetic causes of cancer, and inform him that he had a rare cancer syndrome—all in the remaining 20 minutes.

"Well, Jason. It sounds like you have been giving this a lot of thought. You're right that most cancers are caused by exposures to carcinogens. Carcinogens are agents in the environment that have been proven to cause cancer. The major carcinogens are cigarettes, alcohol, and excessive sunlight. Now, it's true that direct contact with high doses of chemicals can cause cancer, but I don't think this would explain why you and your brother developed cancer, do you?

"No, I guess not," Jason agreed reluctantly. "That's what our doctor said too."

"And I very much doubt that eating microwaved food increases one's cancer risks. Microwaves have been around long enough to know whether they cause cancer. So I think it is okay to cook your food for more than 2 minutes."

"Well, that's a relief. The frozen foods didn't taste very good only half-cooked," grinned Jason.

"Lots of people have wondered about power lines. I have to tell you that most scientists do not think that power lines increases the risks of cancer, but not everyone is convinced that we know for certain. It can be difficult studying possible carcinogens because cancer is such a common disease. You mentioned that you have two neighbors who developed cancer. Unfortunately, 1 of 3 people will develop some type of cancer over their lifetime, so it is not unusual to know of people who have had cancer. The truth is, Jason, that cancer is usually caused by a combination of factors."

"Oh, so you mean my brother and I got cancer because of the chemicals *and* the power lines?" said Jason, furrowing his brow in thought.

"Well, the exposure to carcinogens may be part of the answer. But I think there is another risk factor in your family. An inherited risk factor called an altered gene. Genes are passed on from generation to generation. Altered genes don't work right and can cause members of a family to be predisposed to developing a disease, like cancer. The predisposition to disease is passed on like other family traits."

"You think my family has one of these altered genes?" asked Jason.

"Yes, I do." The counselor went on to describe genes in more detail. Jason seemed fascinated by the idea that he had an inherited risk of cancer.

"So I could have a mutant gene?" he asked excitedly.

"Well, I guess you could call it that," said the counselor with a smile. "Another way to describe it is to say that your family has a cancer syndrome. There are many different cancer syndromes, but there is only one that fits the pattern of cancer in your family. This syndrome is called LFS or Li-Fraumeni syndrome. It is very rare. Have you ever heard of LFS?"

Jason shook his head 'no', and the counselor provided a brief overview of the syndrome, adding that many families with LFS had an alteration in a gene called *TP53*. Jason asked several questions about LFS and eagerly accepted the fact sheet about it. The counselor also mentioned their hospital's previous *TP53* research project and commented that some of his relatives might even have participated in it. She did not feel as though she could disclose his family's involvement in the project or the *TP53* result without obtaining permission to do so.

"It's now time for your next appointment, but I'd like to schedule a follow-up visit in a few weeks so that we can talk more about this. Other members of your family would be welcome to join you." Jason agreed to this plan and said he would invite his brother to come along. At the end of the visit, Jason said, "I guess that doctor was right. It probably is a million to one odds that my family would have this syndrome."

Key Points of Case:

1. Elements of counseling session—see Section 7.2, especially 7.2.2 and 7.2.3

2. Issues for survivors of childhood cancer - see Section 7.4.3

3. Counseling techniques—see Chapter 8, Section 8.2.2

7.6. REFERENCES

Baker, D. 1998. Interviewing techniques. In Baker, D, Schuette, J, and Uhlmann, W (eds) A Guide to Genetic Counseling. John Wiley & Sons, New York, NY, 55–74.

Baker, N. 1991. Relative Risk. Living With a Family History of Breast Cancer. Penguin Books, New York, NY, 221.

Baty, B, Venne, V, McDonald, J et al. 1997. BRCA1 testing: genetic counseling protocol development and counseling issues. J Genetic Counseling 6:223–244.

Claus, E, Risch, N, and Thompson, W. 1994. Autosomal dominant inheritance of early-onset breast cancer. Cancer 73:643–51.

Croyle, R and Lerman, C. 1999. Risk communication in genetic testing for cancer susceptibility. Monogr J Nat Ca Inst 25:59–66.

Gail, M, Brinton, L, Byar, D et al. 1989. Projecting individualized probabilities of developing breast cancer for white females who are being examined annually. J Natl. Cancer Inst 81:1879–86.

Greenstein, R (ed). 2000. Manual on reimbursement for medical genetics services. Copyright American College of Medical Genetics.

Hallowell, N, Statham, H, Murton, F et al. 1997. Talking about chance: the presentation of risk information during genetic counseling for breast and ovarian cancer. J Genetic Counseling 6:269–286.

Keene, N, Hobbie, W, and Ruccione, K. 2000. Childhood Cancer Survivors: A Practical Guide to Your Future. O'Reilly Publishers, Sebastopol, CA.

Kessler, S. 2000. Advanced counseling techniques. In Resta, R(ed) Psyche and helix: psychological aspects of genetic counseling. Wiley-Liss New York, NY

McKinnon, W, Guttmacher, AE, Greenblatt, MS et al. 1997. The familial cancer program of the Vermont cancer center: development of a cancer genetics program in a rural area. J Genetic Counseling. 6:131–146.

Meier, S and Davis S. 2001. The Elements of Counseling, 4th edition. Wadsworth Publishers, Toronto, Ontario, Canada.

Penson, R, Seiden, M, Shannon, K et al. 2000. Communicating genetic risk: pros, cons, and counsel. The Oncologist. 5:152–161.

Peters, J. 1998. Genetic counselling. In Inherited Susceptibility to Cancer. Eds.: Foulkes WD and Hodgson SV. Cambridge Univ. Press, New York, NY, 60–95.

Peters, J, Graham, J, Stadler, M et al. 1999. Components of a genetic cancer risk clinic. In Shaw (ed) Cancer genetics for the clinician. Kluwer Academic/Plenum Pub. New York, NY, 1–26.

Peters, J. 1992. When a history of breast cancer is identified during a counseling session. Perspectives in Genetic Counseling 14(3):2–3.

Peters, J and Stopfer, J. 1996. Role of the genetic counselor in familial cancer. Oncology. 159–175.

Prouser, N. 2000. Case Report: genetic susceptibility testing for breast and ovarian cancer: a patient's perspective. J Genetic Counseling 9:153,155.

Schneider, K and Marnane, D. 1997. Cancer risk counseling: how is it different? J Genetic Counseling 6:97–110.

Uhlmann, W. 1998. In Baker, D, Schuette, J, and Uhlmann, W (eds) A Guide to Genetic Counseling. John Wiley & Sons, New York, NY 199–230.

Weil, J. 2000. Cancer risk counseling. In Psychosocial Genetic Counseling. Oxford Univ. Press, Oxford, UK, 168–180.

Weitzel, J. 1999. Genetic cancer risk assessment: putting it all together. Amer. Cancer Society Second National Conference on Cancer Genetics. Cancer Supplement. 86:2483–2492.

PSYCHOLOGICAL ASPECTS OF CANCER COUNSELING

Counselees give direct information about themselves that a genetic counselor can utilize to form a psychosocial answer to the question: "Who is this person?" It also helps the counselor to address two important questions: "Can I understand this patient, and what can I offer beyond didactic information?"

(Djurdjinovic, 1998, p. 129)

The psychological, and educational dimensions of cancer counseling are closely intertwined. To counsel effectively, a genetic counselor must be attuned to the client's emotional well-being and be aware of the potential emotional impact of the genetic counseling interaction. This chapter discusses the psychological aspects of counseling clients at risk for developing cancer.

8.1. EMOTIONAL RESPONSES TO CANCER RISK

Clients' perceptions of their cancer risks often depends more on their emotional well-being and life experiences than on their actual numerical risks. This section discusses the range of emotional responses to cancer risk counseling as well as the influence of personal experiences. Most of the research in this area has focused on women at risk for breast cancer, but these emotional responses are likely to hold true for individuals (men and women) at risk for other forms of cancer as well.

8.1.1. EMOTIONAL STATUS

Individuals at high risk for cancer live with the possibility that one day they might be diagnosed with a malignancy. Clients can have a variety of emotional responses to living with these increased risks of cancer as can clients who have already been diagnosed with cancer. As listed in Table 8-1, clients may display the following emotions or feelings:

1. *Anger*—Clients may feel angry or frustrated about the uncertainty of their future because of the possibility that they will develop—and perhaps die of—cancer. This anger may be nonspecific or may be directed at a particular person, such as the parent who passed on the risk or a physician who minimizes the client's worries about cancer. Some clients may express their anger as distress or depression, which are more socially acceptable emotions. Anger is also a natural part of the grief process and thus, may also be expressed by individuals who are still grieving for relatives who have died.

2. *Anxiety*—All high-risk individuals experience some degree of anxiety about developing cancer. It may be beneficial to have a certain level of anxiety, since it can motivate people to undergo appropriate cancer surveillance. Too much anxiety, however, can have a paralyzing effect, leading to an avoidance of screening practices or denial of symptoms. It is customary for people to experience some anxiety when seeing their physician or waiting for the results of a screening test. However, for some clients, worries about cancer are constant and, at times, overwhelming. Anxiety disorders include generalized anxiety, obsessive thoughts, compulsive behaviors, and various phobias. Generalized anxiety about cancer can be mani-

TABLE 8-1. COMMON EMOTIONAL RESPONSES TO HIGH RISK STATUS

Anger
Anxiety
Fear of disfigurement
Fear of becoming a burden
Fear of dying
Grief
Guilt
Loss of control
Negative body image
Sadness
Sense of isolation
Shame

fested in various forms, including depression, sleeplessness, loss of appetite, excessive withdrawal from daily activities, physical pain, inability to trust oneself, and denial of reality. In extreme cases, clients may have displacement anxiety, which means that they have made their high-risk status the focal point of all that is wrong in their lives. Thus, they may blame their unhappiness on their fears of cancer rather than the actual source of anxiety (for example, loss of job, unhappy marriage).

3. *Fear of disfigurement*—Many people equate cancer with disfigurement. The disfigurement may be temporary or permanent. The most obvious source of disfigurement is the surgical removal of tumors and surrounding normal tissue. Other treatments can also leave their marks, such as rashes from radiation therapy, hair loss from chemotherapy, and scars from invasive procedures.

4. *Fear of becoming a burden*—High-risk individuals may also express fears about the physical and mental limitations which can result from cancer and its treatment. They may worry about being a burden to their families, because they would no longer be able to work or would have greatly decreased strength or mobility. These fears may be heightened if individuals have been involved in taking care of relatives with cancer.

5. *Fear of dying*—Fears about developing cancer are often entangled with fears of death. Thoughts of death naturally become stronger as people age; it is less common for children or young adults to focus on their mortality. Yet this is frequently the case within families with inherited forms of cancer. Fear of death may lead to vigilance about monitoring practices or preventative strategies or, in contrast, may result in a resigned attitude about their probable fate (that is, dying of cancer someday) and unwise risk-taking. Fear of dying may be strongest in those who have watched relatives die from cancer or who are themselves parents of young children.

6. *Grief*—Feelings of grief are common for people at increased risk for cancer. They may grieve for the relatives who have died from cancer, as well as for those who are at risk for developing cancer, including themselves. Some clients have not come to terms with the death of a family member, either because the loss was too sudden or overwhelming, or because family members discouraged discussion of the illness or death. An incomplete grieving process can lead to one of the unresolved grief reactions described in Table 8-2. Unresolved grief reactions can, over time, lead to the development of a chronic sadness that can overshadow all other everyday activities. This has been termed chronic sorrow and is not uncommon in families that have suffered multiple losses due to cancer.

TABLE 8-2. TYPES OF UNRESOLVED GRIEF REACTIONS

Chronic and prolonged grief	Intense grief reactions triggered by events throughout the person's life.
Delayed grief	An initial absence of grief due to numbness or other factors, followed by an intense grief reaction weeks, months or even years later.
Exaggerated grief	An overly excessive grief reaction that can be disabling.
Masked grief	Denied grief that manifests itself as physical or other emotional symptoms.

Source: Burton and Watson, 1998, p. 95–96.

7. *Guilt*—Guilt feelings are often present in people with family histories of cancer. Clients may feel that they could have done more for family members who have developed cancer, especially relatives who have died. Survivor guilt may occur if clients contrast their own good health with relatives who have developed cancer or even their own access to genetic testing or cancer prevention options not previously available to other relatives.

8. *Loss of control*—No one has control over whether or when a malignancy will occur. However, unlike most people, individuals at high risk have reason to believe that cancer is likely to occur in their lives, especially at earlier than usual ages. Living with such uncertainty can lead to feelings of extreme vulnerability. This in turn may cause lowered self-esteem and an inability to cope with day-to-day activities. In an effort to gain back control, some individuals may turn away from the traditional medical community and practice alternative therapies.

9. *Negative body image*—Clients who continually worry about the development of cancer may be less satisfied with their bodies than those who do not have these concerns. Having a negative body image has a direct impact on a person's self-esteem and may also lead to difficulties with interpersonal relationships and sexual satisfaction.

10. *Sadness*—High-risk individuals may live with underlying feelings of sadness or depression. This sadness might be the cumulative effect of the grief, isolation, and helplessness that is experienced by the individual. Clients may also have general feelings of sadness that their families face such trials and tribulations while other families do not.

11. *Sense of isolation*—Individuals who are dealing with fears of cancer and other issues may feel that their concerns are unique from those

of friends, co-workers, or even other cancer survivors. They may feel that no one understands their situation, which only worsens their feelings of isolation. These feelings of isolation may also stem from an inability to describe their situation to others due to uncertainty about medical terminology or a desire to keep such concerns private. Although many support groups exist for patients being treated for cancer and cancer survivors, there are surprisingly few options for high-risk individuals to meet others in similar situations outside of their own families. Some high risk individuals have also expressed frustrations that even their physicians are not taking their cancer concerns seriously enough.

12. *Shame*—Cancer continues to be a condition that can be stigmatizing. Individuals may feel a sense of shame about their family history of cancer, which influences their reactions to being at increased risk themselves. This sense of shame may result in their inability to openly discuss the family cancer history with health care professionals or other family members. In extreme cases, this can lead to decreased self-esteem or even self-loathing.

8.1.2. Past Experiences Color Present Perceptions

... a woman who has had personal experience with breast cancer is more sensitive to the disease. She is not acting irrationally, is not a hypochondriac, and does not have "cancer phobia." Instead she is responding in a rational manner to her own life experience.

(Kelly, 1991, p. 17)

The various emotional responses to cancer risk may be partially explained by the clients' past experiences with cancer. Although high-risk individuals have almost always had some direct experiences with cancer, there are certain aspects that will have the greatest impact on their perceptions of cancer risk.

1. *Proximity of affected relative*—The client's degree of relatedness to a relative with cancer greatly influences the emotional impact of the diagnosis. Thus, cancer diagnosed in a parent or sibling will generally be more emotionally devastating than cancer in an uncle or cousin. Of course, the impact is also influenced by emotional bonds within the family. Clients may feel especially close to a certain family member, so that a diagnosis of cancer in that person will be especially distressing. Cancer in a child, for example, may be particularly devastating to the parents even when the child is an adult. In addition, the geographic proximity of the relative is important to consider. The diagnosis of cancer in a grandparent living in another state has a very

different impact from an affected grandparent who lives in the same house or town. In families with adult-onset cancer syndromes, the first cancer to be diagnosed in the client's generation (for example, sibling or first cousin) may be more anxiety provoking than cancers in older relatives.

2. *Other cancer experiences*—Clients may also be influenced by the diagnoses of cancer in other important people in their lives. For example, a woman who recently inquired about genetic counseling revealed that she was very concerned about developing cancer, not due to her striking family history but because her best friend had recently been diagnosed with uterine cancer. Another female client who carried a *BRCA1* mutation reversed her decision not to have prophylactic mastectomies when a friend's wife died from metastatic breast cancer. A cancer diagnosis in a person who is famous, such as Suzanne Somers (breast cancer) or Katie Couric's husband (colon cancer) can also affect an individual's awareness and perception of the disease.

3. *Timing issues*—There are certain times when clients seem to be acutely affected by their personal experiences with cancer (see Table 8-3). The emotional impact of cancer in a relative is also influenced by the client's age. For example, a child or adolescent may have an especially difficult time dealing with a parent's cancer diagnosis.

4. *Outcome of cancer diagnosis*—Hereditary cancer syndromes have widely variable expression, yet clients tend to define the syndrome by their own families' experiences. For example, clients who relate that all affected relatives have died of their disease are likely to consider the cancer syndrome lethal. Conversely, a client whose affected relatives have lived fairly normal life spans may perceive a cancer diagnosis with greater equanimity.

5. *Family's communication style*—In some families, cancer is openly discussed, whereas in others it is seldom mentioned. In fact, some families try to ignore the occurrences of cancer altogether. Clients in

TABLE 8-3. TIMEPOINTS THAT CAN TRIGGER MEMORIES OF CANCER EXPERIENCES

Any major life transition (i.e., change of jobs, birth of child)
When a relative is newly diagnosed with cancer
The anniversary of the client's cancer diagnosis
The anniversary of a relative's cancer diagnosis or death
When the client approaches the age at which a parent, sibling, or other close relative was diagnosed with or died from cancer
When the client's child approaches the age the client was when a parent, sibling, or other close relative was diagnosed with or died from cancer

---

families with open communication styles may be better at discussing issues regarding inherited risks or testing options.

8.1.3. IMPACT OF CANCER FEARS ON BEHAVIOR

Having a family history of breast cancer impacts on us in many unfortunate ways ... The powerful legacy we've inherited affects our self-esteem, our sexuality, our career choices, our relationships with our husbands and children—virtually every aspect of our lives.

(Baker, 1991, p. 221)

The concerns and fears about impending disease can have an important impact on people's lives. This can influence how clients conduct their daily activities, lifestyle behaviors, medical care practices, and even how they make major life decisions.

1. *Daily activities*—Cancer worries can, at a severe level, interfere with a person's ability to conduct or enjoy normal daily activities. This refers to a person's daily schedule, such as school or work responsibilities, family obligations, and social activities. For example, clients may have difficulty concentrating at school or work or may have less interest in getting together with friends or doing routine tasks. Clients may also complain of altered sleep or eating habits, both of which can impact on daily functioning. Clients who perform their day-to-day activities with undercurrents of cancer worries may feel that it is not a matter of *if* they will develop cancer but *when* they will develop it. Specific events can sometimes trigger anxieties about cancer, such as visiting a friend in the hospital or reading about cancer research in the newspaper. Clients who can discuss their anxieties openly with family members or friends tend to be less affected by their high-risk status in their daily lives.

2. *Lifestyle behaviors*—Clients are generally eager to reduce their cancer risks in any way they can. One way people may be able to reduce their risks of some forms of cancer is through lifestyle changes, such as eating more fruits and vegetables and exercising more frequently. It may also involve avoiding risky behaviors such as smoking or excessive sun exposure or, at the least, moderating such activities. Making lifestyle changes may give clients a greater sense of control despite little (if any) evidence that changing one's lifestyle can substantially alter one's risk of hereditary cancer. This is also an area in which clients may feel guilty that they are not doing all that they could. A certain amount of guilt is acceptable if it helps motivate people; however, too much guilt can be paralyzing.

3. *Medical care practices*—Recommendations about surveillance range from routine clinical examinations to more specialized procedures, such as colonoscopy or magnetic resonance imaging (MRI). Some individuals at high risk will consider all available monitoring tests and prevention strategies, whereas others are less eager to implement any additional medical practices. The differences in attitude can be at least partly explained by their past experiences with cancer and the medical care system. For example, client attitudes may be influenced by whether relatives ultimately survived cancer. The adherence to monitoring practices depends on many other factors as well including the level of concern about developing cancer, faith in the monitoring procedure, logistical issues, and the discomfort involved in the procedure. The range of interest in prophylactic measures, whether prophylactic surgery or chemoprevention, may also be grounded in the client's prior experiences with cancer.

4. *Major life decisions*—High-risk individuals may make major life decisions based on the certainty that they will someday develop cancer. Examples of major life decisions include educational goals, choice of career, and whether to marry and/or have children. In making these decisions, some clients will be only minimally influenced by their high-risk status. However, for others, the fear of developing cancer is a central concern, making it difficult to aspire to long-term career goals, sustain a long-term relationship, or feel comfortable having children.

8.1.4. COPING RESPONSES TO CANCER FEARS

Individuals develop specific coping strategies for dealing with stressors such as their high-risk status. Coping strategies are acquired in response to past problems that have been encountered. Ideally, individuals abandon strategies that did not help and adopt ones that do. However, some individuals continue to use strategies that are not helpful, either because they do not recognize the ineffectiveness of the coping strategy for the particular situation or they feel helpless to change.

Clients may utilize several different coping strategies depending on the current problem or crisis situation. As listed in Table 8-4, coping strategies can be considered "adaptive" or "maladaptive." Adaptive coping strategies are healthy responses to a stressful situation, that is, living in a family with an inherited form of cancer, whereas maladaptive strategies are inappropriate and potentially harmful. The genetic counselor's role might be to reinforce the adaptive strategies that are working for the client and helping the client to recognize and potentially let go of some of the maladaptive strategies.

TABLE 8-4. TYPES OF COPING STRATEGIES ADOPTED BY HIGH-RISK INDIVIDUALS

Adaptive Coping Strategies	Maladaptive Coping Strategies
Accepting responsibility	Anxious preoccupation
Cognitive avoidance	Confrontational
Fighting spirit	Denial
Humor	Displacement
Intellectualism	Distancing
Magical thinking	Escape-avoidance
Planning	Fatalism
Positive reappraisal	Projection
Seeking approval from caregivers	Rationalization
Seeking social support	Regression
Stoic acceptance	Self-controlling

Source: Greer et al., 1979; Watson et al., 1994; and Burton and Watson, 1998, p. 34–42.

This section discusses examples of adaptive and maladaptive strategies. Keep in mind that the lines between adaptive and maladaptive strategies can be blurred. Thus, an adaptive strategy can actually be maladaptive if used in excess. Conversely, a maladaptive strategy may be a reasonable short-term coping mechanism in certain situations.

The following adaptive coping strategies have been observed in high-risk individuals.

1. *Accepting responsibility*—Individuals who seek appointments in high-risk clinics are dealing responsibly with their high-risk status. Thus, they faithfully maintain their surveillance schedules and carefully avoid cancer risks whenever possible. This strategy allows people to feel more in control of their situation.

2. *Cognitive avoidance*—In this strategy, individuals suppress thoughts about the topic that is frightening or overwhelming to them. People frequently utilize this strategy when faced with potentially frightening experiences. For example, some individuals may "forget" that certain relatives have been diagnosed with cancer. Cognitive avoidance may be an appropriate response that allows one the space to avoid thinking about a subject until emotionally ready to handle it. It is important to note that this strategy differs from denial in that the individual is aware of the issue but consciously elects not to think about it.

3. *Fighting spirit*—Watching close relatives die from cancer can act as a powerful motivator to avoid a similar fate. This "fighting spirit" might involve keeping careful vigilance to screening or continually

searching for better strategies for cancer prevention or early detection. In some cases, individuals might even decide to become cancer researchers themselves or to advocate on behalf of cancer causes.

4. *Humor*—Individuals may utilize dark humor to help them cope with their series of adverse experiences. As one client joked, "We don't call them funerals anymore, we call them family reunions." The ability to speak humorously about cancer and one's own high-risk status can be a valuable coping strategy. Clients may also interject jokes or sarcasm into the genetic counseling session to relieve their rising anxiety or tension.

5. *Intellectualism*—Some clients feel that the key to controlling their cancer fears is to learn all the information they can. For these individuals, the standard discussion of risk estimates is inadequate; they will want to know how these figures were derived and may insist on seeing the journal citations. In fact, they may come to the counseling session with printouts from various internet sites. This thirst for information is generally a helpful coping strategy because it can lead to high adherence to screening protocols. However, over-intellectualism can be problematic because it implies that the person knows all the facts but is not acknowledging any emotional impact.

6. *Magical thinking*—Superstitious beliefs are common among people at increased risk of cancer. Clients may demonstrate magical thinking in describing why they perceive their risks to be significantly higher or lower than their actual risks. For example, "I know I'll get breast cancer like my mother because I look just like her." This coping strategy may be employed to make sense out of a series of frightening experiences.

7. *Planning*—Some individuals deal with their high risk status by focusing on the logistics of scheduling physician appointments and monitoring tests. The focus on planning may help clients feel more in control of their situation. Clients who undergo genetic testing are likely to have plans for what they might do once they know their test results and may even have made plans for when or if they are diagnosed with cancer. For example, parents may spend time figuring out how their children would get to and from school in the event of a cancer diagnosis.

8. *Positive reappraisal*—Certain individuals find that their experiences with cancer have altered their lives in a positive way. Their high-risk status may make them appreciate how precious life is, allow them to enjoy what they have, and truly value the people around them. This is similar to what many cancer patients have described as a positive outcome of having cancer.

9. *Seeking approval from caregivers*—High-risk individuals may be "model patients," carefully following all suggestions set forth by

their health care providers. This attitude may be viewed as prudent given their cancer risks but might also reflect a need to obtain approval from their caregivers. This is generally a useful coping strategy because it increases compliance with screening guidelines but can exacerbate feelings of dependence and vulnerability, which can be maladaptive if carried to an extreme.

10. *Seeking social support*—Some high-risk individuals surround themselves with a strong network of relatives and friends in addition to a spouse or partner. They might speak of being especially close to family members because of the tragedies they have shared. Because of the losses a client has experienced, he or she may have a heightened need to be loved. Clients might also be subconsciously planning for when they are diagnosed with cancer and will need family members and friends to help them. Individuals may also seek support outside of their circle of family or friends by joining support or advocacy groups.

11. *Stoic acceptance*—Over time, clients may view their risks with a greater degree of acceptance. This implies that they have incorporated the information about their risks into their lives, but have not let the increased risks monopolize their lives.

The following maladaptive (potentially harmful) coping strategies have been observed in some high-risk individuals.

1. *Anxious preoccupation*—Some clients seem to define themselves by their high-risk status. They are obsessed with their risks of cancer and spend enormous amounts of time and energy worrying about minor physical symptoms and the possibility they will develop cancer. These activities, when done in excess, can interfere with daily activities and may also lead to panic attacks or depression. This coping style might also lead to excessive physician visits or to even a sense of disappointment if the counselor does not confirm that they are at high-risk.

2. *Confrontational*—High-risk individuals may decide that the only way for them to get appropriate care is to "fight" their way through the medical system. Such clients will berate staff members scheduling appointments, make frequent demands on health care providers, and argue with information and options presented to them. Although it can be unpleasant dealing with clients who are confrontational or combative, it is important to keep in mind that their underlying motivation is typically fear.

3. *Denial*—Denial is the process of suppressing an unpleasant or unwanted piece of information. Clients who are acutely frightened about developing cancer may ignore or refute any statements suggesting they are at risk. True denial occurs at an unconscious level,

so that clients may not recognize why they are becoming uneasy by the genetic counseling discussion. Manifestations of denial include nondisclosure of information (such as not mentioning all their relatives with cancer when asked about the family history) and opinions as to why certain information is not relevant. For example, "Yes, both my uncles had kidney cancer, but I'm sure it was because they both worked in the same factory."

It is important to realize that a certain level of denial can be a helpful coping strategy (see *Cognitive avoidance* above). For some people, stating that cancer "can't happen to me" is simply an expression of optimism or hope. Such statements may allow clients to proceed through their daily activities and participate in cancer surveillance programs with a modicum of fear. However, maladaptive denial can prevent people from taking action about their cancer risks, because they literally do not see themselves at risk. These clients will not participate in early detection programs, are unlikely to seek out genetic counseling, and may even ignore initial symptoms suggestive of cancer.

4. *Displacement*—In displacement, feelings toward one person (or situation) are directed toward another individual. This is a situation commonly experienced in genetic counseling. Clients who are angry or distressed by their increased cancer risks may direct these emotions toward a particular relative or health care provider. Another instance of displacement is when clients badger relatives to undergo certain monitoring tests but "forget" to make the same appointments for themselves.

5. *Distancing*—Individuals who have experienced a great amount of loss in their lives may utilize a strategy termed distancing, which allows them to remain detached from other people. Clients may utilize this strategy to shield themselves from caring too much about the people around them and from feeling the pain of their many losses. Distancing may make it difficult for people to maintain romantic relationships or relationships with family members, or friends.

6. *Escape-avoidance*—This strategy is used to avoid dealing with unpleasant situations, which might include discussions of cancer risk. Clients employing escape-avoidance tactics might continually interrupt the conversation with amusing anecdotes or questions that are unrelated to the topic. They may also be less likely to make medical appointments or may go through several cycles of setting-up and canceling appointments.

7. *Fatalism*—High-risk individuals may hold fatalistic views about their chances of developing (and dying from) cancer. They may

believe that they are destined to develop cancer regardless of what they do and thus may engage in risky behaviors such as smoking or excessive drinking. Individuals with fatalistic attitudes may also be less interested in pursuing genetic testing or risk-reduction options.

8. *Projection*—Projection may be occurring when individuals ascribe one of their own undesirable traits or feelings to another person. This strategy allows clients to distance themselves from issues that are difficult or overwhelming. For example, clients who are extremely anxious or agitated during the counseling session may project these feelings onto the counselor.

9. *Rationalization*—Rationalization describes the process of giving hypothetically plausible explanations for a specific action, although the real reason for the behavior is to avoid facing an unpleasant reality. Clients may use multiple excuses to explain why they did not schedule appointments that are emotionally difficult or screening tests that are physically uncomfortable. For example, clients may state that they do not want to undergo genetic testing because it is too expensive, but when insurance coverage is obtained, they will provide another reason why they cannot be tested.

10. *Regression*—High-risk individuals may revert to the helpless, dependent behavior typical of childhood. This type of behavior can sometimes be observed in individuals who are newly diagnosed with cancer or those who are highly anxious about developing cancer. For example, "I need to schedule my appointment when my older sister can come with me, because I don't think I can drive to the medical center by myself."

11. *Self controlling*—Individuals with this personality type do not just seek to control themselves but also their environment. This includes anyone with whom they come in contact. Thus, there can be a variety of difficult client-provider interactions, from scheduling appointments on their timetable to writing summary letters to their satisfaction. The interest in control may be an attempt to reduce feelings of vulnerability or helplessness. Unfortunately, self-controlling individuals may experience difficulties maintaining both personal and professional relationships.

8.2. Psychological Assessment

. . . the genetic counselor must work with individuals who face life events with the full range of personalities and experiences and who come from a great diversity of social and cultural milieus. From this diversity of human experience and resources, the genetic counselor must attempt to identify the counselee's strengths and weaknesses, hopes, fears and anxieties in order to craft helpful responses . . . For this reason, there is a professional obligation to probe more deeply into the counselee's thoughts, feelings, and behavior than is consistent with ordinary social interactions.

(Weil, 2000, pp. 1–2)

Assessment of a client's psychological well-being is an integral part of the cancer genetic counseling session. Diagnosing depression or anxiety disorders requires psychological training beyond that of the average genetic counselor and should not be attempted. However, genetic counselors can become adept at identifying clients who are in need of further psychological assessment or intervention. This section describes how to assess the relevant psychosocial features and suggests potentially useful counseling techniques to utilize during the genetic counseling session.

8.2.1. Psychological Features to Assess

A client's psychological profile may affect the understanding of the genetic counseling discussion. If clients do not volunteer information about their emotional well-being, counselors may need to ask directed questions. Sample questions are listed in Table 8-5. This section discusses the five general areas to assess:

1. *Current emotional well-being*—Being at increased risk can lead to a range of emotional problems and can, in extreme cases, impact all facets of people's lives, including daily functioning. Clients may also have other stress factors in their lives that are affecting their emotional well-being, such as marital or job-related problems. It may be helpful

TABLE 8-5. Potential Psychological Assessment Questions to Ask

Current Emotional Well-Being

Over the past few weeks, have you had any problems sleeping?
Have you had any change of appetite?
In the past few weeks, have you felt unusually anxious about anything?
In the past few weeks, have you felt sad or depressed?
Are you crying more easily or more often?
Are you having a harder time getting things done at home or at work?
Do you feel that your worries about cancer affect how well you are able to concentrate?
Do you feel that your worries about cancer affect your relationships with your partner or family?
Do you ever feel hopeless when thinking about your life or future?

Continued

TABLE 8-5. *Continued*

Mental Health History

Are you currently seeing a psychologist or therapist? If yes, how often?
Have you ever met with a psychologist or therapist? If yes, how recently was this?
What led you to meet with a therapist?
Have you ever been told you have clinical depression or anxiety?
Are you currently taking or have you ever taken any medications for psychological
  reasons?
Have you ever tried to commit suicide? Have you ever seriously thought about
  committing suicide?
Is there anything stressful going on in your life right now?

Emotional Response to Family History of Cancer

How often do you think about your cancer risk?
Do you worry about getting cancer?
What worries you the most? Are there specific times when you are more worried?
What do you usually do when you are worried (or upset, angry, etc.)?
How close were you to your relative(s) who had cancer?
Whose cancer experience affected you the most? In what way?
How do you think these experiences have affected you?

Coping Strategies

Is taking a positive attitude something that is difficult or easy for you?
It's not unusual to feel overwhelmed and helpless about being at risk for cancer.
  How do you feel?
Some people feel they want to leave everything to their doctor. Is that how you
  feel?
It sounds like you've been seeking a lot of information about your cancer risks.
Has this helped or do you think it makes you worry more?
Are you the sort of person who tends to accept things as they are or do you
  question what goes on?
Some people find it helps to avoid thinking about their risks of cancer. Are you
  that sort of person?
When you are feeling worried, what do you usually do to feel better?
What strategies seem to work the best for you? Why do you think that is?
Do these strategies make you feel better right away? How about over time?
Who can you talk to about these worries?

Reactions During Counseling Session

How are you feeling about the information we have covered so far?
Is the information I am telling you what you expected to hear? Why or why not?
Is it difficult discussing these issues? Why or why not?
You seem to be worried about something. Did I say something that upset you?

to assess symptoms of depression and anxiety by asking about eating and sleeping habits and recent levels of sadness and hopelessness.

2. *Mental health history*—Asking general questions about the client's mental health history can be a helpful indicator of his/her emotional well-being and attitudes toward psychological counseling. This dialogue gives the client the opportunity to discuss previous psychological encounters and to acknowledge on-going stressors. This helps the counselor better predict how pursuing genetic testing could affect the client's emotional well-being and can pave the way for suggesting that the client meet with a mental health professional. Counselors should ask direct questions about previous episodes of depression or anxiety and any past therapeutic interventions. It might be reassuring, for example, to learn that a client who appears depressed or distraught is already in an on-going therapeutic relationship, although contacting the mental health professional may be advisable if concerns about the client's emotional state are raised during the session. It is also important to ask a few questions about suicidal feelings, intentions, plans or previous attempts. Asking questions about the client's mental health history can be incorporated into a routine series of questions asked of everyone or asked only when concerned about a specific client's emotional well-being.

3. *Emotional response to family history of cancer*—High-risk clients typically have one or more close family members who have been diagnosed with (and perhaps died from) cancer. Clients need to understand the significance of their family history from a genetic standpoint; however, the psychological impact of the cancer history is also important. When collecting medical histories about affected family members, counselors should also ask about the emotional impact of these illnesses or experiences on the clients themselves. Clients at increased risk of cancer should be asked about what their high-risk status means to them. This includes determining the clients' levels of fear and exploring the aspects of their situation that concerns them the most. Some clients will be eager to discuss their emotions and reactions to the cancer in their family, and others will remain reticent. Clients should not feel compelled to discuss their feelings about their cancer risks, but it may be helpful to state that many people find it difficult to talk about these issues. Simply raising the topic may make it easier to generate discussion at a later point.

4. *Coping strategies*—Clients will have developed various ways of coping with the possibility that they might someday develop cancer (refer to Section 8.1.3). Four categories of coping styles are listed in Table 8-6. These coping styles may become evident during the course of the genetic counseling session. Other ways of categorizing coping styles

TABLE 8-6. FOUR CATEGORIES OF COPING STYLES

Emotional strategies	Venting feelings; crying
Interpersonal strategies	Talking with friends; joining a support group
Cognitive strategies	Taking control of one's life; researching the disorder
Action strategies	Keeping busy with other activities

Source: Hainseworth et al., 1994; Hobdell and Deatrick, 1996.

include "information-seekers versus avoiders", "monitors versus blunters", and "task-focused versus emotion-focused problem solvers." It may also be useful to ask clients about how well or poorly their various coping strategies have worked in the past. In addition to these coping strategies, clients might also have strong religious or spiritual beliefs that gives them emotional strength.

It is important to note that a particular coping strategy is not defined by a specific emotion experienced; rather, the emotion will trigger one of the person's coping strategies. For example, a fear reaction to the information presented can invoke quite different responses from abruptly changing the subject to making a joke. It is important to be aware of the influence of the person's coping strategies on the counseling interaction.

5. *Reactions during counseling*—Counseling sessions about cancer typically include discussions about family history of cancer and estimates of cancer risks; both of which can engender feelings of fear, depression, guilt, or vulnerability. Counselors need to continually assess their clients' emotional responses to the information being presented. If clients appear upset or confused, it is important to discover which aspect of the conversation is causing this reaction. Clients also need to feel comfortable admitting and communicating their feelings throughout the counseling session. It is also useful to ask clients how they anticipate the information helping them and how they are prepared to cope with the information.

During a typical cancer risk counseling session, genetic counselors are expected to cover tremendous amounts of information. It may therefore seem daunting to consider how to also monitor the client's emotional well-being during the session. Yet, with experience, this type of assessment can be easily incorporated. As examples, assessment of the factors listed below can provide insight into the psychological well-being of a client during a counseling session:

1. *General appearance*—Two aspects of appearance to consider are grooming and motor activity (that is, whether clients appear quiet or agitated). For example, clients who are poorly groomed may be

exhibiting signs of depression, whereas constant fidgeting may signal anxiety.

2. *Attention and concentration*—Levels of anxiety and depression can be evaluated, in part, by the client's level of attentiveness and concentration. Counselors can also assess whether the client's answers seem appropriate and provide evidence of clear or logical thought. Lack of attention, poor concentration and erratic answers may be indicators of preoccupation, anxiety, depression, or even psychosis.

3. *Mood*—Mood can be defined as a pervasive, sustained behavior. For example, a person's mood may be described as depressed, anxious, euphoric, or neutral. Almost everyone experiences upward or downward mood swings, but it may be useful to determine whether the client's apparent mood is uncharacteristic or of long-duration.

4. *Affect*—Affect refers to immediately expressed emotional responses to a specific situation. It is particularly important to assess the appropriateness, intensity, and duration of a person's emotional responses given the situation. Examples of affect include sadness, anger, or fear.

8.2.2. COUNSELING TECHNIQUES TO USE DURING SESSION

Counseling is not about listening to and tut-tutting about the other's adversities. It is basically about understanding the other person and providing appropriate help in the form of how to think about and work through life problems.
(Kessler, 2000, p. 139)

The educational aspects of cancer genetic counseling should not be separated from the client's psychological issues and potential impact of the information discussed in the session. This section offers suggestions for attending to the psychological needs of clients during a cancer counseling session. Counselors need to identify the techniques they are comfortable using, recognizing that the same strategies will not work with every client.

1. *Set "counseling" goals*—Cancer genetic counseling has two sets of goals; the informational goals and the counseling goals. The counseling model set forth by Dr. Seymour Kessler provides a framework of the "counseling" goals in a genetic counseling interaction (see Table 8-7). Cancer risk counselors should consider these goals during each client encounter.

2. *Convey empathy*—Empathy can be defined as having an unconditional positive regard for one's clients. Establishing empathetic attunement is a necessary foundation for successful client-counselor interactions. To convey empathy, the counselor should listen carefully to the client's story and assess the client's affective state as the

TABLE 8-7. "Counseling" Goals of a Genetic Counseling Session

To understand the other person
To bolster their inner sense of control over their lives
To promote a greater sense of control over their lives
To relieve psychological distress, if possible
To support and possibly raise their self-esteem
To help them find solutions to specific problems

Source: Kessler, 2000, p. 137.

story unfolds. Counselors can convey empathy by their facial expressions and posture and in the way they frame responses and follow-up questions. It is important to recognize the difference between sympathetic and empathetic responses. Sympathetic reactions derive from our own perspective or responses, whereas empathy involves appreciating the client's responses to the story. As Luba Djurdinovic, a certified genetic counselor advises, "Don't break down defenses, melt them with empathetic responses." The use of empathy can help clients to

- make sense of what has happened in the family,
- accept any dilemmas and ambivalence surrounding the core issue,
- appreciate the significance of the problems they have experienced, and
- formulate options and solutions.

3. *Ask direct questions*—Clients will come to the genetic counseling session with different cancer experiences and a variety of coping styles. It should not be assumed that all high-risk individuals are anxious about developing cancer or are motivated by similar factors. Asking questions about the client's emotional well-being should be a routine part of cancer counseling sessions (refer to Table 8-5). The extent to which these issues need to be explored varies according to client needs. However, counselors should refrain from asking questions that are emotionally-laden, value-laden, or confrontational. For example, asking clients "You were told to have a colonoscopy last year, so why didn't you make an appointment?" is likely to lead to defensive responses. A better strategy is to say, "Let's talk now about the colonoscopy exam. I see that you had it done two years ago. What was your experience like?" This introduces the topic in a way that allows clients to describe their previous experiences and explore possible barriers to continued screening.

4. *Stay attuned to verbal and nonverbal cues*—Throughout the counseling session, pay attention to the client's linguistic, paralinguistic, and nonverbal cues. Linguistic cues includes the client's vocabulary and specific questions asked. One technique is to adopt the language or word choices that the client uses and monitor the discussion's level of sophistication. For example, describing the carcinogenic process in detail will confuse the average client as much as simplistic analogies will annoy those with backgrounds in science. Counselors can also strive to match clients' paralinguistic cues, such as the volume, tone, and timing of their responses. Also important are the nonverbal aspects of conversation, including facial expressions, gestures, body position, and eye contact.

5. *Allow clients to express emotions*—The client's high-risk status or the genetic counseling session itself can engender a variety of emotions in clients. It is important to allow and encourage clients to freely express their emotions. It may be tempting to change the subject if the topic becomes too emotionally charged, but continued discussion on the topic or a few moments of empathetic silence can be much more effective. Then, when appropriate, the genetic counselor can guide the conversation back to the topic being discussed.

6. *Maintain inter-personal boundaries*—Respecting and maintaining appropriate inter-personal boundaries with clients are important parts of the counselor-client relationship. Some clients will freely discuss their fears and anxieties, whereas others will be much less forthcoming. It may be that the topic is much too powerful or intensely private for them to discuss. By their use of verbal and non-verbal cues, clients will indicate when their boundaries have been reached and it is important to respect them. Although the counselor may feel that it would be helpful for a client to "talk it out," a wiser course of action may be to respect the client's boundaries. The genetic counselor should use his/her judgment to decide whether or not to reintroduce certain topics at a later time. It is also important for counselors to recognize and respect their own boundaries. Counselors should not feel obligated to answer personal questions about themselves and should not, as a rule, accept any social invitations from clients.

7. *Discuss client reactions*—Counselors should continually assess whether the topics under discussion are overwhelming, disturbing, or distressing. Client's reactions to the information discussed in the counseling session will be influenced by their different coping styles. Some clients may ignore or refute any information regarding increased cancer risks, and others may concentrate on facts and figures as a way of avoiding the emotional implications of their

situation. Still other clients will focus on the cancer risks of other relatives because it is less threatening than thinking about their own risks. In any of these situations, the counselor may find it useful to halt the discussion and address the client's particular reaction. Sometimes, simply acknowledging the client's reaction is helpful in starting a dialogue about these issues.

8. *Ascertain the rationale behind client questions*—Clients are encouraged to ask questions during genetic counseling sessions, yet some questions are focused on issues that seem trivial or irrelevant. For example, the client who spends time discussing whether the BRCA2-related ovarian cancer risk is really closer to 10% or 20%. In these situations, determining the reasoning behind the questions may be more important than continuing the discussion. To know how best to respond, counselors may find it useful to determine why the questions have been asked, what kind of answers clients hope to receive, and how clients feel the information is relevant to their particular situation.

Counselors also need to be sensitive to the fact that clients' cultural or religious belief systems may influence how they and their families perceive the causes of health and illness.

9. *Provide information in general terms*—Discussions about risks and surveillance options may be less threatening to clients if couched in more general terms. Counselors can then proceed from the general discussion to more specific and personal topics. This can then be followed by statements more specific to the client's own situation. For clients who express more concern about the risks of other relatives, it may be useful to explore how they perceive their relatives' situations to be similar or different from their own. This line of discussion may also lead to a more detailed discussion about how clients view their own risk.

10. *Remain professional*—Counselors should maintain an empathetic yet professional demeanor even when faced with intense grief or anger. Welling up with tears in response to a sad story is a human emotion—and cancer counseling is chock full of sad stories. However, crying in front of clients may make it difficult to regain focus of the discussion and may not be of constructive help to clients who already know how tragic their circumstances are. (But debriefing afterward with caring colleagues is a must!) When dealing with anger, the first impulse may be to defend the source of the anger, whether it is the hospital protocol, staff members, or the medical profession in general. However, this tactic will only further entangle the counselor in the conflict and can result in escalating anger on the part of the client. A better strategy would be to allow the client to

vent for a short time, acknowledge their anger (which is different from agreeing with it), and then shift the discussion to the present situation and where to go from here. By doing this, the counselor is more likely to be perceived as an ally not an adversary.

11. *Explore timing issues*—It is useful to ask about important anniversary dates surrounding cancer diagnoses and deaths. It may also be helpful to learn about other previous losses or traumas as well as what is going on in the client's life at present. Some clients will be aware of the connection between previous events and their current emotional status or reactions, whereas others will be less conscious of it.

12. *Recognize one's own reactions*—The provision of cancer risk counseling can be emotionally draining. Genetic counselors may become overly distressed by particular cases or may find themselves unable to provide needed support to clients (burn out). Counselors need to monitor their own emotional well-being and recognize when they need to take a "mental health break." Counselors should also pay attention to whether certain types of cases are more emotionally charged than others and explore possible reasons for this. Perhaps there are features about the client's situation that have particularly resonated with the counselor. Some cases may trigger the counselor's own fears about illness or death. For example, counselors who have had cancer themselves or have had relatives or friends diagnosed with cancer may have intensified reactions to encounters with newly diagnosed or terminally ill cancer patients. It is important for cancer genetic counselors to have a network of empathetic colleagues. Participating in a genetic counseling supervision group can also provide a useful and supportive forum to discuss these types of issues.

13. *Be prepared for clients to ask "What would you do?"*—Occasionally, a client will ask for the counselor's personal opinion about a follow-up option. There are several ways to respond to this type of inquiry and different approaches may be appropriate in different counseling scenarios (for example, decisions about genetic testing versus adherence to standard monitoring). In general, the counselor should acknowledge the question, provide some type of response that does not make the client feel as though the question was inappropriate, and steer the conversation back to the topic under discussion. The counselor should be careful to respond in a way that is not "distancing" from the client, but is also not overly personalized to the counselor's situation or thought process. In summary, an effective response from the genetic counselor should further the discussion, not end it.

As an example, a client may ask, "If it were you, would you have genetic testing?" Possible responses include the following:

- An acknowledgement—"You know, that is a really good question and after all this time I am still not sure what I would do, because I haven't been faced with the decision personally like you are at this time. What I can do is describe the testing process in a little more detail and then we can talk more about whether or not testing might be helpful to you—how does that sound?"

- A general response—"Some people in your situation do decide to be tested and others decide not to be tested. We find that people make very different choices and what works for one person may not work for another. What are your thoughts about being tested?"

- A pros and cons approach—"Some people decide to be tested because they feel the result would help them make medical decisions. Others feel there is no medical benefit to having this information and choose not to be tested. When you think of being tested, what do you see as the advantages and disadvantages?"

- A focus on process—"If it were me, I'd be asking myself questions like: What would I gain from the information? Is this the right time to be tested? How would my family feel about me being tested? Let's discuss which of these questions seems most relevant to you as you are making this decision."

- A reflective response—(a) "If I were you, I'd probably hold off on being tested for awhile. You were diagnosed with cancer so recently and from everything you've told me over the last half hour, regarding your treatments and the problems with your marriage, it sounds like you have enough to deal with right now. Does this describe how you're feeling or am I way off base?" OR (b) "If I were you, I guess I'd consider proceeding with the test. From what I have heard you say in the last half hour, it sounds as though you are ready to learn your genetic test results. You have a sense of how this might impact you and realize that, although it could be difficult for your father, you are prepared to talk with him about the results. Does this describe how you are thinking about this decision or are there other important factors that I've left out?"

- A self-disclosing response—(a) "I would probably choose to get tested. But remember, I'm in the genetics field and I also haven't had the experiences with cancer that you and your family have had. Your choice may be very different than mine. As you think about being tested, what do you see as the important issues to consider?" OR (b) "I would probably choose not to get tested, but then I don't have reason to believe that my family has an alteration in this gene. Families differ in the kinds of health problems they need to be concerned about and they may hold different views about genetic testing. Let's talk about how to help you make the testing decision that is right for you and your family."

8.2.3. THE USE OF GENOGRAMS

Family evolution is like a musical composition, in which the meaning of individual notes depends on their rhythmic and harmonic relationship with each other and with the memories of past melodies, as well as those anticipated but not yet written.

(McGoldrick and Gerson, and Shellenberger, 1999, p. 125)

Genograms are a way of organizing and analyzing families by use of a family systems approach. Family systems therapists believe that chronic diseases or other stressors can affect the entire family system. Individuals are organized within a family structure by generation, age, and gender and these placements, as well as prior and current family events, can affect how the person functions and makes decisions. Family systems therapists further contend that there is a connection between the level of family functioning and the physical and emotional well-being of each family member. A diagnosis of cancer in an individual family member will therefore disrupt the family's ability to function in the short term and may have long-term ramifications as well. Genograms can be used as a tool to specifically look at the emotional impact of having close relatives diagnosed with cancer and assess the family's overall supportiveness and communication style, and to look for any repetitive patterns of behavior in the family. A genogram is constructed from the genetic pedigree by jotting down additional facts next to the family member's pedigree symbol and drawing the appropriate relationship lines between each family member. Consider the following example.

The client, Susan, is a 25-year-old graduate student in law school. She lives alone but is engaged to be married. Her main reason for seeking genetic counseling is to learn if her future offspring could have increased risks of cancer. Susan reports having a close relationship with her fiancé but maintains little contact with her parents and has a contentious relationship with her sister, Lisa. Susan reports somewhat bitterly that Lisa has a solid relationship with both parents and that their mother continues to smother Lisa with attention and concern. Susan was 7 years old when her younger sister was diagnosed with cancer and she has vivid memories of the impact this diagnosis had on the household. In contrast, her father's cancer diagnosis last year seems to have had little impact on her. A genogram depicting this family information is shown in Figure 8-1.

Genograms can take as little as 15 minutes to construct if kept to a narrow focus; sample questions for a cancer counseling session are listed in Table 8-8. Obtain the following types of information when constructing a genogram:

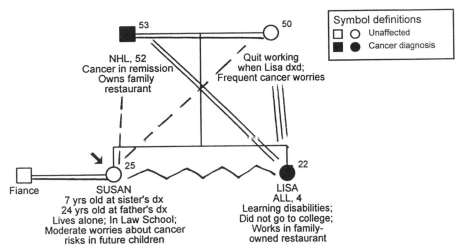

FIGURE 8-1. Genogram of a nuclear family. See accompanying text for details of case and Figure 8-2 for a review of the relationship lines. NHL = non-Hodgkin's lymphoma; ALL = acute lymphoblastic leukemia.

1. *Demographic data*—This is information that is typically collected during the construction of the pedigree, such as the current age or age at death, dates of birth and death, and cancer status for each close relative. The cancer status of key non-relatives, such as in-laws or friends, may also be important information to include. The counselor may also wish to inquire about the client's level of education and current or past occupation.

2. *Functioning level*—This relates to how well the person is functioning in life, from physical limitations or prowess to emotional problems and inner strength. The counselor should ask about family members' responses to being at high risk, both emotionally and in terms of their cancer monitoring practices.

3. *Critical family events*—These events may overlap with the demographic data collected but typically includes more detailed information. For purposes of cancer counseling, it would be important to learn how each cancer diagnosis or death impacted the client. To do this, it is important to ascertain how old the client was at that time because a person's stage of emotional and cognitive development will influence the overall impact of the event. It is also useful to ask about crucial dates to assess potential reactions to an anniversary that may be driving decisions. It may also be helpful to document separations, divorces, major moves, losses, or successes and learn how each family member dealt with these life events.

TABLE 8-8. SAMPLE QUESTIONS TO ASK WHEN ASSEMBLING A GENOGRAM, FOCUSING ON CANCER EXPERIENCE AND CURRENT STRESSORS.

Who lives in your household?

Of the people you have listed, who do you feel
  especially close to?
  distant or in conflict with?
  overly dependent on?

Who helps out when help is needed? In whom do family members confide?

Now I would like to ask a few questions about your relatives who have had cancer:
  When was your relative diagnosed with cancer? How old was your relative at that time?
  How old were you when your relative was diagnosed with cancer?
  How old were you when your relative died from cancer?
  What did you understand about the diagnosis?
  How involved were you in the care of your relative?
  How much did this relative's cancer diagnosis impact you?

How did the family react when a particular family member died? Who took it the hardest? The easiest?

Have there recently been any major changes in your life?

Are there any other major events or changes going on in your life right now?

Are you thinking about making any major changes in your life?

How often do you drink alcohol? Do you take any recreational drugs?

Do you smoke cigarettes? How many cigarettes do you smoke a day?

How stressful would you say your life is right now? What do you think are the factors contributing to your level of stress?

Source: McGoldrick et al., 1999.

4. *Family relationships*—Family relationships among family members are illustrated by specific types of lines drawn between two family members (as shown in Fig. 8-2). This indicates how communicative and supportive family members are to one another.

5. *Current stressors*—This includes major problems or changes that are contributing to the stress level in the client's life or the family unit. It may also pinpoint stressors that are influencing the client's attitudes about cancer surveillance and prevention strategies.

Genograms can be incorporated into the genetic counseling discussion or done afterward as a way of conceptualizing family issues. Most clients appreciate the opportunity to talk more about themselves and their families,

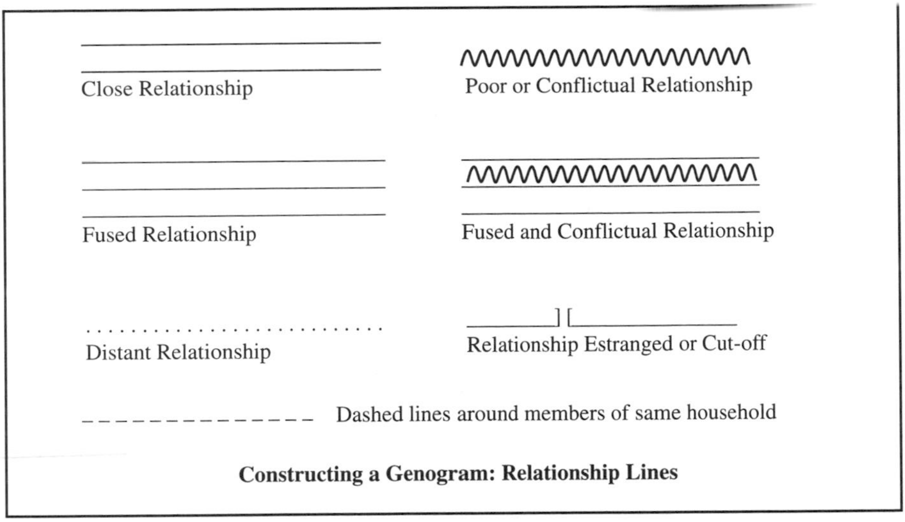

————————	∿∿∿∿∿∿∿∿∿∿∿
Close Relationship	Poor or Conflictual Relationship
═══════════════	∿∿∿∿∿∿∿∿∿∿∿
Fused Relationship	Fused and Conflictual Relationship
· · · · · · · · · · · · · · · · · · ·	——————] [——————
Distant Relationship	Relationship Estranged or Cut-off

– – – – – – – – – – – – – Dashed lines around members of same household

Constructing a Genogram: Relationship Lines

FIGURE 8-2. Genogram Constructing a genogram: relationship lines. [Source: McGoldrick et al., 1999, p. 30]

and the discussion can strengthen the counselor-client bond. This discussion might also uncover issues that would benefit from more in-depth psychological counseling.

8.3. MENTAL HEALTH REFERRALS

For some individuals, it will be sufficient to explore psychosocial issues within the genetic counseling session; others will be in need of more in-depth psychological counseling and should be referred appropriately.

8.3.1. WHEN TO MAKE A MENTAL HEALTH REFERRAL

Some individuals will want to meet with a mental health professional to discuss strategies for dealing with any of the issues that could arise around their at-risk status, such as fears about screening appointments, distress about a genetic test result, family communication problems, or impending decisions about prophylactic surgery. A few clients may have reached a "crisis point" in their lives and could benefit from short-term counseling to help them through a difficult time. Still others may need counseling on a long-term basis to help resolve issues surrounding their experiences with cancer, delayed grief reactions or general unhappiness about life. Although most high-risk clients would benefit from at least one meeting with a mental health professional, few cancer risk programs routinely provide this service. It is therefore important for genetic counselors to recognize clients who are in need of psychological support or intervention. Counselors should have a strategy for how to assess the client's level of distress and how to determine the source of the distress (that is, is it related to the cancer history or due to other life events). Psychological counseling services should be offered to clients who appear to have high levels of anxiety or depression regarding their cancer risks, have adopted poor coping responses to their risks, or seem to be having significant difficulties in other aspects of their lives. Table 8-9 lists examples of situations that would warrant psychological referrals.

In general, genetic counselors should refer any client whom they do not feel comfortable handling. Clients may not openly disclose their distress, so it is also important to pay attention to common warning signs of psychological distress (see Table 8-10). Even well-functioning clients may wish to talk in greater depth with someone outside their family about their risk status or cancer experiences. Cancer genetic counselors should have a system of referral in place so that they are not scrambling to identify a mental health provider when the need arises. Counselors would also benefit from having consultations with mental health providers regarding difficult cases and decisions about referral.

TABLE 8-9. CLIENTS WHO SHOULD BE OFFERED REFERRALS FOR PSYCHOLOGICAL COUNSELING

Clients who become particularly distraught during the genetic counseling session.
Clients who express extreme or constant anxiety at the thought of developing cancer.
Clients who verbalize thoughts of suicide or violence.
Clients who need to discuss psychological issues at greater depth than you can handle.
Clients who have no one to share their concerns about cancer.
Clients with cancer worries that interfere with enjoyment of daily activities.
Clients with cancer worries that interfere in their work or personal lives.
Clients who express great dissatisfaction with other aspects of their lives.
Clients who appear to have converted psychological distress into physical ailments.
Clients who are experiencing major disruptions in eating or sleeping patterns.
Clients with exacerbated fears of cancer due to recent transitions in their lives.
Clients who appear to have signs of major depression whether or not related to cancer.
Clients who seem to have unresolved feelings about the death of a relative.
Clients who seem to have difficulty differentiating themselves from a relative with cancer.

TABLE 8-10. Possible Warning Signs of Psychological Distress

> Increased sleep disturbances
> Less energy or effectiveness at completing tasks
> Changed eating habits
> Crying more easily or more often
> Increased irritability
> Decreased enjoyment in activities
> Increased feelings of hopelessness

8.3.2. How to Make a Mental Health Referral

All cancer genetic counselors should establish alliances with mental health professionals who can suggest strategies for dealing with psychosocial issues, review challenging cases, and assist in the referral process as needed. Ideally, the mental health professional will have experience with families dealing with chronic or acute illnesses and will possess fundamental knowledge about the inheritance pattern and cancer risks associated with hereditary cancer syndromes.

Suggesting that the client seek further psychological counseling can be raised in the genetic counseling session or during a follow-up interaction. Obviously, the discussion needs to be handled with sensitivity and tact, and it is not unusual for the suggestion to be ignored the first time it is mentioned. After ascertaining that the client is interested in meeting with a mental health provider, the actual referral can be accomplished by either contacting the mental health provider and asking him or her to call the client directly or providing the client with the provider's telephone number and encouraging him or her to call and make an appointment.

When making a referral, it is important to consider what type of mental health provider would most benefit the client. Possible mental health providers include psychiatrists, psychologists, social workers, family therapists, and grief counselors. Other factors that may be important in making a referral include geographic location, gender preferences, and coverage by the client's health insurance. Client may need mental health referrals from their primary physicians, especially if they are in health maintenance organizations.

8.3.3. A Few Words about Support Groups

No matter how caring and supportive health care professionals are, they cannot match the benefits of speaking to people who have been through it themselves. Support groups, if available, can be a valuable way for people to connect with others in similar situations. As shown in Table 8-11, support group organizations exist for several of the hereditary cancer syndromes. These organizations can provide a wealth of support and resources to families.

Just as prenatal genetic counselors saw a need for support groups to help people cope with genetic terminations, cancer genetic counselors have begun to set up support groups specifically for people at high risk for cancer. In establishing such a group, there are several issues that should be considered.

1. *Leader*(s)—Support groups can be peer-led or facilitated by one or two health care providers. Groups led by two co-leaders work especially well because one person can moderate the discussion while the other tracks group dynamics. Genetic counselors may benefit from coleading a group with a mental health professional or cancer survivor. At least one of the co-leaders should be trained and/or experienced in facilitating a support group.

2. *Group composition*—Groups are most successful when participants have similar needs and can empathize with one another. Thus, it is important to decide whether the group will be open to everyone or limited to people interested in a particular topic, such as individuals contemplating genetic testing, members of families known to have a hereditary cancer syndrome, or individuals with positive genetic test results.

   Group leaders also need to decide whether group membership will be open or closed. In an open group, people come to as many meetings as they like. This allows participants greater flexibility but can be logistically challenging for facilitators and frustrating for some participants. In a closed group, advanced registration is required, and the group stays the same for the entire series of meetings. This format facilitates group bonding and may increase participants' comfort in sharing with the group. However, counselors would need to be prepared to deal with the difficult group dynamics that can arise in closed groups. Examples include when there is continual friction between two participants or when participants begin to resent a group member who frequently monopolizes the discussion.

3. *Timing*—Groups can take place on a regular basis, such as the first Tuesday of every month. With this format, the expectation is to offer a forum for interested individuals to come together for discussion and mutual support. Support groups can also be offered as a fixed number of meetings (for example, 4 weekly meetings). The latter format is probably more useful for short-term crisis intervention.

4. *Format*—Group participants are usually seeking both support and information. Facilitators need to allow sufficient time for participants

TABLE 8-11. Contact Information for Hereditary Cancer Syndrome Support Groups

Cancer Syndrome/Support Group	Contact Information
Ataxia-telangiectasia	
National Ataxia Foundation	www.ataxia.org
A-T Children's Project	www.atcp.org
Beckwith-Weidemann	
Beckwith-Weidemann Support Network	www.beckwith-wiedemann.org
Breast and ovarian	
FORCE: Facing our risk of cancer empowered	www.facingourrisk.org
National Alliance of Breast Cancer Organizations	www.nabco.org
National Breast Cancer Coalition	www.natlbcc.org
Y-ME National Breast Cancer Organization	www.y-me.org
Gilda Radner Familial Ovarian Cancer Registry	www.ovariancancer.com
Conversations! The newsletter for women who are fighting ovarian cancer	www.ovarian-news.org
Cancer survivors	
National Coalition for Cancer Survivorship	www.cansearch.org
Childhood cancers	
Candlelighters Childhood Cancer Foundation	www.candlelighters.org
Colon cancer	
Familial Gastrointestinal Cancer Registry	www.fascrs.org/ascrs cancerreg.html
Hereditary Colon Cancer Association	www.hereditarycc.org
Intestinal Multiple Polyposis and Colorectal Cancer Foundation	PO Box 11, Conyngham, PA 18219
Fanconi anemia	
Fanconi Anemia Research Fund, Inc.	www.fanconi.org
Multiple endocrine neoplasia, 1	
Canadian Multiple Endocrine Neoplasia type 1 Society	PO Box 100, Meota, SK SOM 1X0 CANADA
Neurofibromatosis	
National Neurofibromatosis Foundation, Inc.	www.nf.org
Neurofibromatosis, Inc.	www.nfinc.org
Tuberous sclerosis	
Tuberous Sclerosis Alliance	www.tsalliance.org
Von Hippel Lindau syndrome	
VHL Family Alliancewww.vhl.org	www.vhl.org
Xeroderma pigmentosum	
Xeroderma Pigmentosum Society, Inc.	www.xps.org

Source: Genetic Alliance. www.geneticalliance.org

to share stories and vent frustrations. This time can be structured around a specific theme or kept unstructured, depending on the facilitator and/or group's preference. To meet the informational needs of group members, the facilitators can devote part of the meeting time to learning about a specific topic. This may consist of listening to a lecture or panel discussion, watching an educational videotape, or even participating in self-help or role-play exercises.

5. *Setting*—Participants are more likely to attend a support group if the meetings are held in a convenient location with ample parking The group meetings can be held in a hospital conference room or in a more neutral setting, such as a community center. On the one hand, participants will be familiar with the hospital which is an advantage and the facilitator may find it easier to arrange a conference room and refreshments within his/her own hospital setting. However, hospitals can also evoke strong emotional responses from group members and might affect overall attendance or the group dynamics.

Counselors who do not have the interest or resources to begin a support group should consider other ways of offering support, such as recommending specific internet sites or maintaining a list of clients who are willing to speak to others in similar situations.

8.4. Case Examples

The following four cases illustrate some of the psychosocial issues that can arise during a cancer genetic counseling session.

8.4.1. Case 1: I Just Want My Life Back

John, age 38, was an avid bicyclist who consulted with his internist after feeling unusually winded after a 15K race. John was found to have alarmingly high blood pressure, leading to the discovery of a pheochromocytoma (which is an adrenal gland tumor). Because this was his third pheochromocytoma to be diagnosed his physician referred him for genetic counseling. John met with a genetic counselor 1 week before his surgery and opened the session by announcing that his family almost certainly had some type of cancer syndrome. His tumors were diagnosed at ages 28, 31, and 38, and his father had died from a brain tumor at age 35. In addition, his paternal grandmother had died from some type of cancer in her forties. Neither he nor his father had any siblings, and he had no information about more distant relatives.

As John was talking, the genetic counselor was running through the possible hereditary cancer syndromes associated with multiple pheochromocy-tomas and brain tumors. The differential diagnosis included neurofibro-matosis, hereditary paraganglioma syndrome, multiple endocrine neoplasia 2A, and von Hippel Lindau syndrome (VHL). When John added that he had recently been found to have two small renal cysts, the counselor felt that VHL was the most likely explanation for the pattern of cancers in the family. The genetic counselor told John that there was likely to be an inherited basis to his multiple tumor diagnoses and that he might have von Hippel-Lindau syndrome (VHL). John asked several questions about VHL and the possible implications for his two children. He appeared more intellectually curious than emotionally distressed at the possibility of having VHL and seemed eager to clarify whether or not this was the case. John was told he should undergo specialized screening tests to look for additional features of VHL and that more family history information would be helpful. He was asked to obtain medical records on his father and paternal grandmother to clarify the exact types of tumors they had. When the geneticist joined the conver-sation, she corroborated the possibility of VHL and arranged for John to undergo additional screening tests to rule out other features of VHL.

John was a licensed child psychologist with a successful private prac-tice. He conversed easily during the session and frequently smiled or laughed. He displayed a philosophical attitude about his upcoming opera-tion to remove the tumor and expressed eagerness to get it over with so he could "get his life back to normal." He spoke of his commitment to his patients and talked enthusiastically about an upcoming bicycle race for charity he had entered. The session ended with John agreeing to obtain the requested information and come in for a follow-up session. He was encour-aged to bring his wife to the next appointment.

About 3 months later, John came in alone to the follow-up genetic coun-seling session. He brought documentation confirming that his father's brain tumor was a hemangioblastoma and that his grandmother had had renal cell carcinoma. In addition, John had undergone a careful eye exam that revealed two retinal angiomas. Together with the geneticist, the genetic counselor explained that this pattern of tumors was consistent with VHL and reviewed information about the features and inheritance pattern of VHL. John had already alerted his surgeon of the possibility he had VHL, and they had dis-cussed appropriate follow-up. The option of genetic testing was briefly dis-cussed but was not something John wanted to pursue at this time. At John's request, the geneticist agreed to contact John's surgeon directly. After the geneticist left the room, the counselor began to close the session. She asked John how he felt about having the VHL diagnosis confirmed. He said that it came as no surprise and expressed his appreciation of having this informa-tion and being able to plan accordingly.

John had been politely attentive during the entire conversation but seemed subdued and downcast, a marked contrast from his demeanor during the previous visit. The counselor felt awkward about asking a licensed psychologist about his emotional well-being but felt she could not ignore the issue. At a lull in the conversation, she tentatively asked, "You seem sort of down compared with the last time we met. Is something going on?" Far from being annoyed by the question, John seemed to welcome the opportunity to unburden himself. He tearfully described his inability to work or bicycle due to unforeseen surgical complications and continued erratic blood pressure. He now faced the prospect of additional surgery and the possibility that his bicycling days were over. John stated bitterly, "My entire life is taken up by doctor's appointments, and they can't even fix the problem," and also complained about his wife's lack of support, "She never asks about my health anymore. I don't think she even cares about me." The counselor listened and empathized with how his life had been dramatically altered and gently asked if he had considered meeting with someone to discuss what he had been through. John agreed that it would be helpful and was given an appointment to meet with the program psychologist the next day. The session ended with the counselor explaining that she would send him a letter summarizing their discussion and that she would stay in touch.

John met with the program psychologist and talked openly about the issues that were troubling him. He was referred to a psychologist with experience helping people cope with chronic health problems. This psychologist continued to meet with John weekly for several months. In follow-up telephone conversations, the genetic counselor was relieved to find John in much better spirits. He had started back to work part-time and remained hopeful that he would someday be able to race again. He also mentioned that both he and his wife had become active in the VHL Family Alliance and that they had found it helpful to speak with others who had gone through similar—or even worse—ordeals.

Key Points of Case:

1. Impact of new diagnosis on client's emotional well-being—see Section 8.1.1

2. Paying attention to changed demeanor—see Section 8.2.1

3. Making decision that a mental health referral was warranted—see Section 8.3.1

8.4.2. CASE 2: I NEVER GOT TO SAY GOOD-BYE

Joanie, age 40, came to the genetic counseling session with her arms filled with medical records documents and a detailed drawing of her family tree with the causes of death written out in calligraphy. Joanie explained that her mother had died from colon cancer in her forties as had her grandfather and two uncles. She also brought a letter from her cousin, which stated that he carried a deleterious *MSH2* mutation. Joanie's motivation for meeting with a genetic counselor was to obtain information on behalf of her two young children. The genetic counselor discussed Joanie's 50% risk of carrying the familial *MSH2* alteration, described the features of hereditary nonpolyposis colon cancer (HNPCC), and briefly discussed the logistics and pros and cons of genetic testing. The genetics aspects of the counseling session were straightforward, but the counseling issues were more complex.

Joanie had just entered high school when her mother became ill and was 17 years old when her mother died. At one point, she overheard that her mother had colon cancer, but no one in the family openly spoke of it. She reminisced about how tough it was to visit her mother in the hospital and not be able to acknowledge her declining health. Joanne related that whenever she became tearful, her grandmother would pull her out of the mother's hospital room. "I had to pretend everything was fine if I wanted to stay with my mother." Because the family never acknowledged that her mother was going to die, Joanie felt she was never given the opportunity to say good-bye to her. Even though her mother had died over 20 years ago, Joanie's grief was palpable and she cried frequently during the genetic counseling session.

Joanie also spoke of how difficult it was to come to a cancer hospital and see people who were obviously undergoing treatment. She talked candidly about her own fears of developing cancer, which centered around leaving her children motherless. In fact, she seemed obsessed with the possibility that she could die while her children were young and even quoted statistics related to highway fatalities. She mentioned that before making the 1-hour trip to the genetic counseling appointment, she had written out good-bye letters to each of her children "just in case she died in a car crash." In response to the genetic counselor's query, Joanie said she assumed she would get cancer someday and just hoped it was when her children were grown.

The counselor was concerned about the intensity of Joanie's grief and worried that it might become even greater as she approaches age 45—the age her mother died of cancer. Another important "anniversary reaction" could occur when Joanne's children reach the age she was when her mother became ill. An additional concern was whether Joanie would view a positive *MSH2* gene test result not only as confirmation that she had HNPCC, but also that she would eventually die from cancer. Because Joanie was not really interested in being tested, this issue was not explored in depth. However, the counselor did mention that her mother's death still seemed to be affecting her and suggested that she speak to a therapist or grief counselor. Joanie did not seem interested in a referral and expressed concern that such a meeting would only exacerbate her grief. The session ended with the counselor telling Joanie to contact her if she had any further questions, desired *MSH2* testing, or "just wanted to talk."

Joanie called the genetic counselor several times over the next few months. During the second conversation in which Joanie could not mention her mother without crying, the counselor again suggested she meet with a grief counselor. Joanie seemed more amenable to the suggestion this time and was given the name and phone number of a local grief counselor. About 1 month later, Joanie called back to request the grief counselor's phone number, which she had misplaced. She mentioned that she was dreading the upcoming week because it was the anniversary of her mother's final hospitalization and death. At this point, the counselor asked if it would be okay for the grief counselor to call Joanie, stressing that Joanie did not have to meet with her if she did not feel comfortable. Joanie agreed to this plan and the counselor made the referral. The genetic counselor called the grief counselor and described the case to her. The grief counselor agreed that the referral was appropriate and an appointment was set-up. Joanne continued to meet with her every other week over the next several months and, as part of the healing process, wrote a personal good-bye letter to her mother, which she shared with the genetic counselor.

Two years later Joanie chose to undergo genetic testing and was found not to carry the familial *MSH2* mutation. She rejoiced in the news, mainly for the sake of her children. Beaming, she said, "For the first time in my life, I feel I can dream about holding my grandchild in my lap." Joanie admits she will probably always worry about death more than the average person but feels it no longer consumes her. She also talked excitedly about her latest project for her children—creating an elaborate memory book about their grandmother.

Key points of case:

1. Delayed grief reaction—see Section 8.1.1
2. Impact of cancer experience on risk perception and coping strategies—see Sections 8.1.2 and 8.1.4
3. Strategies for making a referral—see Sections 8.3.2

8.4.3. Case 3: What Good Are Doctors, They Couldn't Save My Brother

Mr. Lewis Tarrington, a 47-year-old businessman, made an impression on the hospital staff even before coming in for his genetic counseling appointment. He berated the clinic coordinator when he could not obtain an appointment for a particular day, blasted the clinic manager about the billing procedures, and harassed the registration staff on arrival at the hospital. Unfortunately, the genetic counseling encounter did not start out well either; the clinic was running 30 minutes late, and the medical records documenting the family history (which had been mailed to the clinic) could not be located.

The genetic counselor, who had been warned about his explosive temper, hurriedly apologized when she entered the consult room and, in hopes of avoiding his wrath, plunged into the review of his family history. Mr. Tarrington related that three relatives had died from pancreatic cancer— his maternal grandmother, a maternal uncle, and, most recently his younger brother. There was also a maternal history of insulin-dependent diabetes. Although Mr. Tarrington answered the questions asked of him, he was obviously still fuming about his prior encounters with the hospital staff. The counselor eventually realized that she would never gain rapport with him until she at least acknowledged his anger. So she halted the discussion, put aside his file, and said (not without trepidation), "Maybe we should start at the beginning. Sounds like you had a trying time getting in to see us." Mr. Tarrington immediately began his litany of complaints, speaking in a loud, furious tone. The genetic counselor let him speak his piece, acknowledged the hassles he had encountered, and only minimally defended the hospital staff and procedures. She apologized again (more sincerely this time), thanked him for bringing these issues to her attention, and promised to address his complaints at the next clinical staff meeting.

As the counselor began to transition the discussion back to the review of his family history, Mr. Tarrington launched into a tirade against incompetent physicians and barbaric cancer treatments. Knowing that his younger brother had died less than 1 month ago, the counselor wondered whether the client's acute grief was the underlying cause of his anger. The counselor responded that it sounded like his family had had some bad experiences with hospitals and invited him to tell her about his brother's diagnosis. Mr. Tarrington's brother, Joe, had few symptoms when diagnosed with advanced-stage pancreatic cancer at age 45; he died 8 weeks later. Mr. Tarrington described Joe's initial workup and diagnosis but focused more on the unsuccessful course of treatment and the illness' unrelenting downward spiral. As he described his brother's illness and death, his sadness at losing his brother became much more prominent than his anger.

When the medical oncologist joined the discussion, he pelted her with detailed questions about conventional and experimental treatment for pancreatic cancer. It was almost as if he were seeking a postmortem second opinion on behalf of his brother. He said that his brother had consulted with several oncologists when first diagnosed but ultimately chose to be treated at the local community hospital. More than once, Mr. Tarrington asked whether it would have made any difference had his brother been treated at a larger cancer center. He was assured that nothing could have altered the course of his brother's disease, but Mr. Tarrington seemed to find this difficult to accept. Although he was concerned about his own risks of cancer, the clinic visit seemed much more a way of coming to terms with his brother's death.

The oncologist and genetic counselor discussed the high likelihood that the family had a hereditary form of pancreatic cancer, described the few options for monitoring, and stated that hopefully someday better options would be available. The session ended with a promise to contact him when his family records were reviewed and to also provide him with information about on-going research protocols, in which he had expressed interest.

Follow-up interactions were businesslike; Mr. Tarrington remained demanding but less hostile, and the counselor counted it as a victory when he finally gave her permission to address him by his first name. Months later, the counselor and other staff members were astonished to learn that he had given a generous donation to their high-risk cancer program—although he did not pass up the opportunity to recount the problems with his initial clinic visit in the accompanying letter!

Key points of case:

1. Client's anger masks underlying grief—see Sections 8.1.1
2. Timing of appointment is important—see Section 8.1.2
3. Counseling techniques to work through client's anger—see Section 8.2.2

8.4.4. CASE 4: I DON'T NEED COUNSELING, JUST GIVE ME THE FACTS

When the genetic counselor entered the exam room, Paula was standing by the window with her arms crossed tightly across her chest. In response to his greeting, Paula said flatly that she did not need any "counseling;" it was the breast oncologist she expected to meet. (Not the most auspicious beginning to a session!) The genetic counselor explained the nature of the multidisciplinary clinic and that his role was to quantify Paula's risks of cancer based on her family history. Keeping his tone of voice friendly but sincere, he assured her that he would not subject her to any psychological counseling. Paula seemed to relax during this explanation and accepted the invitation to sit down.

Paula recited her family history in a precise, semidetached manner. At age 42, Paula was the oldest of six siblings; she had one brother and four sisters. Over the past 6 months, two sisters had been diagnosed with breast cancer. Despite two paternal aunts and a cousin with premenopausal breast cancer, Paula and her sisters had never considered themselves at increased risk. Even when the first sister was diagnosed with breast cancer at age 38, the family attributed it to her obesity and other health problems. However, when the second sister (Sara) was diagnosed with breast cancer at age 32, the family became more alarmed and began seeking answers as to why this had happened. Paula's expressionless recital of the history was evidence that she was profoundly affected by her sisters' diagnoses, but a question about how she was coping with it seemed to annoy her. She also brushed aside the counselor's comment that her family had been through a lot over the past few months, stating that "every family has difficult things to deal with, you can't dwell on it."

Paula knew she wanted to have BRCA1/2 testing. The genetics discussion was at a sophisticated level because Paula was a biochemist currently working, ironically in a genetics biotechnology firm. She had a good understanding of the implications of a positive BRCA1/2 result from reviewing the literature and speaking to colleagues. Paula said she would definitely undergo prophylactic mastectomy if her results were positive and carefully outlined her reasoning for coming to this decision, insisting "it's the only logical thing to do." The counselor told Paula that testing could be done through their program but that it made more sense to first test one of her affected sisters.

Near the end of the session, Paula casually mentioned that her father had walked out on the family when she was 13 and that her family had not had much contact with their paternal relatives since then. She acknowledged that the current interactions with her paternal relatives were a bit awkward but predictably minimized the impact of her father's desertion, "We did just fine without him. It taught me to be self-reliant." The counselor felt concerned that Paula's emotional state was more fragile than she was admitting (and that perhaps she had never fully dealt with the emotional blow of her father's desertion). But he recognized that asking more questions would only serve to alienate her and would also betray his earlier promise that she would not be subjected to any "counseling."

Paula called to make a testing appointment the day after her sister Sara was told she carried a BRCA2 mutation. Paula seemed surprisingly shaken by the news, confessing that she had never truly believed that her sisters' cancers were linked with the paternal history of cancer. However, once again she made it clear she did not want to discuss the emotional impact of this news. Paula asked if she could just come in to have her blood drawn but seemed resigned to another meeting with the genetic counselor and oncologist.

The informational portion of the pretest session was straightforward and Paula's only questions centered around the logistics of scheduling a prophylactic mastectomy. Paula seemed a little more distressed at the visit but refused to openly discuss or even acknowledge any emotional ramifications of a positive test result, making the encounter somewhat frustrating for the genetic counselor. The counselor did mention the option of meeting with one of the hospital social workers to discuss psychosocial issues and Paula conceded that other people might find this helpful, but that she would not.

Paula came to the results disclosure visit with her husband. After learning that she did carry the BRCA2 mutation, she immediately talked about scheduling her prophylactic mastectomies. Her husband concurred that the surgery should be done as soon as possible. This launched a lengthy discussion about the logistics of surgery. After agreeing on an appropriate plan of referral with the oncologist, the counselor interjected and gently asked her what it was like to hear this news. Paula said curtly that she had expected it, but then immediately dissolved into tears and described how overwhelmed she felt. The counselor listened empathetically, but was careful to avoid any counseling-type remarks. He noted that she rebuffed her husband's efforts to comfort her and at one point, got up and turned away from the group until she composed herself. When Paula sat back down, she seemed embarrassed about her tears and wanted to re-focus on the medical management issues. At the end of the session, the genetic counselor mentioned the possibility of meeting with the program social worker, not as something that was necessary but as an option that might be helpful. Paula did not agree to meet with the social worker, but the genetic counselor was encouraged that she did not refuse it outright.

Over the next several months, Paula called the genetic counselor several times. Sometimes she had a specific question, but other times she just seemed to want to talk. During one of these conversations, Paula expressed guilt that she had not recognized the predisposition to breast cancer in her family and "warned" her siblings about it. She commented that it had always been her responsibility to take care of her younger brother and sisters. At one point she remarked sadly, "I guess I'm not doing a very good job," but then caught herself and changed the topic before the genetic counselor could respond. Paula admitted to feeling both sad and worried about her test result but seemed to have remarkably little insight into why she might be feeling this way. At her husband's urging, Paula did finally make an appointment with the social worker but ended up canceling it at the last minute.

Paula underwent prophylactic bilateral mastectomies and recovered nicely from surgery. She continues to call the genetic counselor once in awhile. On "bad days" she describes feelings of sadness, but, in general, she just doesn't think about it; a strategy that seems to have worked well for her in the past.

Key points of case:

1. Intellectualism as a coping strategy—see Section 8.1.4
2. Conducting a psychological assessment but respecting client boundaries—see Sections 8.2.1 and 8.2.2
3. Encouraging a referral, but also providing support—see Section 8.3.2 and Chapter 9, Section 9.3

8.5. REFERENCES

Audrian, J, Schwartz, M, Lerman, C et al. 1998. Psychological distress in women seeking genetic counseling for breast-ovarian cancer risk: the contributions of personality and appraisal. Ann Behav Med 19:370–377.

Baker, N. 1991. Relative Risk: Living With a Family History of Breast Cancer. Penguin Books, New York, NY.

Baum, A, Friedman, A, and Zakowski, S. 1997. Stress and genetic testing for disease risk. Health Psych 16:8–19.

Burton, M and Watson, M. 1998. Counselling People With Cancer. John Wiley & Sons, West Sussex, UK.

Carter, E and McGoldrick, M (eds). 1999. The expanded family life cycle: individual, family, and social perspectives. Allyn & Bacon, Boston, MA.

Djurdjinovic, L. 1998. Psychosocial Counseling. In A Guide to Genetic Counseling Wiley-Liss, New York, NY, 127–170

Gilbar, O. 1997. Women with high risk for breast cancer: psychological symptoms. Psychol Reports 80:800–802.

Greer S, Morris, T, Pettingale, K. et al. 1979. Psychological responses to breast cancer: effect on outcome. Lancet 785–787.

Hainseworth, M, Eakes, G, Burke, M. 1994. Coping with chronic sorrow. Issues Ment Health Nurs 15:59–66.

Hobdell, E and Deatrick, J. 1996. Chronic sorrow: a content analysis of parental differences. J Genet Counseling 5:57–68.

Hopwood, P, Keeling, F, Long, A et al. 1998. Psychological support needs for women at high genetic risk of breast cancer: some preliminary indicators. Psycho-oncology 7:402–412.

Kelly, P. 1991. Understanding Breast Cancer Risk (health, society, and policy series). Temple University Press, Philadelphia, PA.

Kessler, S. 2000.. Teaching and counseling. In Resta, R (ed) Psyche and Helix. Wiley-Liss, New York, NY 135–142.

Lerman, C, Daly, M, Sands, C et al. 1993. Mammography adherence and psychological distress among women at risk for breast cancer. J Natl Cancer Inst 85:1074–1080.

Matloff, E. 1997. Generations lost: a cancer genetics case report. J Genet Counseling 169-172, 1997. [In same issue, see commentaries by Eunpu, D (173-176) and Djurdjinovic, L (177–180).]

McGoldrick, M, Gerson, R, and Shellenberger, S. 1999 Genograms Assessment and Intervention, 2nd edition. W.W. Norton & Company. New York, NY.Richards, M, Hallowell, N, Green, J et al. . 1995. Counseling families with hereditary breast and ovarian cancer: a psychosocial perspective. J Genet Counseling 4:219–233.

Rolland, J. 1994. Families, Illness, and Disability: An integrative treatment model. Basic Books, New York, NY.

Tarkan, L. 1999. My mother's breast: daughters face their mothers' cancer. Taylor Publishing, Texas.

Walsh, F. 1998. Strengthening family resilience. Guilford Press. New York, NY.

Watson M et al. 1994. The Mini-MAC: further development of the Mental Adjustment to Cancer Scale. J Psycholonc 12:33–46.

Weil, J. 2000. Psychosocial Genetic Counseling. Oxford Univ. Press, Oxford, UK.

Worden, J. 1991. Grief counseling and grief therapy, 2nd edition: A handbook for the mental health practitioner. Springer Pub Co. New York, NY.

PREDISPOSITION TESTING AND COUNSELING

For many people at risk for a genetic disorder, the question of whether to pursue genetic testing is particularly troubling. The possibility of learning that one is not at high risk for breast cancer or Huntington disease must be tempered by the prospect that one must live with the opposite result.

(Smith, 1998)

Cancer genetic counselors are frequently asked to describe and arrange genetic tests. Chapter 9 describes the major elements of the testing and counseling process, which includes arranging a test, providing pretest counseling, and providing results disclosure and follow-up. This chapter ends with three genetic counseling cases.

9.1. ARRANGING A TEST

The initial steps of the testing process include determining the client's eligibility, choosing the right laboratory, assessing the client's interest in and readiness for testing, and explaining the logistics of the testing program.

9.1.1. DETERMINING CLIENT ELIGIBILITY

Because only 5–10% of cancer cases have a strong hereditary component, genetic testing is not appropriate for every family. Determining eligibility for a specific genetic test relies on a thorough assessment of personal and family histories of cancer. Families offered genetic testing should have moderate or high risks for having a particular hereditary cancer syndrome. And, of course, there needs to be a genetic test that is available. Currently available cancer susceptibility genetic tests are listed in Table 9-1.

Once it has been deemed that genetic testing is appropriate for a specific family, the next issue is to decide which family member to test first. Before testing at-risk family members, it is important to establish that cancers in the family are associated with a specific gene mutation. Testing should, therefore, begin with the person in the family most likely to carry the gene mutation. This is either an individual who has had one of the syndrome-related malignancies or an individual who is deemed an obligate carrier (has a parent and a child who have developed cancers associated with the syndrome). Identifying the exact mutation for the family will allow other at-risk relatives to have a targeted, definitive test. The rationale for initially testing an affected relative before testing at-risk relatives may seem obvious to genetic providers, but this concept can be puzzling to families and even other health care providers. Of course, there may not be an affected member of the family available to test. In these cases, testing should be offered to a first-degree relative of an affected family member. Again, from a genetics standpoint, the goal of testing is to identify the underlying cause of cancer for the family, that is, by obtaining a positive test result. Therefore, it makes more sense to test an affected individual's sibling or child who is at 50% *a priori* risk of having a gene mutation than a cousin who may only be at 12.5% risk. Part of the rationale for this approach is the financial burden on the family; while full gene analysis can cost upward of two thousand dollars, single site analysis is usually less than $400.

In determining a client's eligibility, counselors should consider the following factors:

1. *Client's cancer status*—If there is no known mutation in the family, then testing should begin with an individual who has had a syndrome-related cancer. This individual will be helpful in defining the mutation for the family. If the client has not had cancer, then it is preferable to delay testing until an affected family member has been tested.

   If there is a known mutation in the family, then other relatives will have the option of being tested. In syndromes with rare or unusual tumor types, such as von Hippel-Lindau syndrome or neurofibromatosis, affected individuals probably do not need to undergo confirmatory gene testing. In general, a family member who displays clinical features of a rare cancer syndrome can be assumed to carry the familial mutation. This is not the case for syndromes with more common tumor types, such as colon or breast cancer. Affected relatives should be offered testing to distinguish between hereditary and sporadic cases.

TABLE 9-1. CANCER SUSCEPTIBILITY GENETIC TESTS THAT ARE CURRENTLY AVAILABLE

Gene (location)	Syndrome	Available
APC (5q21)	Familial adenomatous polyposis	Clinically
ATM (11q22.3)	Ataxia-telangiectasia	Research
BLM (15q26.1)	Bloom syndrome	Clinically
BRCA1 (17q21)	Breast-ovarian cancer syndrome	Clinically
BRCA2 (13q12)	Breast-ovarian cancer syndrome	Clinically
BWS (11p15)	Beckwith-Weidemann syndrome	Clinically
CDK1 (12q14)	Melanoma, familial	Clinically
CMM1 (1p36)	Melanoma, familial	Clinically
FACA (16q24.3)	Fanconi anemia	Clinically
FACC (9q22.3)	Fanconi anemia	Clinically
FACD (3p26)	Fanconi anemia	Clinically
MEN1 (11q13)	Multiple endocrine neoplasia, type 1	Clinically
MLH1 (3p21)	Nonpolyposis colon cancer	Clinically
MSH2 (2p22)	Hereditary nonpolyposis colon cancer	Clinically
MSH6 (2p16)	Hereditary nonpolyposis colon cancer	Clinically
NF1 (17q11.2)	Neurofibromatosis, type 1	Clinically
NF2 (22q12)	Neurofibromatosis, type 2	Clinically
PMS1 (2q31)	Hereditary nonpolyposis colon cancer	Clinically
PMS2 (7p22)	Hereditary nonpolyposis colon cancer	Clinically
PTC (9q22.3)	Basal cell nevus syndrome	Clinically
PTEN (10q23)	Cowden syndrome	Clinically
RB (13q14.1)	Retinoblastoma	Clinically
RET (10q11.2)	Multiple endocrine neoplasia, type 2	Clinically
SMAD4 (18q21.1)	Juvenile polyposis	Research
STK11 (19p13.3)	Peutz-Jeghers syndrome	Clinically
TP16 (9p21)	Melanoma, familial	Clinically
TP53 (17p13)	Li-Fraumeni syndrome	Clinically
TSC1 (9q34)	Tuberous sclerosis	Clinically
TSC2 (16p13.3)	Tuberous sclerosis	Clinically
VHL (3p25)	von Hippel-Lindau syndrome	Clinically
WRN (8p12)	Werner syndrome	Research
WT1 (11p13)	Wilms' tumor, familial	Research
WT2 (11p15.5)	Wilms' tumor, familial	Research
XPA (9q34.1)	Xeroderma pigmentosa	Clinically
XPB (2q21)	Xeroderma pigmentosa	Clinically
XPC (3p25.1)	Xeroderma pigmentosa	Clinically
XPD (19q13.2)	Xeroderma pigmentosa	Clinically
XPE (11p12)	Xeroderma pigmentosa	Clinically
XPF (16p13.2)	Xeroderma pigmentosa	Clinically
XPG (13q32)	Xeroderma pigmentosa	Clinically

Source: Online Mendelian Inheritance in Man, OMIM (TM), 2000.

2. *Client's a priori risks*—If there is a known mutation in the family, the risk for other family members to carry the mutation is based on their placement in the pedigree. For example, if the syndrome follows a dominant inheritance pattern, clients with an affected first-degree relative will have a 50% risk of carrying the mutation and should be offered testing. Individuals at 25% risk of carrying the mutation are also eligible for testing if their at-risk parent is not available or not interested in testing. In general, testing a branch of the family is most informative if it begins with the oldest living at-risk family member. Thus, testing a grandparent will determine whether it is necessary to offer testing to his or her children and grandchildren.

3. *Age of the client*—The age of the client when diagnosed with cancer may be important in sorting out the likelihood that it is a hereditary or sporadic case. Malignancies diagnosed at younger than usual ages are more likely to represent hereditary forms of cancer. For example, if there is no known mutation in the family and two sisters have had breast cancer, one at age 32 and one at age 55, then it makes sense to initially test the sister who was diagnosed at the earlier age. The sister with pre-menopausal breast cancer has a higher likelihood of having a hereditary rather than sporadic form of breast cancer.

   It is also important to distinguish between clients who are over age 18 and those under age 18. In general, children should undergo predisposition testing only if knowledge of the gene status will confer medical benefit.

4. *Ethnicity of the client*—The client's ethnic background may play a role in determining which cancer susceptibility gene to assess or whether it is possible to order a more targeted test. Founder mutations are prevalent in populations which have been historically isolated due to geography (e.g. Iceland) or religious beliefs (e.g. the Amish). A founder mutation is one that originated in a single ancestor and, due to the closed gene pool, was passed on to multiple descendents. It is conceivable that founder mutations will be identified for every cancer susceptibility gene. Individuals in communities or ethnic groups with known founder mutations can be tested for the common mutation(s) rather than the full gene.

   Because genetic counselors in the United States frequently counsel individuals of Ashkenazi Jewish heritage, it is worth discussing the *BRCA1/2* and *APC* mutations in a bit more detail. See text below.

   - *Panel BRCA1/2 testing*—This test looks for three specific mutations: the 187delAG and 5385insC mutations in the *BRCA1* gene and the 6174delT mutation in the *BRCA2* gene. It is estimated that Ashkenazi Jews have a 2% probability of carrying one of these three mutations; Sephardic Jews may also have increased risks. Clients of Jewish heritage who have ovarian or pre-menopausal breast cancer are at greatly increased risk of having one of these three mutations even in the absence of additional family history. There are two possible results from panel testing: a positive result or an indeterminate negative result. Clients with indeterminate negative results can consider undergoing analysis of the entire BRCA1 and BRCA2 genes. This can determine whether their families are among the small subset (less than 10%) of Ashkenazi Jewish families with hereditary breast/ovarian cancer who have mutations elsewhere in the BRCA1/2 genes. Clients with a known mutation in the family are recommended to undergo panel testing rather than single site analysis because of the small chance they could also have inherited a mutation from the other parent of Jewish heritage. There have been reported cases of Ashkenazi Jewish clients who carry two separate BRCA1 and BRCA2 mutations.

- *I1307K mutation*—This test looks for a specific mutation in the *APC* gene mutation. The I1307K mutation may be associated with two- to threefold increased risks of colon polyps or cancer. Unlike mutations in other regions of the *APC* gene, the I1307K mutation does not lead to polyposis or other extracolonic tumors. The estimated frequency of the I1307K mutation in the Ashkenazi Jewish population is about 6%. Because the clinical significance of this mutation is uncertain, not all programs are in favor of offering I1307K testing, especially to families with negative histories of colon cancer.

9.1.2. CHOOSING THE RIGHT LABORATORY

Identifying a laboratory to perform a specific genetic test is not always easy. Because most cancer syndromes are rare, the genetic tests are usually performed by only a few laboratories. One of the best resources for identifying a molecular laboratory within North America is the Gene Tests internet site (www.genetests.org). Asking other cancer genetic colleagues is another excellent way of identifying potential laboratories, especially if the test is only available through a research laboratory. A final strategy for finding a laboratory is to conduct a literature search and contact the researchers who have published work on the gene(s) in question.

Genetic testing can be done on a research or clinical basis. The major differences between research and clinical laboratories are described below.

1. *Research laboratory*—The interests of research laboratories include locating and characterizing the disease gene, perfecting the best method of analysis, and determining the gene frequency within specific populations. These efforts are important in furthering the

understanding of inherited forms of cancer and often lead to the development of a clinical test. Participation in a research study may require extensive documentation of the family history, completion of questionnaires, and collection of blood and/or tissue specimens. There is typically no charge for the DNA analysis. In certain preliminary research studies, laboratories have no provisions for disclosing results to individual study participants, which is important for individuals to know before enrollment. If the research laboratory does agree to disclose results when available, participants need to be aware that it may take several months (or years) for the laboratory to generate a reportable result. A research result needs to be confirmed in a clinically-certified laboratory before the result is disclosed.

2. *Clinical laboratory*—Clinical laboratories are service laboratories that offer molecular analysis for a fee. Clinical laboratories generally have their own requisition forms that must be completed by the provider. Several also have their own consent forms and specimen kits. In most cases, full payment must accompany the specimen unless prior insurance authorization has been obtained and approved by the laboratory's billing department. Results are generally available within three to six weeks.

Providers ordering a test for a cancer susceptibility gene may have little choice in the laboratory they use. However, if there is more than one laboratory providing DNA analysis, then counselors should consider the following features as they select which laboratory to use:

1. *Clinical certification*—All laboratories in the United States performing clinical tests are required to have certification. There are two levels of certification for DNA-based tests which are The Clinical Laboratory Improvement Amendments of 1988 (CLIA) and the voluntary proficiency program through the College of American Pathologists and the American College of Medical Genetics (CAP/ACMG). The CAP certification is more rigorous but either is acceptable.

2. *Technique and accuracy*—Laboratory techniques vary and include linkage analysis, Southern blotting, single-strand conformational polymorphism (SSCP), analysis and DNA sequencing. The type of analysis that is used depends on the gene in question and whether there is a known mutation in the family. Accuracy rates also vary depending on the technique used. Ideally, the genetic test should have close to 100% sensitivity, meaning that a positive result is really positive. The specificity of a test (whether a negative result is truly negative) is usually lower than the sensitivity. Ascertaining the specificity rate is difficult because it means estimating the number of mutations that were missed. Members of families with known mutations can be

reassured that single-site analysis has close to 100% sensitivity and specificity.

3. *Cost and payment flexibility*—The cost of molecular-based tests can be quite expensive, ranging from a few hundred dollars to a few thousand dollars. Health insurance plans may not consider genetic testing to be necessary, especially if the person has already had cancer. In addition, some health insurers distinguish between in-network and out-of-network laboratories, which might also influence coverage. Plans that do cover testing may actually pay for only a portion of the total costs. As an example, *BRCA1* and *BRCA2* full gene analysis costs around $2,700. The client assures you that his or her insurer has promised to cover the expense of testing. But what does this really mean? In many cases, the insurer has actually agreed to cover 80% of the costs, which means that the client will need to submit a $460 co-payment with the specimen. When the insurer later receives the bill from the laboratory, it may decide that $1,800 is what is "usual and customary" for this test and will send a check to the lab for that amount. The laboratory will then bill the client for the $340 that was not paid for by the insurer, which is termed "balanced billing." Thus, for a test that was "covered by insurance," the client still had to pay $800. All clients undergoing genetic testing should be warned about potential charges even if they have prior approval from their insurance company.

Some laboratories do not accept prior insurance approval and require that clients send the total amount of payment with the specimen. Clients can then submit the bills to their insurance company with hopes of being reimbursed. For clients with limited financial means, this may be prohibitively expensive. Some laboratories are more flexible than others in terms of requiring upfront payment, and a few allow clients to set up a monthly payment plan.

9.1.3. ASSESSING THE CLIENT'S INTEREST AND READINESS

Clients request predisposition testing for a variety of reasons, ranging from "I don't want to keep having colonoscopies if I don't need them" to "I just have to know." Counselors should ask clients whether they are undergoing testing in order to make specific medical decisions or for the sake of other family members. Ascertaining why clients are interested in testing can provide valuable insight into the individual's concerns as well as their understanding of the test. Clients may need to be reminded that DNA testing looks for the presence of a cancer susceptibility gene, not the presence of cancer. A client who undergoes predisposition testing should not ignore any symptom that could be a warning sign of cancer.

The option of genetic testing should be discussed in a nondirective manner. One of the main counselor roles is to describe the option of testing impartially and to help clients reach their own decisions about whether or not to pursue it. Counselors are, however, encouraged to assist clients in thinking through the issues. It may be helpful, for example, to review the possible test results (see Section 9.2.2), discuss the potential risks and benefits of testing (see Section 9.2.4), and ask how they might use the information to make medical management decisions.

The interest in genetic testing is in part influenced by the hereditary cancer syndrome itself. Although there are exceptions, interest in genetic testing tends to be low for syndromes in which

- gene mutation carriers are reliably detected by physical exam (e.g. Nevoid basal cell carcinoma syndrome),
- occurrences of cancer are rarely familial (e.g. Wilms' tumor), and
- there are no effective early detection or prevention strategies available (e.g. Li-Fraumeni syndrome).

Interest in genetic testing tends to be higher for syndromes in which

- recommended surveillance is burdensome, invasive, or expensive (e.g. Hereditary nonpolyposis colon cancer syndrome),
- there are potentially effective early detection or risk-reduction strategies available (e.g. Multiple endocrine neoplasia, 2), and
- it is rarely possible to detect gene mutation carriers by other means (e.g. Breast-ovarian cancer syndrome).

The interest in testing also varies among families and even within families. Some clients greet the availability of testing as an opportunity, whereas others see it as more of a threat. Perhaps even more important than ascertaining clients' interest in testing is assessing their readiness to be tested. Important factors that may influence both interest and readiness are listed below.

1. *Personality type*—Individuals may be more likely to seek genetic testing if they feel that they are in control over whether they develop cancer and believe that the more information they have the better. In addition to having an internal locus of control and being an information seeker, the client may also have greater faith in available monitoring or prevention strategies and deal better with certainty (even if bad news) than uncertainty. An individual's coping strategies may also influence decisions about testing.
2. *Current events*—Clients are frequently galvanized into making decisions about testing because of events that are going on in the family.

This may be a cancer-related incident, such as experiencing a cancer scare that turned out to be benign, reaching an age at which others were diagnosed, or watching yet another relative be diagnosed. Other non-cancer-related events can also trigger testing decisions. Examples include the birth of a first grandchild, changed life circumstances, or the imminent loss of health insurance.

3. *Religious/cultural beliefs*—Individuals who hold strong convictions that their destiny is in "God's hands" or as "Allah wills it" may be less interested in genetic testing. Clients with certain religious or cultural beliefs may not see any importance or usefulness in learning their genetic test results. And some may feel that the act of learning their genetic test results is contradictory to their beliefs. It is important for counselors to be aware of and respectful of client's beliefs and recognize that some people place much less emphasis on obtaining this type of information. However, if the client expresses a viewpoint that makes the counselor uncomfortable (for example, the genetic condition is seen as retribution for some past misdeed), it might be useful to seek information or assistance from someone who is knowledgeable about the client's religious or ethnic culture.

4. *Understanding of the test*—It has been said that the more individuals learn about a genetic test, the less they will be interested in having it. Regardless of whether this is true, clients who are ready to be tested should have a clear understanding of what testing can and cannot tell them. Alerting clients of all possible implications and consequences of being tested is sometimes referred to as devil's advocate counseling. Clients who are ready to be tested will be able to articulate the reasons for wanting to learn their test results and will be aware of, but not swayed by, the potential risks of testing.

5. *Family composition*—Clients may be more motivated to consider testing if they have siblings or children who are potentially at increased risk. For example, clients who have sisters or daughters may be more inclined to pursue *BRCA1/2* testing than women who do not. The age of the client and/or these relatives may be important factors as well, especially if the genetic test result would alter medical management recommendations.

9.1.4. EXPLAIN THE LOGISTICS OF THE TESTING PROGRAM

Interested clients need to be told the logistics of the testing program so that they can make final decisions about being tested. This discussion should include the following simple yet important details:

1. *Number and length of visits*—Clients need to be told how many appointments they will be expected to make should they decide to be

tested. Most cancer programs require two genetic counseling visits: a pretest visit and a results disclosure visit. A pre-test session can last upwards of two hours whereas results disclosure visits tend to be less than one hour. Some programs also require a follow-up visit after results are given, and a few require an additional visit prior to making the decision to be tested.

2. *Team of providers*—Clients should be aware of whom they will be meeting at each of their testing appointments. The team of providers usually consists of a genetic counselor, nurse, and/or physician. It is obviously preferable for clients to have met with each of these providers before the disclosure visit . Some programs also require that clients meet with a social worker or psychologist; again, it is important for clients to be aware of this beforehand.

3. *Informed consent procedure*—Each client who undergoes a genetic test should sign a written consent form. This consent form can originate from the testing laboratory or from the testing program. Testing programs should check with the hospital's institutional review board (IRB) for guidance about developing testing consent forms. Many medical centers require that consent forms follow a specific format and may also require that certain language be included. The consent form should describe the possible test results, implications of the results to the client and family, accuracy and limitations of testing, and potential risks and benefits of testing. It is also important that clients have ample opportunities to ask questions about the test. Thus, the testing program needs to include an informed consent process; handing clients a form to sign is not sufficient.

4. *Results*—One question that clients invariably ask is when results will be available. For clinical genetic tests, the answer usually lies somewhere between 2 and 8 weeks. Obtaining results from research laboratories can take much longer. Because DNA testing often takes longer than anticipated, it is prudent to provide a range of time rather than specifying an exact date. Clients should also be informed that second blood samples are sometimes necessary and that this is not usually indicative of carrier status. The method of disclosure should also be discussed beforehand. Most programs require that results be disclosed in person unless there are extenuating circumstances (for example, client is too ill to travel).

5. *Billing practices*—Clients have sometimes complained that they receive information about every aspect of genetic testing—except how much it will cost. The total cost of testing may include the genetic counseling services (for 1–3 visits), the blood draw, and the labora-

tory analysis. Clients need to be aware of all major testing-related charges because they may need to find out ahead of time whether these costs will be covered by their health insurer.

6. *Confidentiality practices*—Counselors will want to reassure clients that their results and other information shared during the testing process will remain private. It may be helpful to discuss the specific mechanisms to maintain confidentiality. If the standard testing protocol includes releasing results to anyone other than clients (for example, their physicians) or placing the result in their medical records, they should be informed of this policy at the outset. Clients who receive positive results should be asked for verbal or written permission before results are released to anyone, including other family members. When testing terminally ill cancer patients, ask them to designate one or two individuals to whom the result can be released in the event of the patient's demise.

7. *Special circumstances*—At times, it will be necessary to deviate from the testing program's normal protocol. Counselors and other program personnel need to discuss and agree on changes to the standard testing protocol. These situations are usually handled on a case by case basis and any modifications to the testing protocol should be resolved before the client is tested. Special circumstances include the following:

- *Clients who do not live locally*—Genetic counselors who work at tertiary medical centers may be asked to arrange testing for patients who live in other states or countries. Whenever possible, the disclosure of results should be coordinated around repeat visits. However, there will be situations in which clients are not planning to return. For example, a client is eligible for and interested in genetic testing but he is returning to Greece before the results are available. In this situation, the counselor will need to make arrangements to disclose the results over the telephone or in a letter. It may also be important to enlist the help of an interpreter during the pretest counseling session and to translate the results letter into Greek.

- *Terminally ill clients*—Another special circumstance is when clients are terminally ill. The logistics of arranging testing for someone who is dying involves discussing the logistics and implications of testing with the client's spouse and close family members, arranging how the test will be paid for, and determining who will be receiving the results. If the client is not able to consent to the test, the next of kin (typically the spouse, followed by first-degree relatives) needs to provide written consent. Families of an individual who is terminally ill may not agree upon the need for genetic testing, but might be willing to store a blood specimen in case this option is something they want to pursue in the future.

• *Clients with intellectual limitations or mental illness*—Clients who have mild to moderate mental retardation will require simplified discussions of the genetic test and may not be able to articulate how they will react to learning the result. Clients with mental illness, such as schizophrenia or dissociative disorder, may not be able to logically follow a discussion and may not have a clear understanding of why testing is being done. Providing genetic counseling and testing to individuals with intellectual limitations or mental illness can be challenging and will require modifications to the testing protocol. A mental health professional should be involved in the case to provide both assessment and guidance. Counselors may also want to involve the client's support person, therapist, and/or physician into the testing process. As a separate issue, counselors will need to ascertain whether the client is legally competent to consent to the testing procedure or whether the individual's next of kin or guardian needs to provide consent.

9.2. PRETEST COUNSELING

The purpose of pretest counseling is to give people sufficient information to make an informed decision about whether to proceed with testing. The pretest session should include the following: possible test results, accuracy and limitations of testing, the implications of testing for the client and relatives, and potential risks and benefits of learning this information (see Table 9-2). The amount of time spent discussing each topic will vary depending on the client's prior knowledge about testing, number of questions asked, and any special issues that are of concern to the client or counselor. Refer also to Section 8.2.2 for suggestions of counseling techniques to use during the session.

TABLE 9-2. LIST OF TOPICS THAT SHOULD BE DISCUSSED BEFORE PREDISPOSITION TESTING

Logistics of testing program
Basics about cancer genetics and probability
Possible test results and implications
Accuracy and limitations
Potential risks and benefits of testing
Possible emotional reactions

9.2.1. BASICS ABOUT CANCER GENETICS AND PROBABILITY

Many clients will have had little to no exposure to genetics or statistics in school. And it is safe to say that the genetics taught before 1990 will not have included information about cancer genetics. Clients who have been educated through the media or internet may have gained some information, but may also be misinformed. Clients may better comprehend their results if they are given basic information about cancer genetics and probability. These complicated concepts can be reinforced through the utilization of simple visual aids.

Counselors may want to educate clients about the following concepts:

1. *Genes and chromosomes*—It seems reasonable for clients undergoing genetic testing to have some basic understanding of genes and chromosomes. This can include the following concepts:

   - basics about DNA, genes, and chromosomes,
   - functioning of genes,
   - the types of gene mutations that can occur, and
   - the impact of a gene mutation.

2. *Autosomal dominant inheritance*—Clients at risk for a dominantly inherited cancer syndrome should be told how the gene mutation can be passed to the next generation. This will help them to understand how the counselor has determined the risk estimates for themselves and other family members. Clients at risk for dominantly inherited gene mutations need to be reminded that the gene mutation could be passed on from either parent (and could be passed on to sons and daughters).

3. *Carcinogenesis*—Explaining the multistep process of carcinogenesis will help underscore the point that a germline mutation is not sufficient to cause cancer. Clients can be told that a series of genetic errors are necessary for a malignant tumor to form. This concept brings up the importance of environmental risk factors and explains the differences and similarities of inherited and sporadic forms of cancer.

4. *Statistics and probability*—Clients may have a poor grasp of statistics and probability, which can pose a problem for counselors since the implications of genetic test results are usually described in statistical terms. Clients may not completely understand the quoted cancer risks or may display disbelief when both siblings have the gene mutation instead of just one. Teaching probability concepts can be difficult, especially in a limited amount of time, but it may be helpful to review certain math concepts (1% = 1 in 100) and basic tenets of probability.

TABLE 9-3. POSSIBLE GENETIC TESTING RESULTS

If known mutation in family:	Positive result
	True negative result
If no known mutation in family:	Positive result
	Indeterminate negative result
	Variant of uncertain significance

9.2.2. POSSIBLE TEST RESULTS AND IMPLICATIONS

Clients should be aware of the different answers they might receive from a genetic test. The *a priori* likelihood of finding a germline mutation depends on whether there is a known mutation in the family. As shown in Table 9-3, the possible results also differ depending on whether there is a known mutation in the family.

If there is no known mutation in the family, there are usually three possible results:

1. *Positive result*—A positive result is one in which a specific germline mutation has been identified or proof of such a mutation (for example, protein truncation) has been established. Examples of germline mutations include frameshift mutations or deletions, splice-site mutations or missense mutations that have been shown to affect the function of the gene. A positive result will likely explain the pattern of cancer in the family and means that the client has increased risks of specific malignancies. Other relatives will also be at increased risk for carrying the mutation but now have the option of undergoing a targeted genetic test.

2. *Indeterminate negative result*—An indeterminate negative result is one in which no mutation or variant has been identified in either copy of the gene. This result may decrease the likelihood that the client has an inherited predisposition to cancer but does not eliminate the possibility. The family could have a mutation in the analyzed gene that cannot be detected by current technologies or could have a mutation in another gene that has not yet been identified. It is also possible that a combination of genetic and environmental factors have caused the pattern of cancer in the family. In families with a high likelihood of having a cancer syndrome, an indeterminate negative result should not alter the client's estimated cancer risks or recommendations about enhanced monitoring. Other relatives will not have the option of predisposition testing, because no deleterious mutation was identified. However, another relative with a syndrome-related tumor can undergo full gene analysis. It is possible that the initial person tested

did not have the syndrome, which would explain why the individual tested negative.

3. *Variant of uncertain significance*—It is possible that the laboratory analysis will reveal a novel DNA change, which is a missense mutation of unknown functional significance. This type of result is termed a variant of uncertain significance. The result could either turn out to be a functional, deleterious mutation (that is, positive result) or a polymorphism of no clinical significance (that is, negative result). Receiving a variant result should not alter estimates of risk or recommendations about screening, although clients may want to delay decisions about prevention strategies until the variant result has been clarified. However, this can take months or years. Other family members should not be offered predisposition testing until the variant result has been determined to be a deleterious mutation. The laboratory may request blood samples from additional family members as part of their efforts to determine the significance of the variant. Family members asked to donate samples for such a study need to be aware that these efforts may still not yield a definitive answer. Additional laboratory tests might include linkage studies, functional assays, and observations of the variant in other families or in the presence of a known deleterious mutation.

If there is a known mutation in the family, two results are usually possible:

1. *Positive result*—A positive result is one in which the familial mutation or proof of the mutation (for example, protein truncation) has been identified. A positive result means that the client has increased risks of specific malignancies. The client's offspring are now at increased risk (usually 50%) for carrying the mutation. However, this result does not alter the likelihood that the client's siblings carry the mutation unless this is the first positive result in their branch of the family. If there is evidence that the client inherited the mutation from a parent, then each of the client's siblings and offspring have a 50% chance of carrying the mutation. If the mutation represents a new (*de novo*) genetic event, then the client's siblings are not at increased risk for carrying the mutation, but the client's offspring are at 50% risk.

2. *True negative result*—A true negative result is the absence of the familial mutation in either copy of the gene. The client does not have the increased risk of cancer due to family history. The client's descendents are no longer at risk for carrying the mutation and do not ever need to be tested. The client's result does not alter the likelihood that his or her siblings could carry the mutation.

9.2.3. ACCURACY AND LIMITATIONS

DNA testing is never 100% accurate due to the nature of testing and the potential for human error. Counselors should inform clients of the test's accuracy rate and describe mechanisms in place to prevent or minimize errors, such as careful labeling of samples and confirming that results make sense given the pedigree. Although single-site DNA analysis should be close to 100% accurate, full gene analysis is less accurate given the potential for false negatives.

For example, *BRCA1* full gene analysis is a highly accurate test, in that it is unlikely to reveal a false positive result or miss a mutation that is detectable by conventional means. However, within the group of individuals who receive negative *BRCA1* results, some probably do have a *BRCA1* mutation. The Dutch population, for example, has two founder mutations in exons 13 and 22, which result in the complete deletion of the exon. These exon deletions will not be detectable by standard technologies.

It is also important that clients understand the limitations of a genetic test result for cancer susceptibility. For a positive result, these include the concepts that

1. A positive result is not synonymous with cancer—Penetrance is high for many of the hereditary cancer syndromes but is rarely 100%. Clients need to understand that a positive result does not guarantee that they will develop cancer. It may also be important to clarify that the absence of cancer does not mean the test results are wrong (which is a separate issue!).

2. Uncertainties about cancer remain—Clients may overestimate the power of DNA testing, so they need to be cautioned that results will still leave many unanswered questions. A positive result confers an increased risk of cancer but does not resolve which type of cancer will develop, at what age the cancer will be diagnosed, or how amenable the cancer will be to treatment.

A negative genetic test result carries the following limitations:

1. An indeterminate negative result does not rule out an inherited susceptibility—Families need to be counseled that the absence of a gene mutation does not exclude an inherited predisposition to cancer. For example, about 25% of classic Li-Fraumeni syndrome families do not carry a detectable germline *TP53* mutation. In most cases, the diagnosis of a hereditary cancer syndrome is based on clinical criteria, not a DNA test.

2. A negative result does not guarantee that cancer will not occur—Individuals with indeterminate negative results should still be coun-

seled about their possible increased risks of cancer. Individuals with true negative results can be reassured that their risks of developing cancer are the same as a person in a low-risk family—which are not insignificant risks. This is quite different from other inherited disorders in which noncarriers have disease risks approaching zero.

9.2.4. POTENTIAL RISKS AND BENEFITS OF TESTING

Deciding whether or not to undergo genetic testing is a personal, potentially life-changing decision. Before allowing modern medicine to foretell your future, do your homework so you know what a test will and won't tell you, psychologically prepare yourself for the results—both good and bad—and make sure that you really want to peek into this crystal ball.

(Monson, 1995)

When there are proven strategies to prevent or cure inherited forms of cancer, the emphasis on the risks versus benefits of testing will dissipate. This has been the case for *APC* and *RET* testing, two cancer genetic tests that are routinely offered. For other genetic tests, detailing the pros and cons of testing is a key part of the pretest genetic counseling session (see Table 9.4). Although each risk and benefit deserves mention, it is important to focus on the issues that are of most concern and relevance to the client.

The potential risks of genetic testing include:

1. *A positive result may increase anxiety, sadness, and fear*—For clients, the most frightening aspect of genetic testing is facing the possibility that they have an inherited susceptibility to cancer. Individuals receiving positive results frequently exhibit increased sadness and anxiety that can be of long duration. More serious emotional sequelae include depression, alcoholism, and even suicidal ideation. In short, a positive result can take away the hope that the individual does not have

TABLE 9-4. POTENTIAL RISKS AND BENEFITS OF PREDISPOSITION TESTING

Potential risks:	Increases anxiety and sadness
	Lack of proven prevention strategies
	Concerns about discrimination
	Strain on family relationships
Potential benefits:	Ends uncertainty about status
	Possibility of negative result
	Influences medical management
	Clarifies risks for other relatives

the familial predisposition to cancer and this can have a powerful effect. Counselors should discuss the potential negative sequelae of testing with all clients, regardless of their affect or emotional well-being. Many clients underestimate the emotional impact of learning their results.

2. *Lack of proven prevention strategies*—The ability to identify individuals with inherited susceptibilities to cancer has surpassed our ability to prevent cancer for those at high risk. In some syndromes, there are strategies for reducing one's risks of cancer, but the prevention of cancer is not yet possible. For some clients, their interest in testing decreases markedly when told there is no way to prevent cancer altogether.

3. *Concerns about discrimination*—Fears about insurance discrimination continue to be a major reason why people decide against having a genetic test. Individuals cite concerns about possible uninsurability and other forms of insurance discrimination if test result is positive (for example, higher monthly premiums or exemption from covering cancer-related illnesses). At this time, the perceptions of discrimination far exceed the reality. However, counselors should be prepared to discuss concerns about current or future insurability if the result is positive.

4. *Strain on family relationships*—Genetic testing can detrimentally alter relationships within a family. Family members may make different decisions about testing, and, for those who undergo testing, there is a chance that they will receive disparate results. This may cause awkwardness or strain between certain relatives, which can have a ripple effect throughout the family. Non-blood family members (e.g. spouses, in-laws) are also likely to be impacted by the news. Although some people enter testing with the sole intent of sharing the results with their relatives, others see the task of informing their at-risk relatives as an unwelcome burden.

Potential benefits of genetic testing include:

1. *Ending the uncertainty about one's gene status*—Clients who undergo testing have often lived with their cancer worries for a long time. The burden of not knowing whether one is at increased risk may add to the mystique and terror of the situation, especially within a family in which cancer is so prevalent. Learning one's gene status may provide a sense of control over the cancer syndrome—and one's destiny. There has also been some research to suggest that family members who elect not to be tested actually have higher anxiety scores than those who

were tested and found to carry the genetic predisposition. For some people, it is the "not knowing" that is hardest to live with.

2. *Possibility of learning a negative result*—Clients undergoing testing usually have a 50% or better chance of not having a deleterious gene mutation. A true negative result means that the client is not at increased risk of cancer and that his or her offspring cannot inherit the familial mutation. Thus, learning a true negative result may have both a psychological and a medical benefit. Learning of an indeter minate negative result may also confer some psychological benefit, even though it does not rule out the possibility of an inherited predisposition to cancer.

3. *Result may influence medical management*—One of the purposes of genetic testing is to identify individuals who are at high risk for developing cancer. Individuals who do have an inherited susceptibility to cancer will often be advised to undergo specialized surveillance tests or to undergo monitoring at earlier ages and/or more frequent intervals than is customary. There may also be risk-reduction strategies available, such as chemoprevention or prophylactic surgery. And if the result is negative, the client may be allowed to relax the recommended surveillance regimen.

4. *Result may clarify risks for other family members*—The initial positive result in the family directly affects other relatives, including siblings, children, aunts, uncles, and cousins. Although there are certain cancer syndromes in which gene mutations frequently occur as new genetic events, most are inherited. Thus, a positive or true negative result may clarify the risks for other family members and their descendents. The initial positive result in the family gives other family members the opportunity to undergo a targeted genetic test. For some clients with cancer, this is their main motivation for being tested.

9.2.5. POSSIBLE EMOTIONAL REACTIONS

Predisposition testing should be considered a major event in a person's life. Learning the results of a genetic test—regardless of whether it is positive or negative—can have a significant impact on one's emotional well-being. For this reason, it is important for genetic counselors to discuss the potential emotional ramifications of testing and assess the client's emotional vulnerability. Many research testing programs have monitored the psychological well-being of patients with a combination of standardized measures and structured interview questions. Clinical testing programs should also strongly consider incorporating some type of psychological assessment.

(More detailed information about psychological assessments can be found in Chapter 8.)

Topics to explore with clients undergoing predisposition testing include

1. *Current emotional well-being*—Because the testing process can exacerbate psychological problems, counselors should assess the client's current emotional well-being. This includes asking questions about current or recent

   • changes in eating, sleep, or work habits,

   • episodes of depression or severe anxiety,

   • feelings of hopelessness,

   • past suicidal thoughts or ideation,

   • visits to a mental health provider,

   • use of alcohol or recreational drugs, and

   • use of any psychotropic medications.

2. *Anticipated impact of results*—It may be helpful for clients to verbalize what it might be like to learn they have a positive or negative result. This exercise is a way of initiating discussions about possible medical management decisions, communicating the result to other family members, and the potential impact on the client's self-concept.

   It is also useful to ask clients whether they expect to receive a particular result. Some will be convinced that they do carry a gene mutation, whereas others will admit that they expect the result to be negative. For some, there is a certain rationale to their expectations (the client with polyposis should expect a positive result), but, in other cases, it is due to intuition or perhaps even wishful thinking. Learning whether the client anticipates a certain result, and why he or she expects this result, may be helpful in providing support when the result is disclosed.

3. *Coping resources*—Everyone develops certain coping resources over time, although some strategies are healthier than others (see Chapter 8). It might be useful to discuss the client's coping resources and how he or she has handled other stressful events in the past.

4. *Support network*—Clients who have no close friends or family members may be in need of extra psychological support. This may also be the case when the client's choice of support seems questionable (the clinically depressed sister or the 13-year-old son). Some people tend to be more private and prefer not to turn to others when distressed or worried. It is also possible that clients do have support people in their lives but prefer not to discuss them during the counseling session.

TABLE 9-5. WHEN TO REFER CLIENTS TO A MENTAL HEALTH PROVIDER

Testing situations in which clients should be referred for psychological counseling:
  Client seems unlikely to be able to cope with result
  Client seems to have no close support
  Client has significant, untreated depression or anxiety
  Client equates positive result with cancer diagnosis or death
  Testing has triggered intense delayed grief reaction
  Testing has triggered posttraumatic stress syndrome
  Client seems overwhelmed by other major life stressors

5. *Other major life stressors*—Any number of other stressful life events could be present at the time a client decides to be tested. These events may be cancer related (terminally ill relative) or may be completely unrelated (job woes, marital strife, parenting problems). Cancer-related stressors should be considered carefully as they could greatly influence the client's reaction to the test result. Non-cancer-related stressors should not be ignored because a positive test result could add another potentially overwhelming stressor. A client in the midst of a life crisis is unlikely to have the same reservoir of emotional resources as other clients. Clients should therefore be urged to consider whether this is the right time to undergo testing in light of other events going on in their lives.

It is also important for testing programs to have a protocol in place to deal with clients who require additional psychological support. A client should be referred to a mental health professional if there is any concern about the person's ability to cope with the results due to previous cancer experiences, lack of support, or other major life stressors. Table 9-5 lists testing situations in which psychological counseling should be offered. Deferral or denial of testing should only be considered if providers have evidence that disclosing a test result could lead to suicidality or could cause incapacitating depression or anxiety.

9.3. RESULTS DISCLOSURE AND FOLLOW-UP

An expert in breaking bad news is not someone who gets it right every time—she or he is merely someone who gets it wrong less often, and who is less flustered when things do not go smoothly.

(Buckman, 1992, p. 7)

The goal of the results disclosure session is to disclose the genetic test results and provide immediate information and emotional support as needed.

9.3.1. BEFORE RESULTS DISCLOSURE

The results disclosure can be the most difficult aspect of the testing process for the client—and the counselor.

Before results are disclosed, the following should be arranged:

1. *The proper setting*—Whenever possible, genetic test results should be disclosed in person. An in-person counseling session ensures that clients will be given the appropriate information and support and allows genetic counselors to better assess clients' reactions and needs. Most programs require that results be disclosed in person. Clients should be aware of this policy in advance so that they will not be surprised or anxious about being asked to return for the disclosure visit. Sometimes it is difficult for clients to return to the medical center, due to geographic distance, illness, or transportation problems. In these extenuating situations, counselors may decide to disclose the results by telephone.

   For in-person visits, it is important to consider the setting in which the results will be disclosed. Pay attention to the layout of the room. For example, make sure that there are enough chairs for everyone and that the seating arrangement will allow everyone to feel included in the conversation. If possible, avoid having the client seated on an exam table or the counselor seated behind a desk. The room should also have a door that can be completely shut to ensure privacy and quiet.

2. *The people attending the session*—Results are often disclosed with both the genetic counselor and physician present. This is particularly helpful in cases of positive results because clients are likely to have questions for both providers. In some programs, the physician will join the conversation after the result has been disclosed, either as standard procedure or as needed. Other providers may also be included in the results disclosure visit, such as other program personnel or the client's personal physician.

   Clients should also be encouraged to bring at least one support person with them. This can be their spouse or partner, family member, close friend, or therapist. Sometimes the client's choice of support person can introduce new complexities into the counseling session. For example, if the support person is also at risk for carrying the mutation, then he or she may have additional questions or reactions to the news separate from the client's concerns. In addition, it is not uncommon for the client to bring someone to the results session who did not attend the earlier session(s). This support person might have an incomplete understanding of the test result or may hold an alternative view of what the test result means. As is true of any genetic counseling encounter, it is important to be aware that each person present may have a different agenda.

Some clients bring an entire entourage with them, whereas others prefer to come alone. The number of companions brought to the disclosure session may be influenced by the client's ethnicity or culture. In certain cultures, individuals are expected to handle difficult situations themselves whereas in other cultures, individuals rely on the presence of relatives and friends for support.

3. *Preparations for the session*—Genetic counselors should have a list of topics that they plan to cover, although they need to be flexible in case clients have extreme or unexpected reactions to the news. To prepare for results disclosure sessions, genetic counselors should

- make sure that a consult or clinic room has been reserved and that the appointment time has been confirmed with the client and all providers,
- review the lab report, resolve any questions about the result, and confirm that it is the client's result,
- plan how to handle any anticipated counseling issues (unexpected result, complex family dynamics, vulnerable client),
- prepare materials to give client (lab report, summary letter, fact sheet, support group information), and
- make effort to start session on time.

Clients should also be prepared for the results disclosure visit, by knowing in advance

- how and when results will be disclosed,
- the range of possible results that will be disclosed (e.g. a client in a family with a known mutation will receive either a positive or true negative result.),
- who will be present at the disclosure, and
- where the appointment will be held.

9.3.2. THE RESULTS DISCLOSURE

Although killing the messenger is no longer considered good form, bearing bad news is still a difficult task.

(Lubinsky, 1994, p. 5)

There is more than one right way to disclose a genetic test result, but there are also plenty of wrong ways. This section discusses useful strategies for disclosing the result in a professional yet empathetic manner.

1. *Disclose result early in session*—Only rarely will clients come to the disclosure visit and decide at that point that they do not want to learn their result. Therefore, it is safe to assume that clients who show up for the disclosure visit are there to learn their results. Certainly, the result should not be blurted out before everyone has been seated, but there should be a minimum of preliminaries to get through before the result is disclosed. Clients will be anxious about the news they are about to hear and are unlikely to focus on any sort of in-depth discussion. Therefore, unless absolutely necessary, counselors should hold questions or lengthy explanations until after the result has been given.

2. *Use simple language*—When disclosing the result, counselors should look directly at the client and state the result in simple, straightforward language. Counselors should choose an approach with which they are comfortable and which seems to be appropriate for this client. For example, the counselor can say, "Yes, you do have the *VHL* alteration that is in your family."

    Counselors may also wish to alert clients that they are about to learn their result and/or offer some expression of empathy with the disclosure. For example, "Are you ready to learn your result? Okay. Unfortunately, the test did reveal a mutation in the *BRCA2* gene. I'm so sorry to have to tell you this."

    Other counselors may prefer to give the result in a bit more formal manner: "The university laboratory looked for mutations in two separate genes called *MSH2* and *MLH1*. Their analysis did identify a mutation in the *MSH2* gene. This result helps explain why you developed colon cancer at such a young age." More detailed explanations of the implications or limitations are important but should follow the client's initial reaction to the news.

3. *Allow clients time to react*—After the result is disclosed, pause. This gives clients a chance to consider the news and react to it. Do not launch into detailed explanations or even provide encouragement that a positive result is not that bad. At that moment, it *is* bad news and clients need the opportunity to acknowledge that fact. There is plenty of time later in the session or during other follow-up interactions to qualify the information and offer statements of encouragement. Clients may also appreciate a few minutes of privacy to process the news with their support people.

4. *Be empathetic but professional*—Disclosing a positive result to an unaffected individual can be emotionally difficult for the counselor. It is not as bad as giving a cancer diagnosis but may seem devastating all the same. For some clients, this is the worst news they have ever received. Counselors will want to acknowledge the client's dis-

appointment and sadness by being appropriately empathetic. It is natural for counselors to be affected by the overt grief and emotional pain of the client, but they need to retain a professional manner. Counselors will not be effective providers if they become emotionally distraught themselves.

Some clients will accept and even seek demonstrations of comfort from the counselor (such as a touch on the arm or a hug), but others will become uncomfortable by these gestures. Counselors need to learn to read client signals and respect the counselor-client boundaries.

5. *Let clients set remaining agenda*—The remainder of the counseling session should be tailored to the clients' needs. Upon hearing their results, some clients will have dozens of questions, whereas others may have very little to say. This could be because they are still processing the information or may indicate a state of shock. Attending to the client's needs for information may therefore involve a lengthy, detailed discussion or may mean skimming through the information and offering a follow-up visit.

9.3.3. POSSIBLE CLIENT REACTIONS

The moments before learning the test result are nerve-racking for almost everyone. It is understandable that clients will be nervous in anticipation of learning their results. Common ways of expressing nervousness include abrupt speech, difficulty sitting still, and sudden tears or laughter. However, more extreme demonstrations of anxiety, such as severe agitation or difficulty concentrating, may indicate that the person will need extra support once results have been given.

This section describes the types of emotions and reactions that have been observed among individuals who received cancer genetic test results. Although the majority of reactions are transient or short term, there have been cases of emotional duress that lasted longer. In general, reactions to test results reflect the reasons why testing was done in the first place. For example, the client who underwent testing to determine if her offspring are at increased risk may have a different reaction to a positive result than the cancer survivor who was curious to know what caused her cancer.

1. *Positive result*—Clients who are told they have gene mutations that predispose them to cancer may experience a variety of emotions, including sadness, disappointment, shock, fear, anger, and disbelief. These feelings can be intense in the first few days or weeks following the results disclosure but generally subside over time. A small number of clients become clinically depressed after receiving their positive result and may require therapeutic and/or pharmaceutical

interventions. Some clients have described feeling vulnerable, over-whelmed, or isolated. The test result can also trigger delayed grief reactions or strain family relationships. For some clients, feeling the need to contact relatives and share this information can be emotion-ally burdensome. This is particularly true if the client is the first person in the family to be tested or the relatives are upset or angry by the news.

Reactions to a positive test result are not always adverse ones. Some clients may experience feelings of relief or closure that they have an explanation for the cancer in their families or because they finally know their gene status. Positive results can also lead to increased feelings of control, greater motivation to pursue cancer monitoring, and closer ties to other family members.

2. *Indeterminate negative result*—An indeterminate negative result can lead to conflicting emotions among clients. Clients should experience some relief that their test results were not positive. However, some clients may be so elated that the result was not positive that they ignore the limited value of this information. Other clients may focus so much on the lack of a definitive answer that they do not experi-ence any relief from the negative result. Instead they may feel frus-trated or disappointed that there is still no clear explanation for the cancer in the family.

3. *True negative result*—Clients who receive true negative results typi-cally experience relief, joy, and decreased levels of depression, anxiety, and cancer worry. However, clients may also experience intense sur-vivor guilt, isolation from affected or mutation-positive family mem-bers, and regrets about major life decisions. Clients who have lived for a long time with their elevated cancer risks may find that it takes time to adjust to their altered risk status and may not be willing to let go of increased monitoring practices.

4. *Variant of uncertain significance*—Clients with variant results may be confused more than anything else by this uninterpretable finding. They may also express feelings of frustration, anger, or disappoint-ment that the genetic test did not provide them with a clear answer. It may take months or years for the variant result to be reclassified as a deleterious mutation or benign polymorphism. This waiting period may turn out to cause as much or more emotional turmoil as a positive result.

At this time, there is no standardized measure that can accurately predict which clients will "fall apart" when learning their result. Counselors tend to be most concerned about individuals who learn they have deleterious gene mutations, yet there is great variability in the range of reactions among clients.

General factors that might predict which clients will have greater distress if they are given positive results are described below.

- Client has significant baseline depression or anxiety—Clients who exhibit significant depression or anxiety may be in need of additional support following the results disclosure. This is especially true if the emotional problems are of long duration and are not being currently treated.

- Client has never had cancer—Clients who have had cancer may be quite upset by the news of a positive result but tend to react less emotionally than clients who have never had cancer. This might be because, having already had cancer, they may have less to fear from the test result itself. Cancer survivors have also gone through the experience of being diagnosed with cancer and may find that, in comparison, learning a genetic test result is far less traumatic. For clients who have never had cancer, receiving a positive test result may be the most difficult news they have ever had to face. A result that confirms the client's high risks of developing cancer may cause feelings of extreme sadness, vulnerability, or helplessness.

- Client has first-degree relative who died from cancer—Having one or more close relatives who have died from cancer may intensify the meaning of a positive genetic test result. Clients may identify more strongly with their affected relatives or may experience a delayed grief reaction.

- Client did not expect result—Clients may have a more difficult time adjusting to their gene status if the result they received was unexpected. This includes clients who are shocked to learn they have positive results as well as those who are surprised by negative results. Unexpected test results may cause individuals to readjust their self-image or to question life decisions that they have made.

- Client has children—One of the most distressing aspects of a positive result for clients who are also parents is the realization that their children could also be at risk. Even individuals who are sanguine about their own risks of cancer may have difficulties sharing the news with their offspring or watching them undergo predisposition testing.

9.3.4. Discussion of Result

After the actual disclosure of the result, counselors may want to discuss several topics, including the implications of the result, possible medical management options, significance for other family members, and the adjustment process regarding the result. The number of topics and length of the conversation can greatly vary. Some clients will have dozens of questions, and others will be in too much shock or distress to discuss anything. Regardless of the client's outward appearance, it is a good idea to review information again at a later time, either in a follow-up telephone call or visit. Clients should also be given or sent a letter summarizing the information about the gene result including the following.

1. *Implication of result to client*—Clients have been told, probably more than once, what the results would mean in terms of their cancer risks. Despite this, it is not uncommon for patients to ask for clarification once they know their result, sometimes as though they are hearing this information for the first time. The information can be tailored to the client's actual result as well as their situation. For example, the discussion about a positive *BRCA1* result will vary depending on the client's gender, age, and cancer status.

2. *Medical management options*—Clients with a positive result may need to consider increasing cancer surveillance, whereas those with true negative results can consider decreasing surveillance. In reality, many clients receiving a positive result are already being monitored carefully. There may be other options, such as chemoprevention or prophylactic surgery, that clients will want to consider once they learn their test results. Clients may feel urgency in making decisions but should be reminded that they have time in which to consider all options and to discuss any plans with their primary physicians. Some clients find it difficult or overwhelming to be faced with making decisions about medical management.

3. *Implication of result to client's family*—Testing is performed on an individual basis, yet each result has implications for the entire family. Decisions about being tested will differ within a family, just as family members will display different approaches toward monitoring practices. Some families will operate in secrecy regarding who is being tested, whereas others will be much more open. Clients should be reassured that their test results will remain completely confidential, even though the counselor may be providing testing to other family members.

   Clients with an initial positive result should be encouraged to share the information with close relatives. Disseminating this information to the family can prove to be emotionally difficult, especially if relatives were not initially aware that the client had undergone testing. The client should be the one to decide how to disclose the result to other family members, but counselors can provide assistance and support to clients as they consider how best to do this. Most clients with a positive result do end up sharing the information with at least some of their relatives.

4. *Adjustment to the result*—Although clients frequently become emotional during the results disclosure session, only rarely will they require immediate psychological intervention. Some clients are intensely affected by the news and may need extra support over the first few weeks or months after the disclosure. However, the vast majority seem to be coping well by 1 year post-disclosure. At the time of the disclosure, it is reasonable to ask the client about his or her plans for the remainder of the day and to determine that he or she has at least one person that can be called on for support if needed. This can be a partner, relative, friend, or therapist. Counselors should also plan to call clients within a few days to check how they are doing, regardless of their demeanor during the session. Sometimes, clients who seemed completely calm while learning their result are the ones who have the most difficult time adjusting to the news.

9.3.5. FOLLOW-UP COUNSELING

Genetic counseling services should not end with the results disclosure visit. All clients, regardless of the results, should be given at least one opportunity to discuss the result a few days or weeks after the disclosure visit. Clients with positive results should be called within 1–3 days of the disclosure and again 1–2 weeks later. The level of support should depend on the needs of the client or concerns of the counselor. For some clients, counselors will want to initiate weekly contact, at least for the first few months. All clients should be given the opportunity of coming in for a follow-up visit to review the testing information. Testing programs can make follow-up telephone calls or visits a standard part of the testing process or can offer such services to clients who request or seem to need additional information or support.

Counselors may be asked to arrange appropriate referrals to physician or mental health specialists, review information about the test result, discuss ways to disclose the result to other family members, and provide emotional support. Follow-up can consist of additional in-person visits or telephone interviews. Counseling topics can include the following.

1. *Implications of results*—It is important to review the implications of the result, tailoring the discussion to the client's questions. Counselors may want to open the discussion by asking clients what their understanding is of the results. Another focus of the conversation should be the implications of this result to other at-risk family members and communication of the result. Counselors can discuss

ways in which this disclosure might be done or can even offer to draft a letter that the client could send to other at-risk relatives. Counselors should also offer to field questions from other family members or make referrals to local genetic counseling services. Family meetings might also be a useful forum to discuss complicated or potentially distressing genetic test results. Holding a family meeting allows providers a chance to disclose the same information to each relative in attendance and gives family members an opportunity to ask questions and discuss the implications of the test result with their providers and each other.

2. *Cancer prevention/early detection*—This should be a major focus of follow-up discussions. Clients with positive results may need to make decisions about their monitoring regimen and whether they need to consider any cancer prevention strategies. Clients with indeterminate results will need to consider options based on their uncertain or potentially increased cancer risks. Even clients with true negative results may benefit from a general discussion of cancer monitoring and living a healthy lifestyle.

3. *Coping resources*—It is important to continue assessing how well (or poorly) clients are coping during the weeks and months following the results disclosure. Counselors can ask clients how they have assimilated the information into their lives and the impact it has made on them. Some clients will benefit from meeting with a mental health professional. The emotional response to testing seems to be most intense in the first few weeks or months after learning the results but tends to dissipate over time. However, specific issues and concerns may arise in the future as the client's children become older or when another relative is diagnosed with cancer. It is important for clients to be aware of resources that are available to them.

4. *Review of genetics and cancer*—Despite extensive discussions about the implications of results for themselves and their children, clients may continue to be confused. For example, clients may question a positive result because they are past the age at which other family members developed cancer. Or clients with true negative results may still request predictive testing for their offspring. It may therefore be useful to review the basic concepts of genetics and cancer. Even clients who seem to have a good grasp of these concepts may be unable to relate this information to their own situations.

9.4. CASE EXAMPLES

The following three cases illustrate some of the counseling complexities that can occur with the option of predisposition testing.

9.4.1. CASE 1: WHAT HAVE I DONE?

Rose Goldblum was one of the lucky ones. Her early-stage ovarian cancer had been detected by chance during a routine hysterectomy. She was doing well 7 years after her diagnosis. She had learned about BRCA1/2 panel testing through a lecture series at her temple, and, when a friend's daughter developed breast cancer, it galvanized Rose to request testing for the sake of her two daughters.

Rose was well informed about the BRCA1/2 test, and the only questions she asked were about the monitoring recommendations that would be given to her 25- and 28-year-old daughters. Rose's husband had died a few years ago of prostate cancer, but Rose had a large circle of close friends, one of whom came with her to the pretest counseling session. At age 60, Rose was not anticipating that a positive result would impact her medical care or her emotional well-being. She said that she was curious to know the result since she was the only member of her family to be diagnosed with cancer. Her parents had both died from heart disease and her one 63-year-old brother was doing well. Rose's family is Jewish, originally from Poland.

Rose has close relationships with both of her daughters. Her older daughter lives out of state, but they speak often by phone, whereas her younger daughter still lives at home while she attends graduate school. Rose had spoken to her daughters about the option of genetic testing, but neither was aware that Rose was being tested at this time. The counselor suggested that Rose inform her daughters about the impending BRCA1/2 result, but Rose preferred to wait until there was a concrete result to share. She signed the testing consent form and had blood drawn for the analysis.

Three weeks later they once again sat together in the consult room, this time to discuss the result. Rose sat down next to her friend, folded her hands together in her lap, and looked expectantly at the counselor, "Well?"

"Yes, the analysis did find a mutation in one of the genes. The BRCA1 gene."

Rose had no visible reaction to the news except mild curiosity. "Okay, which one is that. Is that the one linked with breast cancer?"

The counselor reviewed information about the 5385insC mutation and showed her the laboratory report. Rose said that she had anticipated this news and was almost glad the result was positive because now her daughters would be able to be tested and do everything they could to avoid getting cancer. She planned to tell her younger daughter right away but thought she might wait until her older daughter's visit at the end of the month to tell her. Although Rose was sanguine about being found to carry the mutation, she hoped fervently that neither daughter had inherited it. The counselor ended the session with a reminder that she and other program personnel were there if Rose needed them and that her daughters were welcome to call if they had any questions.

The counselor called Rose the following day to check in with her. Rose said that she was doing fine and seemed somewhat amused that the counselor would be worried about her. They chatted for a bit longer—more about a local art gallery exhibit than about the result; in closing, the counselor reiterated that Rose should feel free to contact her if she had any other questions or concerns.

Over the weekend, the counselor was surprised to receive a page through the hospital operator and even more surprised to hear Rose on the other line. Rose was so distraught that it was difficult at first for the counselor to understand what had happened. The counselor eventually learned that, earlier in the day, Rose had shared the result with her younger daughter, who had become hysterically upset by the news. After spending the day calming down her younger daughter, Rose decided to call her older daughter, who could always be counted on to be rational and supportive. Not this time. Her older daughter was horrified to learn that her mother had been tested and furious that her mother had just blurted out the result without any warning. The conversation ended with her hanging up on her mother, something she had never done before. Rose was distraught that she had caused her daughters such grief and worried aloud that they might never forgive her. "What have I done?" she said repeatedly. She was also somewhat bewildered that an act she had done on their behalf had resulted in this situation and was uncertain about how to repair the damage. The counselor spent most of the conversation just listening. When Rose seemed a bit calmer, the counselor commented that it was not uncommon for people to become upset and angry when hearing news like this. She reassured Rose that her daughters' panicked responses did not mean that they hated her nor that this result had permanently ruined their lives. They simply needed more time to adjust to it. The counselor and Rose then discussed what she could do to help her daughters adjust to the news. The counselor agreed with Rose's plan to acknowledge that she should have involved them more in her decision to be tested and to assure them that she would not bring up the topic again unless they wanted to talk about it. The counselor and Rose made plans to speak again the next day and ended up talking often over the next several months.

Rose did patch things up with her daughters, although it took months before either was interested in learning more about the test result. The older daughter eventually decided to be tested and Rose accompanied her to both genetic counseling visits. The daughter tested negative for the 5385insC mutation but, to everyone's surprise, was found to carry a 6174delT mutation. This result had repercussions not only for Rose's daughters but also for their paternal relatives. Rose had the hardest time coping with this result, perhaps because it fell to her to disclose the result to her relatives by marriage, most of whom did not take the news well. "Why did I ever start this?" she moaned to the genetic counselor during one of their many follow-up phone conversations.

Over time, things settled down for this family and Rose came to accept and even appreciate the genetic test information. Rose reported proudly that her older daughter has coped well with her positive result and even started a support group for other high-risk women in her city The younger daughter was being carefully monitored for breast cancer and planned to have her ovaries removed when she is older but remains comfortable with her decision not to be tested.

Two years later, Rose sent the counselor a picture of her new grandson with the message, "Life is good. Here is our latest genetic experiment. Turned out pretty good, didn't he?"

Key Points of Case:

1. Client eligibility and motivations for *BRCA1/2* panel testing—see Sections 9.1.1 and 9.1.3

2. Reactions to a positive result—see Section 9.3.3

3. Importance of follow-up interactions—see Section 9.3.5

9.4.2. Case 2: The One Thing I Don't Have Is Time

The genetic counselor answered the page from the breast oncologist who asked whether she would arrange *BRCA1/2* testing for one of her patients. As the genetic counselor greeted Ana, she noted that the woman did not look well. Her pale face was drawn in pain, and her body seemed frail and emaciated. In reviewing Ana's thick medical folder, the counselor learned that Ana was just 31 when found to have a 4-cm mass in her left breast. She was diagnosed with invasive ductal carcinoma; 13 of 14 lymph nodes were positive. Unfortunately, after 22 months of intensive therapy, including a bone marrow transplant, she had exhausted all medical options.

Ana was joined by her two sisters who flanked her on the consult room sofa. The sisters, with their olive skin and robust figures, were pictures of contrast next to Ana, except for their eyes, which were identical shades of luminous brown. Most of their relatives still lived in Lebanon, but Ana and her sisters had lived in the United States for the past 5 years. After greeting the client and her two sisters, the counselor explained that Ana's oncologist had wanted them to meet to discuss the option of genetic testing.

In accented but perfect English, Ana opened with, "My doctor said you could arrange for me to have gene therapy."

"You mean gene *testing*. Yes, I can arrange that for you. Let's talk about what testing could. . ."

"No, no—I mean gene therapy," interrupted Ana, " Like in this article." She handed over a clipping of a recent newspaper article detailing the potential wonders of gene therapy and cloning. With a sinking feeling, the counselor took the article and scanned it quickly. When she looked up, she saw three pairs of eyes staring hopefully at her. The counselor's heart sank further. She knew she had to clarify the misunderstanding but felt like she was taking away the family's last hope.

As gently as she could, the counselor said, "I read this article too. And it does talk about gene therapy as a potential strategy for treating cancer. Unfortunately, this isn't possible right now. There is a lot of research going on in the area of gene therapy and maybe in another 10 or 20 years it will be an option for cancer patients."

This speech was greeted by silence, then the older sister spoke up, "So you cannot arrange gene therapy?"

The counselor shook her head. "No, I can't. At this time, gene therapy is not available. I'm sorry."

"But the work is going on at this hospital," the sister pointed out forcefully, clearly not willing to give up. "Look, the article mentions this doctor who works here. Maybe we could speak with him."

"You are right; this doctor does work here, and he is one of the researchers trying to perfect gene therapy. But he is not treating patients yet. The researchers need more time before they can offer gene therapy as a treatment option."

"The one thing I don't have is time," interjected Ana softly. She turned to her younger sister who patted her hand and murmured comforting phrases to her in Lebanese. The older sister glared at the counselor before putting her arm around Ana and joining their conversation. The counselor waited uncertainly while the three of them quietly conversed and thought her best bet would be to say a few words about genetic testing and then exit gracefully.

"I am so sorry about the misunderstanding. There is a lot we still cannot do in genetics. What we can do is find out if families have an inherited predisposition to breast cancer. This is called genetic testing. But we don't have to talk about this now if you would rather not."

The younger sister spoke up tentatively, "I guess I would like to hear more about this genetic test. My doctor has also mentioned it to me. What do you think, Ana?"

Ana thought for a minute and then nodded, "Yes, I think we should find out more about this. It could be important information for the two of you to have. Not to mention my five nieces." The older sister did not openly disagree with her, but her silence spoke volumes.

The counselor explained that she would like to begin the testing discussion by assessing the pattern of cancer in the family. Ana was the only member of her large family ever to develop cancer. Ana asserted that illnesses were discussed openly in their family and that they would almost certainly have learned of other cancer diagnoses had they occurred. Once the pedigree was completed, the counselor explained that, despite Ana's unusually young age at diagnosis, it was likely that her breast cancer was a random occurrence. This was reassuring to all three sisters but also seemed to underscore how unfair it was that Ana had developed breast cancer in the first place.

The counselor then detailed the logistics of the testing process. The usual discussion about the risks and benefits of testing and potential impact of the result seemed less useful under these circumstances. When the counselor mentioned that the results would be available in about 4 weeks, both sisters looked uneasy but did not say anything. Ana signed the testing consent form, and her sisters agreed to cover the costs of testing if her insurance plan did not. The counselor then handed Ana a one-page form and matter of factly requested that she designate whom should be given the results in case she was no longer available to receive them. The sisters looked even more perturbed by this direct reference to her terminal illness, but Ana took the form without comment and signed permission for either of her sisters to receive the genetic test results.

The counselor felt as though Ana's impending death was the proverbial "elephant in the room"—the topic that everyone was conscious of but no one wanted to admit. The counselor was not sure whether Ana wanted to talk about it either but did not feel right about continuing to talk around the issue. As Ana handed the completed form, the counselor gently asked her, "Is it hard answering questions like this?"

Ana smiled wanly and said, "Not really. I've made my peace with dying—at least, I've tried to. And then again, who knows? A year ago, I was given a few months to live and yet I'm still here. My doctor says I defy predictions." Her smile grew stronger.

"Sounds like you have a very strong will to live," commented the counselor smiling back.

"Yes, I am a fighter. But I also have a strong faith. I'm not afraid of dying." Her sisters both burst into speech at this point, chiding her for sounding like she was giving up, and Ana looked wryly at the counselor. "I guess you could say we are a family of fighters. My family keeps searching for a miracle." She said it in a light voice, but her eyes held such sadness that the counselor knew she herself did not hold out the same hope.

The counselor did not feel comfortable agreeing with either the client or her sisters about the likelihood of a miracle cure so she decided to shift the conversation; "You certainly have a very supportive family around you."

"Yes, it helps a lot. To have to go through something like this alone, I can't even imagine it. I guess that's why I want to do the genetic test—it is one more thing I can do for my family." Ana squeezed both her sisters' hands as she spoke. The nurse then took Ana to draw her blood, while the counselor sat with the two sisters. They asked a few more questions about the possible genetic test results but did not seem eager to have testing themselves. The counselor then walked them back to the oncologist's office where they were to discuss options of hospice care.

The counselor received Ana's negative *BRCA1/2* result 1 week after Ana's death. The counselor waited a few weeks and then sent both of Ana's sisters a note saying that the result was available. The older sister called right away, and the counselor disclosed the result to her over the phone. She expressed relief that the result was negative, although the reaction was muted by her numbing grief over her sister's death. They spoke of Ana for several minutes; in closing, the counselor said that she would send a summary letter and copies of the result and a computerized pedigree.

The younger sister called a few days later. She had learned of the result from her sister but wanted to make sure that Ana would still be included on the computerized pedigree being sent to them. The counselor assured her that Ana would always be part of their family tree, and, at her request, the counselor did not indicate that Ana had died on the pedigrees sent to the family.

In addition to sending the information to both sisters, the counselor also sent handwritten condolence notes to each of them. The counselor eventually filed away the client's folder, but the image of sad brown eyes stayed with her for a long time.

Key Points of Case:

1. Client eligibility and motivation—see Sections 9.1.1 and 9.1.3
2. Client's understanding of genetics—see Section 9.2.1
3. Counseling a terminally ill client—see Section 9.1.4 and Chapter 7, Section 7.4.5

9.4.2. Case 3: Welcome to Genetic Limbo

Jeri had the frazzled appearance of a mother trying unsuccessfully to occupy her young children in a public place. As she wheeled the stroller into the conference room, she apologized to the genetic counselor for having to bring along her two sons (ages 2 and 4); her babysitter had cancelled at the last minute. The counselor assured her that it was alright but mentally condensed her agenda as she eyed the giggly boys—the chances of making it through a 1-hour conversation were slim. When the two boys were seated at the desk with paper and crayons and bribed with a future promise of ice cream, Jeri turned back to the counselor, pushed her uncombed hair away from her face, and said "Ready, set, go."

The counselor began by reviewing what they had discussed over the phone prior to the visit. Jeri had been diagnosed with bilateral breast cancer last year at age 35 and had undergone bilateral mastectomies. She had a significant family history of breast cancer, as shown in Figure 9-1. Jeri had also faxed the counselor a copy of a paternal cousin's genetic test result, which had revealed a *BRCA1* variant of uncertain significance. The cousin, Sandra, had never had cancer herself, but Sandra's sister, Tina, had died of breast

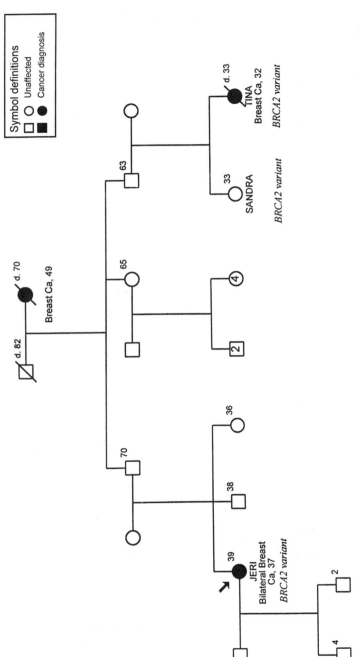

FIGURE 9-1. Jeri's pedigree. Family history is consistent with a hereditary breast cancer syndrome. Jeri, Sandra, and Tina carry a variant of uncertain significance.

cancer at age 33. Jeri was now undergoing BRCA1 and BRCA2 full gene analysis to determine whether she had a separate deleterious mutation that could explain the history of cancer in the family.

Jeri had a good understanding of why she was being tested and seemed keen on learning the information. The counselor described the three possible results she could receive: a positive result, an indeterminate negative result, or a variant result (the same as Sandra). The counselor explained further that the clinical significance of the variant result would not be proven were she to have it, but, if the variant were absent, it would reduce the likelihood that it was the underlying cause of breast cancer for their family.

The counselor then asked Jeri about what she saw as the main risks and benefits of testing. By this point, the younger son had crawled under the desk and was throwing crayons at his brother who was squealing gleefully each time he missed. After Jeri pulled them away from the desk and settled them together in an armchair with crackers and juice boxes, she answered that the primary benefit of identifying a mutation would be to give her sister an opportunity to be tested. She said that the downside to this information would be having to make a decision about having her ovaries out. Jeri's oncologist had informed her about the possible increased risk of ovarian cancer and had recommended a prophylactic oophorectomy. After all she had been through over the past year, she was reluctant to undergo additional surgery. Jeri, a certified yoga instructor, said that one of the most difficult aspects of the cancer experience was having to limit her physical activities for so long.

The conversation came to an abrupt halt when the boys' wrestling match ended with the younger one tumbling to the floor. Jeri dried his tears and cuddled him in her lap as she reviewed the testing consent form. The older boy began pushing the stroller around the room, singing cheerfully. "You can see why I need to meditate," commented Jeri as she signed the consent form. They all walked down to the blood-drawing laboratory, and Jeri made an appointment to come back in 4 weeks. The counselor encouraged her to bring someone (preferably an adult) to the results session. Jeri said that she would ask her husband to come with her—and would try hard to leave her sons at home next time.

A month later, the counselor shared with Jeri that she had the same BRCA1 variant as her cousin. They reviewed what this result meant and what it did not mean. Her husband, who did come to the appointment, asked few questions but made several humorous observations. After listening to a lengthy explanation of the genetic test result, he said, "So basically the message is 'Hi, folks. Welcome to Genetic Limbo.'" The counselor conceded that this was about right.

When the program oncologist joined the session, Jeri's husband shook his hand and said that their jobs were similar—as a tax accountant, he too was used to seeing people in pain. The oncologist laughed while Jeri rolled her eyes and said, "Please, don't encourage him." They discussed options for medical management, including prophylactic oophorectomy, and the oncologist acknowledged that it was difficult to know whether Jeri was at increased risk for ovarian cancer.

They then returned to discussing the variant result and explored possible strategies for clarifying the meaning of the test result. One option was to obtain a tissue specimen from Tina, the cousin who had died from early-onset breast cancer, to see whether the variant was tracking with the cancer in the family. Jeri said she would talk to Sandra about this option but thought she would be interested in doing this.

The following morning, the counselor had a voice mail message from Sandra who wanted to proceed with obtaining the tissue specimen from her sister, Tina. This turned out to be a more difficult process than anticipated (and required the cooperation of their parents); however, after 3 months, the counselor finally received the specimen and sent it to a laboratory for the single-site analysis. Two months later, the laboratory reported that Tina also carried the *BRCA1* variant. The counselor disclosed this result to both Sandra and Jeri and spent a great deal of time trying to decipher the meaning of the three family test results. When additional relatives began asking for clarification, the counselor offered the option of a family meeting. Both Sandra and Jeri liked this idea, and a meeting was scheduled.

The family meeting was held at the hospital in a paneled conference room that held an oval-shaped oak table and a large chalkboard. After greeting the family members, the counselor opened the meeting by formally introducing herself, the program oncologist, and the program social worker. Nine family members were in attendance: Jeri and her husband, Sandra and her female life partner, Jeri's brother and his wife, Jeri's sister; and Sandra's parents. The counselor opened the meeting by asking for the main questions or concerns that each person wanted clarified. The responses of the blood relatives were as follows:

Jeri: Should I have a prophylactic oophorectomy?

Sandra: Should I have a prophylactic mastectomy?

Jerri's brother: Am I at any increased risk? What about my daughters?

Jerri's sister: Should I be tested for this variant?

Sandra's father: Is there a surefire way of preventing breast cancer?

The first part of this meeting was spent reviewing basic information about the *BRCA1* and *BRCA2* genes, causes of breast cancer, features of hereditary breast cancer, and the principles of dominant inheritance. The counselor then described the test result itself, stressing that its clinical significance remained unproven. She explained the probability that three family members could carry the same *BRCA1* variant by chance alone. The counselor reiterated that the variant result would need to be clarified before offering testing to other family members. She explained that a positive variant result would confer uncertain cancer risks, and a negative variant result would not rule out any increased risk. She promised to send the family any amended information about the variant result received from the laboratory.

The oncologist then led the discussion about medical monitoring and the options of chemoprevention and prophylactic surgery. He stressed that the family met criteria for a hereditary breast cancer syndrome and thus screening recommendations were being based on the family history rather than the variant test result. Making decisions about prophylactic surgery was trickier because Jeri's sister and even Sandra had uncertain risks of breast cancer, and the risk of ovarian cancer among any of the women was unclear. He assured Jeri's brother that there would be much more information, as well as better interventions, by the time his young daughters reached adulthood.

Lastly, the social worker talked about what it was like to receive this type of result, and the family freely admitted its frustration that testing had not yielded a definitive answer. Because it was possible that this test result would not be resolved for several months or even years, they also talked about what it would be like to continue living with this type of uncertainty. This led to a discussion of their collective and individual worries about cancer and possible strategies for helping them cope with these fears. One suggestion from Jeri's husband was that Jeri buy him a really expensive set of golf clubs. When Jeri asked him how this would be helpful, he said, "Well, it would make me feel better. Why should we both be upset?" Everyone laughed, and Sandra whispered loudly to her cousin, "I sure hope the kids got your sense of humor."

Each family member received a letter summarizing the 2-hour discussion; 12 months later, they continue to wait for clarification of the genetic test result.

Key Points of Case:

1. Elements of the pre-test counseling session—see Sections 9.1.3 and 9.2
2. Possible strategies for clarifying a variant result—see Section 9.2.2
3. Disclosure session and follow-up—see Sections 9.3.4 and 9.3.5

9.5. REFERENCES

American Society of Clinical Oncology. 1996. Genetic Testing for Cancer Susceptibility [www.asco.org]. Adopted February 1996.
Baum, A, Friedman, A, and Zakowski, S. 1997. Stress and genetic testing for disease risk. Health Psychol 16:8–19.

Bernhardt, B, Geller, G, Doksum, T et al. 2000. Evaluation of nurses and genetic counselors as providers of education about breast cancer susceptibility testing. Oncol Nurs Forum 27:33–39.

Botkin, J, Croyle, R, Smith, K et al. 1996. A model protocol for evaluating the behavioral and psychosocial effects of BRCA1 testing. JNCI. 88:1872–1882.

Buckman, R.. 1992. How to Break Bad News: A Guide for Health Care Professionals. Johns Hopkins University Press, Baltimore, MD.

Clark, S, Bluman, L, Borstelmann, N et al. 2000. Patient motivation, satisfaction, and coping in genetic counseling and testing for BRCA1 and BRCA2. J Genet Counseling 9:219–235.

Croyle, R, Smith, K, Botkin, J et al. 1997. Psychological responses to BRCA1 mutation testing: preliminary findings. Health Psych 16:63–72.

Cummings, S and Olopade, O. 1998. Predisposition testing for inherited breast cancer. Oncology 12:1227–1242.

Dorval, M, Patenaude, A, Schneider, K et al. 2000. Anticipated versus emotional reactions to disclosure of results of genetic tests for cancer susceptibility: findings from p53 and BRCA1 testing programs. J Clin Oncol 18:2135–2142.

DudokdeWit, A, Tibben, A, Duivenvoorden, H et al. 1998. Predicting adaptation to presymptomatic DNA testing for late onset disorders: who will experience distress? J Med Genet. 35:745–754.

Emmons, K, Kalkbrenner, K, Klar, N et al. 2000. Behavioral risk factors among women presenting for genetic testing. Ca Epidem Biomarkers Prev. 9:89—94.

Evans, D, Maher, E, Macleod, R et al. 1997. Uptake of genetic testing for cancer predisposition. J Med Genet 34:746–748.

Giardiello, F, Brensinger, J, Peterson, G et al. 1997. The use and interpretation of commercial APC gene testing for FAP. NEJM 336:823–827.

Geller, G, Botkin, J, Green, M et al. 1997. Genetic testing for susceptibility to adult-onset cancer: The process and content of informed consent. JAMA 277:1467–1474.

Grosfeld, F, Lips, C, Beemer, F et al. 2000. Who is at risk for psychological distress in genetic testing programs for hereditary cancer disorders. J Genet Counseling 9:253–266.

Jacobsen, P, Valdimarsdottir, H, Brown, K et al. 1997. Decision-making about genetic testing among women at familial risk for breast cancer. Psychosomatic Medicine. 59:459–466.

Julian-Reynier, C, Eisinger, F, Vennin, P et al. 1996. Attitudes towards cancer predictive testing and transmission of information to the family. J Med Genet. 33:731–736.

Kinney, A, Choi, Y, DeVellis, B et al. 2000. Interest in genetic testing among first-degree relatives of colorectal cancer patients. Am J Prev Med 18:249–252.

Lerman, C, Biesecker, B, Benkendorf, J et al. 1997. Controlled trial of pretest education approaches to enhance informed decision-making for BRCA1 gene testing. J Natl Cancer Inst 89:148–157.

Lerman, C, Hughes, C, Lemon, S et al. 1998. What you don't know can hurt you: adverse psychologic effects in members of BRCA1-linked and BRCA2-linked families who decline genetic testing. J Clin Oncol 16:1650–1654.

Lerman, C, Hughes, C, Trock, B et al. 1999. Genetic testing in families with hereditary nonpolyposis colon cancer. JAMA 17:1618–1622.

Liede, A, Metcalfe, K, Hanna, D et al. 2000. Evaluation of the needs of male carriers of mutations in BRCA2 or BRCA2 who have undergone genetic counseling. Am J Hum Genet 67:1494–1504.

Lubinsky, M. 1994. Bearing bad news: dealing with the mimics of denial. J Genet Counseling 3:5–12.

Lynch, H, Lemon, S, Durham, C et al. 1997. A descriptive study of BRCA1 testing and reactions to disclosure of test results. Cancer 79:2219–2228.

McKinnon, W, Baty, B, Bennett, R et al. 1997. Predisposition genetic testing for late-onset disorders in adults: a position paper of the National Society of Genetic Counselors. JAMA 278:1217–1220.

Metcalfe, K, Liede, A, Hoodfer, E et al. 2000. An evaluation of needs of female BRCA1 and BRCA2 carriers undergoing genetic counseling. J Med Genet 37:866–874.

Monson, N. 1995. Family Affairs. Weight Watchers Magazine April Issue, p.64.

Petersen, G, Brensinger, J, Johnson, K et al. 1999. Genetic testing and counseling for hereditary forms of colorectal cancer. Cancer 86:2540–2550.

Schneider, K. 1997. BRCA1/2 testing. Genetic Testing. 1:91–98.

Schneider, K, Kieffer, S, and Patenaude, A. 2000. BRCA1 testing and informed consent in a woman with mild retardation. J Genet Counseling 9:411–416.

Smith, D, Quaid, K, Dworkin, R et al. 1998. Early Warning: Case and Ethical Guidance for Presymptomatic Testing in Genetic Diseases. Indiana University Press, Bloomington, IN.

THE ETHICAL ISSUES

As genetic possibilities become realities, it is imperative that professionals, clients, policy makers, and the general public scrutinize the values inherent in the health care system and the social and ethical consequences of communicating genetic information. [T]his examination can also serve as a foundation from which to begin to address some legal, ethical and policy considerations in the expanding universe of clinical genetics, one that will profoundly affect the future of us all.

(Bartels, 1993, p. xii–xiii)

This chapter reviews the primary ethical principles that should guide genetic counseling interactions. Adhering to these principles while balancing the rights of individual clients and families can be challenging. This is demonstrated by five case discussions that illustrate some of the ethical dilemmas that can be raised by predisposition testing.

10.1. BASIC ETHICAL PRINCIPLES

Cancer genetic counseling and testing programs should be guided by four basic ethical principles (see Table 10-1).

1. *Autonomy*—The principle of autonomy has three tenets. First, no one should ever be coerced into having a predictive genetic test. Second, individuals need to be able to decide for themselves whether or not to undergo testing. Third, to reach decisions about testing, individu-

TABLE 10-1. THE BASIC PRINCIPLES OF ETHICS IN THE CONTEXT OF
PREDISPOSITION TESTING

Autonomy	Testing decision should be autonomous and informed.
Beneficence	Testing should cause no emotional harm.
Confidentiality	Testing program should respect confidentiality.
Justice	There should be fairness in testing options and decisions based on results.

als need to be counseled about all potential implications of either agreeing or refusing to be tested. This principle underscores the importance of the informed consent process. It should be noted that this a principle of Western culture. In other parts of the world, there may be a much greater emphasis on family decision-making or deference to the decisions of a few family members, such as parents or grandparents.

2. *Beneficence*—The phrase in medicine primum non nocere (first do no harm) summarizes this principle. In terms of predictive genetic testing, this means that genetic counselors, along with other health professionals, have a responsibility to avoid harming people who are not emotionally able to handle the testing process or results disclosure. To avoid potential harm, programs should assess the psychological and emotional well-being of participants before disclosing results. In addition, genetic counseling and other support services need to be available throughout the testing process.

3. *Confidentiality*—There should be careful mechanisms in place to ensure that results and other sensitive information, such as nonpaternity, are not inadvertently disclosed to third parties. Some programs, for example, disclose results to the client's primary physician, whereas others disclose results only to the client. Either of these policies is acceptable as long as clients are aware, from the outset, who will have access to their testing results.

4. *Justice*—This principle implies fairness. Thus, individuals should be eligible for predictive genetic testing regardless of ethnic background, geographical location, or ability to pay. Also, no one should experience discrimination based on the test results.

Not infrequently, counseling interactions lead to ethical dilemmas or challenges. In resolving these situations, genetic counselors may find it useful to review professional position papers and other ethical guidelines listed at the end of this chapter. Members of the National Society of Genetic Counselors (NSGC) are also expected to follow this code of ethics, which

TABLE 10-2. Ethical Guidelines for Genetic Counselors

The counselor-client relationship is based on values of care and respect for the client's autonomy, individuality, welfare, and freedom. The primary concern of genetic counselors is the interests of their clients. Therefore, genetic counselors strive to:

Equally serve all who seek services.

Respect their clients' beliefs, cultural traditions, inclinations, circum stances, and feelings.

Enable their clients to make informed independent decisions, free of coercion, by providing or illuminating the necessary facts and clarifying the alternatives and anticipated consequences.

Refer clients to other competent professional when they are unable to support the clients.

Maintain as confidential any information received from clients, unless released by the client.

Avoid the exploitation of their clients for personal advantage, profit, or interest.

Source: The National Society of Genetic Counselors' Code of Ethics.

can be found on the NSGC website (www.NSGC.org). Members of NSGC who face difficult ethical dilemmas in the workplace can also obtain confidential consultations from the Ethics subcommittee. Table 10-2 lists the NSGC guidelines related to patient care. Table 10-3 summarizes another useful set of guidelines for genetic counselors, developed by David Smith and colleagues (1998). Consider these guidelines while reading the cases discussed in the next section.

10.2. Case Examples and Discussion

We have enormous responsibilities to our patients, to the institutions in which we work, to our profession, and to ourselves. The process of upholding these responsibilities while serving our patients comprises the "art" of genetic counseling.

(*Weinblatt et al., 1998, pg. 391*)

This section consists of five hypothetical cases. These cases have been chosen because they represent the different ethical dilemmas that cancer counselors may face as they provide risk assessment or predisposition testing.

The following cases are discussed in this section:

- Patient autonomy versus rights of the family
- Duty to do no harm versus paternalism
- Duty to warn versus client privacy

Appropriate information	Professionals should consider ethical issues from the inception of every testing, counseling, and research program, and they should provide consultands with information that is appropriately tailored to the stage of the testing-counseling program the consultand has reached. To the extent possible, ethical dilemmas should be anticipated, and the counselor should try to prevent them from arising.
Pre- and posttest counseling	Genetic testing should be accompanied by both pre- and posttest counseling conducted by persons with competencies in medical genetic, laboratory analysis, counseling, and the psychosocial impact of genetic information.
Protocols	Protocols are useful guidelines for the appropriate conduct of presymptomatic testing. Justifications for departure from a protocol must relate to the rationale for that protocol.
Confidentiality	Genetic counselors are ethically obligated to maintain consultands' confidentiality.
Refusing or postponing testing	In deciding whether to refuse or postpone testing, genetic counselors should exercise professional judgment based on clinical observation and the consultand's history.
Freedom to reject disclosure	Consultands should remain free to reject disclosure of test results and other diagnostic information unless their decision not to know their status poses a significant risk to others.
Others' preference not to know	The fact that testing a consultand will reveal the genetic status of other persons, who prefer not to know their status, is not, by itself, a sufficient reason to delay testing.
Testing children	Genetic testing of symptomatic children to make or confirm a diagnosis may be performed subject to general ethical and legal rules governing medical care for children. Presymptomatic genetic testing should only be performed on children when all of the conditions set out in paragraphs A, B, and C are met. A. A presymtomatic test should be given to a child only if both of the child's parents who are reasonably available have consented to the testing. If only one parent is reasonably available, that parent must consent to the testing. B. If the child has or can be provided with a reasonable understanding of the proposed genetic test and its implications, the child's assent to genetic testing must be sought. C. There must be a reasonable possibility that testing will enable the child to receive a real, demonstrable benefit.

Source: Smith et al., 1998, pp. 131–163. [Printed with Permission]

- Right to know versus not to know
- Concerns about testing minors versus parents' right to decide

10.2.1. Case 1: Patient Autonomy Versus Rights of the Family

A 35-year-old female client is concerned about her cancer risks because her mother had both breast and ovarian cancer in her forties and her grandmother had breast cancer in her thirties. Both relatives are deceased. A maternal aunt survived her premenopausal breast cancer and is in her seventies. The family is of mixed European heritage, and are not Jewish.

The client has two younger sisters and seven female first cousins who are also potentially at increased risk of cancer.

You tell the client that she is eligible for BRCA1 and BRCA2 analysis based on this family history but that predictive genetic testing would be more accurate if the familial mutation was identified. This would involve testing her maternal aunt. The client says she will contact her aunt and ask her to be tested.

The aunt eventually comes in to be tested. During the conversation, she tells you that she has no personal interest in learning her genetic test results and wishes aloud that she did not need to be tested. You assure her that the decision to be tested is up to her and that she does not need to proceed with testing. She seems greatly relieved by this and leaves without having her blood drawn. She gives you permission to inform her niece that testing was not performed.

When you tell the niece that testing was not done, she becomes very upset. You remind her that she can still undergo BRCA1 and BRCA2 testing, but she only wants testing if a mutation has been identified in the family. Two weeks later, the aunt returns to the testing center and says she is now willing to be tested. She admits to having received angry phone calls from three of her nieces and her brother-in-law, a physician. It seems obvious that the family has convinced her to be tested. The aunt reiterates that she would prefer not to learn her genetic test results but is willing to do so to keep peace in the family. She insists that she is ready to sign the consent form and proceed with testing.

Do you test the aunt despite your concerns that she appears to have been coerced into testing?

CASE DISCUSSION.   One of the central tenets of predisposition testing is that clients have freely and autonomously made the decision to be tested. In fact, a primary goal of the informed consent process is to ensure that clients have made their own decisions about being tested after learning about the parameters of the test. Autonomous decision making further implies that the final decision to be tested rests with the client, not with other interested third parties (such as physicians, insurers, or even other family members).

In this case, at-risk family members have a vested interest in having the option of a targeted, definitive genetic test. Such a test would accurately identify the relatives at high risk for breast and ovarian cancer and would lead to specific recommendations about monitoring and prevention, including the prophylactic removal of ovaries. Because of the high likelihood that the aunt carries an identifiable *BRCA1* or *BRCA2* mutation, she is the logical person to initially test. The alternative of offering full gene analysis to all at-risk relatives is feasible but is an expensive proposition and may not yield definitive answers. Therefore, it is in the family's best interest that the aunt undergo testing.

However, if the aunt had continued to decline testing, her right to refuse would have superseded the family's wishes. An adult of sound mind clearly has the right to decline an optional, invasive procedure, such as genetic testing. It can also be argued that the female members of this family are already aware of their potentially increased risks of breast and ovarian cancer and can make medical management decisions accordingly. The aunt's refusal to be tested would not, therefore, preclude anyone from obtaining appropriate medical care.

What makes this case difficult for the genetic counselor is that the aunt is willing to sign a consent form and proceed with testing even though she has vocalized her preference not to learn her genetic test results. If the counselor agrees to test the aunt, is she aiding and abetting the coercive efforts of the family? And yet does a counselor have the right to deny a test that a client will consent to have? Whose rights are more important—the aunt's or the family's?

COUNSELOR STRATEGIES.   To help resolve this case, the genetic counselor should consider the following issues:

1. *Who is the primary client?*—One of the complexities of this case is that both the niece and the aunt have been seen by the genetic counselor, which means that the counselor has some obligation to both parties. However, during the pretest counseling session, the aunt is the main client and her needs should take precedence over the wishes of her niece. It is therefore appropriate for the counselor to inform the aunt that she has the option of not being tested.

2. *Is it possible to satisfy both parties?*—The counselor did remind the niece that she could be tested directly but to no avail. Perhaps other at-risk relatives would be more amenable to being tested. A positive test result in any family member would allow the at-risk client to undergo a targeted, definitive test. This strategy would also negate the need for the aunt to be tested. Without the family pressure, it seems likely

that the aunt would choose not to be tested. Another possible strategy is to have the aunt authorize the testing center to disclose the results to her family, not her. This would satisfy the family's desire for information while upholding the aunt's preference not to learn her test results.

3. *Would testing cause harm?*—Because the aunt has agreed to be tested, the onus is on the counselor to prove that this course would be detrimental. The counselor should explore the possible ramifications of obtaining the genetic test results and conduct a psychological screening assessment. However, unless there is evidence of significant emotional distress, this test result is not likely to cause great harm to her. On the other hand, denying the test could seriously strain the relationships within this family.

4. *Is it really coercion?*—Had the aunt indicated that it was her health insurer, employer, or even physician who was demanding that she be tested, the genetic counselor would be within her right to question the validity of the request. However, demands from family members are more difficult to sort out. The bonds of family members are usually closer than that of other relationships, and, presumably, the aunt has some vested interest in the health and well-being of her nieces. The fact that the aunt wants to "keep peace" further implies that she is not willing to break from the family over this issue. In addition, although the family has clearly pressured her to be tested, the aunt has not been threatened or harmed in any way nor did anyone force her to come to the testing appointment. Thus, the family interactions are unlikely to constitute actual coercion.

BOTTOM LINE. The genetic counselor should first explore other avenues of testing for this family that do not involve the aunt's participation. If this is not successful, the counselor should proceed with testing the aunt. The pretest counseling session should include implications of the test result and a standard assessment of emotional well-being. The aunt has stated her willingness to be tested for the sake of her family, and the counselor should accept that family obligations rather than coercion have led her to this decision. Thus, if the aunt signs the consent form, it is ultimately her decision and her agreement to be tested.

10.2.2. CASE 2: DUTY TO DO NO HARM VERSUS PATERNALISM

A 23-year-old male client is at 50% risk of having the familial *VHL* mutation. His mother has had several benign tumors removed from her spine and currently has end-stage renal cell carcinoma and has been diagnosed with von

Hippel Lindau syndrome (VHL). His brother carries a *VHL* mutation and recently had surgery to remove a large brain lesion. The client has yearly abdominal and head CT scans, which have always been normal.

You take a psychological assessment as part of the testing protocol at your center. The client dropped out of college a few years ago and has been working as a waiter since that time. Over the past year, he has held five different jobs. He admits that he often feels like a failure and makes several disparaging remarks about his abilities and intelligence. He also acknowledges that he has had long-standing depression and made two suicide attempts as a teenager. He denies any suicidal ideation at this time, although his depression is not being currently treated. The client also seems to have little social support. He has no close friends and still lives at home. He lists his mother as his main source of support but does not plan to burden her with his result if positive. He does not get along well with his brother, and his father deserted the family several years ago.

The client denies that a positive *VHL* result will cause him any additional emotional distress and assures you that his depression is at a manageable level. He further expresses hope that obtaining his genetic test result will mark a new beginning for him. He feels that a true negative result will help motivate him to make something of his life, and a positive result will motivate him to enjoy life while he can. He declines a referral to your program psychologist.

Do you test this client despite concerns about his emotional well-being?

CASE DISCUSSION.   Rates of suicide tend to be higher among individuals with serious medical conditions, and concerns about suicidality have been extended to include healthy but genetically predisposed individuals. Although the likelihood that a positive genetic test result will trigger a suicide attempt is low, testing programs need to be aware that this is possible. To address this concern, many testing programs have incorporated certain safeguards into the testing process, such as the use of standardized measures of depression or distress and questions about current emotional stress within the genetic counseling interview itself.

The main purpose of identifying emotionally vulnerable individuals is to provide additional services as needed. However, in rare cases, the extent of baseline distress will invoke discussions of deferring or denying the test. In this case, the client is clearly eligible for genetic testing; there is a known mutation in the family and he is at 50% risk for carrying it. This is also a test that the client himself has requested. However, the counselor in this case is not obligated to provide testing if disclosing the result is likely to have a serious adverse effect. A certain amount of distress is an expected corollary of a positive test result, but harming oneself or others is not.

However, making the decision to defer or deny a genetic test is not something to be made lightly.

The main question for providers is whether testing deferral or denial is a beneficent gesture or an act of paternalism. Acting in a beneficent manner implies that the provider's decision to override the client's wish to be tested was made because of reasonable concerns that testing would cause serious harm to the client. Providers who act in a paternalistic manner believe that they know best what the client should do and will make recommendations accordingly, including that of ordering or not ordering a genetic test.

Denying a test does not seem justifiable under any circumstances, as it implies that the client will never be able to undergo testing. In contrast, deferral means that testing will be delayed until circumstances have changed or certain recommendations have been met. With rare exception, clients are expected to make their own decisions regarding genetic testing or other courses of action. It is for this reason that genetic counselors present options in a nondirective manner rather than advising clients what to do. Therefore, it is only in extreme cases of emotional distress that genetic counselors should consider deferring testing requests.

COUNSELOR STRATEGIES. In deciding whether to test this client for a *VHL* mutation, the genetic counselor should consider the following issues:

1. *What is the client's level of distress?*—Deferral of testing should only be made after careful consideration of the client's emotional state. In this case, there are several "red flags" that raise concerns about the client's ability to cope with his test result. These include his long-standing and currently untreated depression, low self-esteem, lack of social support, and two previous suicide attempts. In addition, the timing of the testing request is concerning, as the client's mother (listed as the client's only support) is terminally ill.

   The genetic counselor should obtain as much evidence as possible regarding the client's level of emotional distress. This can include speaking to the client's other medical providers (with his permission) and obtaining scores from one or more written psychological assessments. Although the client refused to meet with the program psychologist, the counselor would be well advised to discuss the case with him or her. If the psychologist feels that the client is not as distressed as the counselor assessment would suggest, then the counselor should feel more comfortable proceeding with testing. If, however, the psychologist concurs that the client is a high suicide risk given his previous history and current stressors, then the counselor is justified in deferring the test.

2. *What is the potential harm in testing?*—The main concern in this case is whether the disclosure of the test result would cause significant harm to this emotionally vulnerable client. In addition to his emotional problems and lack of support, this client also seems to hold unrealis-

tic expectations that the test result has the power to change his life. His statement that a positive result will cause him to enjoy life more "while he can" makes it seem as though he feels his time would be limited, an attitude that is worrisome given that he has already attempted suicide twice. And although this client may be greatly relieved by a true negative result, it is quite possible that the knowledge he was spared (while his brother was not) could cause survivor guilt and worsen his feelings of being a failure. Therefore, either test result could adversely affect this client's emotional well-being.

3. *What is the potential harm in deferring the test?*—This client has a 50% risk of having the familial *VHL* mutation. Knowledge of his test result may have a medical benefit that outweighs concerns about the psychological impact. Although the client is already being monitored for VHL-related tumors, this test result would clarify the need for such procedures. It is also possible that the test result will have little impact on his emotional well-being, given that his problems are of long duration and, in fact, the testing process might be the impetus for him to seek psychological intervention. There is also a possibility that this client could view the testing program's decision to defer testing as yet another "failure," which could also have a detrimental impact on his self-esteem. In addition, *VHL* testing is clinically available. Therefore, this client could pursue testing through his primary care physician who is unlikely to provide the same level of support as the testing program.

4. *What is the program's deferral policy?*—All cancer genetic testing programs should have established criteria for deferring test requests. The genetic counselor in this case should discuss the case thoroughly with other program personnel and make a joint decision about deferring or proceeding with testing. Some programs will defer testing requests only if the client is deemed to be a high suicide risk, other programs will defer testing if the result could exacerbate significant emotional problems, even in the absence of suicidal ideation. The program should also consider alternatives to deferral, such as requiring additional visits with the genetic counselor and/or program psychologist throughout the testing process. Decisions about deferral should be made before the blood draw. Deciding not to disclose an available test result is a morally difficult position to defend and should only be done under rare circumstances.

BOTTOM LINE. The genetic counselor should ascertain whether this client could become suicidal upon learning his genetic test result. If this is the case (and it seems likely), then testing should be deferred. The genetic counselor should be honest with the client about why this decision was made and indicate the parameters under which testing would be resumed. If the client is not deemed to be at risk for suicide, then the genetic counselor should proceed with testing the client. Because of the emotional vulnerability of the client, the counselor should provide increased support throughout the testing process. Determination of the client's current suicidality needs to be made by a licensed mental health professional. If genetic testing is performed, it may be reasonable to require that the client meet with the program psychologist, particularly if he receives a positive result.

10.2.3. Case 3: Duty to Warn Versus Client Privacy

The 27-year-old client in the high-risk breast cancer clinic says she wants to learn more about BRCA1 and BRCA2 testing because two paternal aunts and a first cousin have had breast cancer in their thirties. The client is also concerned about the cancer risks for her 4-year-old daughter. Later in the conversation, the client recalls that the cousin also had a leg removed at age 12 due to bone cancer. When learning the name of the cousin, you realize that you recognize this family as one that has Li-Fraumeni (LFS) syndrome. You are aware that one of her paternal aunts also had childhood adrenal gland cancer and that the cousin has a deleterious TP53 mutation (tested through your center).

   With this client, you discuss the likelihood that the breast cancer in her family could be due to an inherited dominant gene mutation. You briefly describe the features of breast-ovarian cancer syndrome and BRCA1 and BRCA2 testing. You then explain that a BRCA1 or BRCA2 mutation would not explain why her cousin developed both a childhood osteosarcoma and early-onset breast cancer and go on to describe LFS. The client is surprised that her family could have LFS—and does not seem convinced that this is a likely possibility. You tell the client that you would like to rule out the possibility that her family has LFS before arranging for her to have BRCA1 and BRCA2 testing. You encourage her to obtain more information about the diagnoses of cancer in her family and to call back if she obtains any additional information and/or is still interested in genetic testing.

   The client calls back a month later and says that she has spoken to her one living aunt and obtained documentation of her breast cancer diagnosis at age 32. The client was not able to obtain further information about her other aunt (who is deceased) or her cousin. She says that she does not feel comfortable contacting her cousin because they have not been in contact for years. The client reiterates her interest in BRCA1 and BRCA2 testing.

   Do you tell this client about the TP53 mutation in the family?

Case Discussion. Upholding confidentiality is one of the cornerstones of client-provider relationships. Thus, there would need to be a very compelling reason for a genetic counselor to disclose any private information about a client to a third party (even to another family member). Situations in which disclosure to another relative might be considered under rare circumstances are those in which disclosure would confer immediate medical benefits or nondisclosure would cause significant harm.

Counselors may have a moral obligation to inform relatives of their potential risks if the syndrome in question has proven interventions that can prevent or mitigate disease. Examples of syndromes in which there is a clear medical benefit to being aware of one's risks include familial adenomatous polyposis, multiple endocrine neoplasia, 2, and hereditary retinoblastoma. In this case, the syndrome in question is Li-Fraumeni syndrome, which probably lies on the other end of the spectrum; there are few effective detection or prevention strategies to offer at-risk individuals. However, the counselor needs to consider whether any possible medical benefit would justify disclosure.

Another central issue in this case is whether the client is already receiving appropriate cancer monitoring. Genetic counselors may feel less compelled to reveal information about the cousin if the client is already obtaining appropriate care. Sometimes, an awareness of the family history of cancer is sufficient to obtain appropriate medical management. This is often the case when tumor types are also monitored in the general population (such as breast or colon cancer). In contrast, monitoring for less common tumor types, such as brain tumors, would not be done unless the client is known to be at risk for a specific hereditary cancer syndrome. This fact should be taken into consideration when deciding whether to disclose information to this client.

Counselors should also consider the degree of relatedness between the two family members. There may be a greater obligation for counselors to warn first-degree relatives about genetic risks than third-degree relatives, as in this case. It is certainly likely that cousins will not feel the same level of obligation or responsibility toward each other as would be expected between siblings or a parent and child.

COUNSELOR STRATEGIES.   In deciding the best course of action, the genetic counselor should consider the following:

1. *Who is the primary client?*—The genetic counselor has responsibilities to her at-risk client as well as to the cousin who was previously tested. It is very likely that the cousin was assured that her test result would not be shared with any third party without her permission. The counselor needs to decide whether her responsibility to the high-risk client outweighs the moral obligation of keeping this promise to the cousin.

2. *Is there a way to satisfy both parties?*—The genetic counselor should consider ways in which she or he can uphold the cousin's confidentiality but also ensure that the client obtains more information. One pos-

sible strategy is to continue encouraging the client to speak with her cousin or other family members. This is generally the best solution because it allows family members to deal directly with each other. Another strategy is for the counselor to call the cousin, explain that one of her relatives (without disclosing the relative's identity) is seeking information, and request permission to disclose the information to other family members. It may turn out that the cousin is perfectly willing to have the test result released to her relatives. Alternatively, the counselor may learn that the cousin prefers not to share the result with anyone. If this is the case, then the counselor needs to honor this request. A final strategy would be to inform the client that further review of her cancer history has confirmed that her family has LFS. The counselor can then discuss the option of *TP53* testing as though there were no known mutation in the family. This option means that one family member (probably the living aunt) would have to pay for full gene analysis, but it does protect the cousin's confidentiality while providing the client with the option of predisposition testing.

3. *What is the potential harm in disclosure?*—Guidelines about family communication have been clear that client confidentiality should be breached only in rare, extenuating circumstances. Because there are few, if any, effective early detection or prevention strategies available to individuals with LFS, it is debatable whether disclosing this information would confer true medical benefits to the client. Thus, the standards of care may not justify breaching confidentiality in this case. In addition, disclosing the test result after having promised the cousin that this would not occur could have serious repercussions for the counselor as well as the testing program. Therefore, it is easier to justify disclosure of the syndrome in the family than the *TP53* result.

4. *What is the potential harm in nondisclosure?*—In this case, the client knows only about her possible increased risks of breast cancer. She does not know that her family has a hereditary cancer syndrome (LFS) and does not know that she herself has a 25% chance of carrying a *TP53* mutation. By not disclosing this information, the client is denied the opportunity to undergo *TP53* testing. Even more importantly, the lack of awareness about LFS could result in a delayed diagnosis of cancer in her or her daughter. Clients at risk for LFS are recommended to undergo a thorough evaluation of any prolonged somatic complaint. This aggressive work-up of symptoms is quite different from the management of symptoms in the general population. Furthermore, it is unlikely that other providers would recognize that this client is at risk for LFS-related tumors because LFS is a rare syndrome

and the client is unaware of one of the key diagnoses (the aunt's adrenal gland tumor). Another potential problem for the genetic counselor is that he or she has information about the client's family that the client does not have. If the client later learns that the counselor deliberately withheld this information, it is likely to have a detrimental effect on their relationship.

BOTTOM LINE.   The genetic counselor should strive to increase the client's awareness about her cancer risks while upholding the cousin's confidentiality. This might include contacting the cousin to ask for permission to disclose this information to other family members. If these attempts fail within a reasonable time period, then the genetic counselor may have a moral obligation to inform the client that her family meets clinical criteria for LFS. The counselor should not release the cousin's *TP53* test result without permission to do so. However, other avenues of genetic testing could be explored if this is something the client wishes to do.

10.2.4. CASE 4: RIGHT TO KNOW VERSUS RIGHT NOT TO KNOW

An *MSH2* mutation has been identified in a family with hereditary non-polyposis colon cancer. One female relative at 50% risk of carrying the mutation declines testing because she is not sure she could cope with a positive result. However, her 25-year-old daughter, Lisa, has decided that she wants to be tested. Although Lisa acknowledges her mother's viewpoint, she feels it is medically important for her to obtain this information.

In the same family, a pair of 40-year-old identical (monozygotic) twins are counseled about their 50% risks of carrying the *MSH2* mutation. Although both twins are initially interested in the information, only one of the twins, Jerry, decides to be tested. Jerry assures you that he has no plans to tell his brother the test result—unless it is negative.

Do you proceed with testing Lisa and Jerry?

CASE DISCUSSION.   In both of these cases, a positive result in the individual being tested will also reveal the gene status of another family member; an individual who has explicitly declined testing.

These cases illustrate the difficulty of balancing the rights of family members who want to learn their gene status with those who do not. With the advent of direct genetic testing, members of a family with a known gene mutation can make individual decisions about testing without blocking the option of testing for other relatives. Yet situations can still arise in which testing one relative can inadvertently disclose the results for another. The scenarios above describe two of the most common situations: An adult child wants a test that her parent declined, and one identical twin wants testing but the other does not.

The earliest discussions of this issue occurred with individuals tested for Huntington disease (HD), a degenerative neurological genetic condition in which a positive genetic test result confers 100% risks of disease. In a condition that offers no hope of prevention or cure, it seemed compassionate and right to give preference to an individual's right not to learn his or her gene status. Therefore, if Lisa and Jerry were at risk for HD they might well have been denied the option of testing.

Hereditary cancer syndromes differ from HD in several important ways. First, the risk of cancer among gene mutation carriers is usually well below 100%, so that a positive test result does not indicate with certainty that the disease will occur. It is also possible for people to survive a diagnosis of cancer and continue to have a high quality of life. Perhaps most importantly, there may be great medical benefit to learning that one has an altered cancer susceptibility gene. For many of the cancer syndromes, there are potentially effective early detection and prevention strategies that may reduce the likelihood of syndrome-related morbidity or mortality. Thus, cancer genetic testing programs tend to give preferences to those who want to learn their test results over those who do not. However, complicated testing scenarios, like that of Lisa and Jerry, should be considered on a case-by-case basis.

COUNSELOR STRATEGIES.   When faced with this type of ethical dilemma, genetic counselors should consider the following issues:

1. *What is the potential harm in not testing?*—If the genetic counselor were to deny testing to Lisa and Jerry, then they would not be able to learn their *MSH2* gene status. In the worst case scenario, one of them could later develop an hereditary nonpolyposis colon cancer (HNPCC)-related cancer. Whether knowledge of the *MSH2* status would have prevented such a diagnosis is difficult to say. Both at-risk family members should already be undergoing monitoring for colorectal cancer based on their family histories. However, the clients themselves might feel as though knowing the test result would have made a difference. And whether justified or not, the genetic counselor might feel as though he or she had let the client down. Could Lisa and Jerry sue the counselor for malpractice because they were denied the test and later developed cancer? This is unlikely but could conceivably happen. However, it would be difficult for Lisa and Jerry to prove malpractice, provided they were already being recommended to follow HNPCC monitoring guidelines (Burke et al, 1997).

2. *What is the potential harm in testing?*—If Lisa and Jerry proceed with being tested, there is a possibility that this issue could cause them to become estranged from other family members. This is not a very

likely outcome, but the relationships will almost certainly be affected in some way. The extent that this issue damages family ties depends on the closeness of the relationship before testing and how well family members are able to discuss and resolve conflict. The good news is that families tend to be resilient, and therefore differences of opinion about testing rarely cause long-term rifts. Another potential concern is that the family member who did not want the information could become depressed or anxious if they do learn the result. Because this family member was not formally tested, he or she did not receive the continued support and information of the testing program.

3. *Is it possible to keep the result a secret?*—Family members who request testing may plan to keep their result a secret. This allows them to learn the result and honors their relative's preference not to know; everyone is happy. But does this strategy really work? In some families, it will be almost impossible to keep the test result a secret. For example, Jerry does not plan to disclose a positive result to his twin brother. But this does not ensure that his brother will never find out the test result, especially if Jerry shares the news with other relatives. In families that communicate often and openly with one another, keeping this type of secret is not a realistic strategy. Other families may be less communicative and more accustomed to withholding information from one another. Within this type of family, it may be possible for individuals to maintain privacy about their test result. However, clients may feel burdened by keeping their result a secret and must also forego the support that this family member might have typically provided. In addition, if results are positive, Jerry and Lisa may feel compelled to warn their relatives of their increased risks of cancer.

4. *What is the counselor's role?*—Whenever possible, counselors should stay clear of family quarrels, but this is one situation that the counselor needs to address during or before the pretest counseling session. The counselor should make sure that Lisa and Jerry understand how a positive result will disclose the other family member's result and help them to anticipate any possible repercussions. It may also be helpful for the counselor to have contact with the family member who has chosen not to be tested to discuss his or her understanding of and comfort with the situation. It is always better to have discussed these issues before drawing blood for analysis, although clients may prefer to wait and see if it is an issue because they are hoping for a negative result. In Jerry's case, his brother's result would also be negative; in Lisa's case, her mother's status would remain unknown. Although the genetic counselor is unlikely to sway Jerry's mind about sharing a negative result but not a positive result with his brother, it is impor-

tant to have at least discussed with him the possible ramifications of this strategy.

Bottom Line. When it comes to predisposition testing for a hereditary cancer syndrome, an individual's right to know generally takes precedence over an individual's right not to know. Therefore, both Lisa and Jerry should be allowed to proceed with testing even though a positive result will provide information about another family member's gene status. Prior to testing, both clients should be made aware that learning this result could adversely impact their family relationships and should explore ways of lessening the impact that a positive result could have on the family.

10.2.5. Case 5: Concerns about Testing Minors Versus Parents' Right to Decide

The client's wife died of breast cancer last year at age 32, and his mother-in-law died from bilateral breast cancer in her fifties. The family is Ashkenazi Jewish. With the client's permission, you arrange to analyze a tumor specimen from his wife for the BRCA1/2 panel. This analysis reveals a 6174delT mutation in the BRCA2 gene. After being told the result, the client requests predictive testing for two daughters ages 14 and 10.

The client says that his 14-year-old daughter is aware of the test result in the family and has expressed a wish to be tested. His 10-year-old daughter is less aware of her potential risks, and the client would wait until she is older before disclosing the result to her if positive. The client understands that there is no medical benefit to his daughters being tested but feels that there would be great psychological benefit. He says that he would cope better knowing they have positive results than living with the uncertainty of not knowing.

Do you test the client's two young daughters for the familial BRCA2 mutation?

Case Discussion. A precedent was set when presymptomatic testing for Huntington disease (HD) was limited to individuals who are 18 years and older. However, there is much debate (and little consensus) about whether children should have the option of being tested for an adult-onset hereditary cancer syndrome. Consensus statements have cautioned that genetic testing in minors is appropriate only if the condition for which testing is done occurs in childhood and if there is an effective intervention that would be initiated in childhood.

Several hereditary cancer syndromes meet both of the above criteria, including familial adenomatous polyposis, hereditary retinoblastoma, and multiple endocrine neoplasia, 2. Few would argue with the value of testing at-risk minors for any of these syndromes. Not only are the syndromes associated with pediatric-onset tumors, but each has medical interventions that confer clear medical benefits.

The discussion becomes more difficult if there is no clear medical benefit to learning the child's gene status. Li-Fraumeni syndrome, for example, is associated with childhood tumors but has no effective strategies for prevention or even monitoring. Adult-onset cancer syndromes like breast-ovarian cancer syndrome and hereditary nonpolyposis colon cancer do have potentially effective monitoring and prevention strategies—but nothing that is initiated in childhood. Thus, in considering this case, it is important to realize that a *BRCA2* mutation is not associated with childhood tumors nor is there any immediate medical benefit for either daughter to learn this information now. Providers should also keep in mind that parental anxiety does not overrule the lack of medical benefit.

Providers are within their right to refuse to test minors for hereditary cancer syndromes that do not confer immediate medical benefit. However, this may place them in the uneasy position of going against the wishes of the child's guardian or parent. There is a long history within the United States of upholding a parent's right to make treatment decisions for their child. Unless the parent's course of action has potentially life-threatening consequences, medical providers are expected to accede to the parent's wishes. This policy is made under the assumption that parents want what is best for their child and that they are in the position of knowing their child best. Ideally, parents and medical providers will share the decision-making responsibilities regarding the child's care. Thus, an explanation of why *BRCA2* testing is not usually performed on a minor may lessen the client's interest in having his daughters tested.

A separate issue of importance is to consider the age at which a child should be allowed a voice in the decision-making and testing process. At least part of the child's maturity and level of comprehension is dictated by age. Most providers agree that older children and adolescents have at least some complex reasoning skills and should be asked to assent to the test and should be involved in the testing process. The 14-year-old daughter in this case clearly falls into this category and the 10-year-old might as well. The counselor would have to carefully consider the client's request that his younger daughter not be given her test result.

COUNSELOR STRATEGIES.   In considering the best way to handle this case, the counselor should consider the following issues:

1. *What are the potential risks and benefits of testing?*—Possible risks and benefits of predisposition testing in childhood are listed in Table 10-4. It is easy to justify childhood testing for which there is clear, immediate medical benefits. For most of the adult-onset cancer syn-

TABLE 10-4. POTENTIAL RISKS AND BENEFITS OF PREDISPOSITION TESTING

Potential Risks	Potential Benefits
Learning child is at risk could lead to	
Extreme sadness or anxiety	Better cancer monitoring
Hypochondriacal or overprotective behavior of parent	Option of prevention strategies
Altered image of body and self-worth	Altered treatment of tumors
Increased risk-taking behaviors and other maladaptive coping strategies	More comprehensive work-up of symptoms
Altered relationships within the family	Targeting of monitoring and symptom work-up to those at risk
Lowered goals in terms of education, career, or family	Better coping by the child; may be easier to learn result in childhood
Future discrimination	Better coping by the family; certainty may be preferable to uncertainty
Learning child is not at risk could lead to	
Overwhelming survivor guilt	Immense relief and joy for child and other family members
Increased risk-taking behaviors and other maladaptive coping strategies	Reduced fear about the child's cancer risks
Altered relationships within the family	Fewer monitoring tests

dromes, there is no medical rationale for learning a child's gene status. This does not mean that such tests confer no benefit at all. There may be significant psychological benefits to the child and the family. However, there are also very real concerns about the potential risks of testing. These risks include increased anxiety, lowered self-esteem, and changed family relationships. Part of the difficulty in weighing the risks and benefits is that there is very little published information regarding how children and families deal with a predictive genetic test. Not only would it be helpful to have more data about the short-term impact but also the broader impact that this information has over time.

In making decisions about testing a child, it is fair to say that medical benefits trump potential psychological concerns. In the absence of immediate medical benefits, it becomes a matter of weighing psychological risks versus psychological benefits. The counselor should discuss the potential risks and benefits of testing with this client and his daughters and explore whether this is really the right time in their lives to be tested, especially given many teenagers' insecurities about their changing bodies.

One additional concern about offering testing in childhood is that it robs the child of making a future decision about testing. This would be less of an issue if everyone chose to learn their gene status, but this is not the case. Many at-risk adults choose to delay or decline predisposition testing.

2. *What is a child's understanding of testing?*—Children's ages will dictate in large part their involvement in making decisions about testing as well as their counseling needs within a genetic testing program.

Young children do not typically have the reasoning abilities necessary to make decisions about testing. Testing children this age usually involves counseling their parents, who will then have the responsibility for informing them of the result, typically when they become older.

Older children have some degree of reasoning ability and may be capable of providing assent to predictive testing. Assent implies a willingness to be tested but does not preclude the need for obtaining consent from their guardian. Children can be told, in simple language, why testing is being offered and what the results will tell them. The decision about whether to disclose the result directly to the child depends on several factors, including the child's maturity, the wishes of the parents, and the nature of the test result.

Adolescents are increasingly being asked to provide input regarding optional medical procedures. Thus, they should be asked to provide assent to predisposition testing. Providers should honor an adolescent's request not to be tested even though the parent has requested it. A trickier issue is whether adolescents have the right to be tested against their parent's wishes. Assent is not the same as consent, which requires the signature of a parent or guardian. Therefore, in general, predisposition testing should only be performed if the adolescent assents and the parent guardian consents to the procedure.

BOTTOM LINE.   Although there are a few dissenting opinions, the current standard of care is to limit *BRCA2* testing to adults. The genetic counselor should explain to the client that there is no medical rationale for testing his daughters at this time and that it is preferable to wait until they are of an age when they can make their own decisions about testing. The client should also be reassured about the low risk of cancer that his daughters have during adolescence even if they carry a *BRCA2* mutation. The family should also be offered follow-up services, including regular appointments in the high-risk breast cancer clinic. The daughters can reconsider the option of *BRCA2* testing when they reach age 18.

10.3. REFERENCES

American Society of Human Genetics. 1995. Points to consider: ethical, legal, and psychosocial implications of genetic testing in children and adolescents. Am J Hum Genet. 57:1233–1241.

American Society of Human Genetics. 1998. Professional disclosure of familial genetic information. Am J Hum Genet. 62:474–483.

Anderlik, M and Lisko, E. 2000. Medicolegal and ethical issues in genetic cancer syndromes. Seminars in Surg Onc 18:339–346.

Bartels, D. 1993. Prescribing Our Future: Ethical Challenges in Genetic Counseling. Aldine de Gruyter, Hawthorne, NY.

Baumiller, R, Cunningham, G, Fisher, N et al. 1996. Code of ethical principles for genetics professionals: an explication. Am J Med Genet. 65:179–183.

Benkendorf, J, Reutenauer, J, Hughes, C et al. 1997. Patients' attitudes about autonomy and confidentiality in genetic testing for breast-ovarian cancer susceptibility. Am J Med Genet. 73:296–303.

Bloch, M and Hayden, M. 1990. Opinion: Predictive testing for Huntington disease in childhood: challenges and implications. Am J Hum Genet 46:1–4.

Burke, W, Petersen, G, Lynch, P et al. 1997. Recommendations for follow-up care of individuals with an inherited predisposition to cancer. I. Hereditary nonpolyposis colon cancer. JAMA 277:915–919.

Chapman, M. 1992. Canadian experience with predictive testing for Huntington disease: lessons for genetic testing centers and policy makers. Am J Med Genet 42:491–498.

Elger, B and Harding, T. 2000. Testing adolescents for a hereditary breast cancer gene (BRCA1). Arch Pediatr Adolesc Med. 154:113–119.

Garber, J and Patenaude A. 1995. Ethical, social and counselling issues in hereditary cancer susceptibility. Cancer surveys 25:381–397.

Hakimian, R. 2000. Disclosure of Huntington's disease to family members: the dilemma of known but unknowing parties. Genetic Testing 4: 359–364.

Huggins, M, Bloch, M, Kanani, S et al. 1990. Ethical and legal dilemmas arising during predictive testing for adult-onset disease: The experience of Huntington disease. Am J Hum Genet 47:4–12.

Juengst, E. 1995. The ethics of prediction: genetic risk and the physician-patient relationship. Genome Science & Technology. 1:21–36

Knoppers, B and Bodard, B. 1998. Ethical and legal perspectives on inherited cancer susceptibility. In Foulkes, W and Hodgson, S (eds) Inherited susceptibility to cancer: clinical, predictive and ethical perspectives. Cambridge University Press. Cambridge, UK, 30–45.

Michie, S and Marteau, T. 1996. Predictive genetic testing in children: the need for psychological research. Br J Health Psych 1:3–14.

National Action Plan on Breast Cancer. 2000. Position Paper: Hereditary Susceptibility Testing for Breast Cancer. [www.napbc.org] March 24.

The New York State Task Force on Life and the Law. 2000. Genetic Testing and Screening in the Age of Genomic Medicine. November.

Offit, K. 1998. Psychological, ethical, and legal issues in cancer risk counseling. In Clinical cancer genetics: risk counseling and management. John Wiley & Sons, New York, NY, 287–316.

Parens, E. 1996. Glad and terrified: on the ethics of BRCA1 and 2 testing. Cancer Investigation 14: 405–411.

Patenaude, A. 1996. The genetic testing of children for cancer susceptibility: ethical, legal, and social issues. Behavioral Sciences and the Law. 14: 393–410.

Schmerler, S. 1998. Ethical and legal issues. In Baker, D, Schuette, J, and Uhlmann, W (eds) A Guide to Genetic Counseling. Wiley-Liss, New York, NY, 391–421.

Smith, D, Quaid, K, Dworkin, R et al. 1998. Early Warning: Cases and Ethical Guidance for Presymptomatic Testing in Genetic Diseases. Indiana University Press, Bloomington, IN.

Weinblatt, V, Bennett, R, and Reich E. 1998. Putting it all together: three case examples. In Baker, D, Schuette, J, and Uhlmann, W (eds) A Guide to Genetic Counseling. Wiley-Liss, New York, NY, 391–421.

Wertz, D, Fanos, J, Reilly, P. 1994. Genetic testing for children and adolescents: who decides? JAMA 272: 875–881

Wexler, N. 1991. Disease gene identification: ethical considerations. Hosp Pract. 26: 145–8,150,152.

Appendix A   Review of Basic Genetics Principles

A.I. Genes and Chromosomes

1. *DNA*—The human genome is composed of billions of deoxyribonu-cleic acid (DNA) molecules that are present in each cell nucleus. The four DNA bases are adenine (A), thymine (T), guanine (G), and cyto-sine (C). The DNA molecule is constructed of a double helix structure with a ladder-like structure and the nucleotide pairs are bonded together in a predictable fashion, with A and T bonding together and G and C bonding together.

2. *Gene*—A gene is a unit of DNA that codes for a specific protein. The function of the gene is predetermined by its pattern and length of DNA. The estimated 30,000 to 50,000 genes in the human genome are responsible for one's physical appearance as well as conducting the many housekeeping activities of the body. Genes are subdivided into exons and introns (intervening sequences). When the DNA is trans-lated into ribonucleic acid (RNA), only the exons are retained; the introns are spliced out of the sequence. The RNA sequence is then transcribed into protein. The DNA and RNA sequences are read three letters at a time. These three letter words are called codons. Each codon corresponds to an amino acid or a "stop" command.

3. *Chromosomes*—The estimated 30,000–50,000 genes in the human genome are packaged on structures called chromosomes. The chro-mosomes are contained in the nucleus of almost every cell. The human genome consists of 23 pairs of chromosomes; 46 chromosomes

total. The first 22 pairs of chromosomes are numbered 1 through 22 and are termed autosomes. The 23rd pair of chromosomes designates the gender of the individual: XX for a female and XY for a male. The genes are scattered along the chromosomes in a set pattern. Identifying where each gene resides has been the major goal of the recent Human Genome Project, which has been an international, collaborative effort.

4. *Mutation*—A mutation is a DNA error that has occurred in the sequence of a gene and impairs the gene's ability to create a fully functional protein. The mutation can be a missing or extra DNA nucleotide or the substitution of a different DNA letter. The deletion or insertion of a DNA letter into the sequence is termed a frame-shift mutation. This type of DNA change is always deleterious. A DNA substitution may or may not impair protein function. The DNA substitution may be a normal DNA variant (polymorphism) that has no clinical significance or may cause the protein function to be impaired, meaning that it is a deleterious mutation. Examples of possible DNA mutations are below:

Normal sequence:	CAT GAG AAT
Substitution A → T	CTT GAG AAT
Deletion of T:	CAG AGA AT_
Insertion of T:	CTA TGA GAA

A.2. INHERITANCE PATTERNS

1. *Basic Principles*—The nucleus of a human cell typically contains 46 chromosomes, divided into 23 pairs. A notable exception are the gamete cells. The sperm and oocyte each contains 23 chromosomes, which join at the time of conception to give the fetus a total of 46 chromosomes. Each parent has two alleles of every gene, but only contributes one of them to offspring. This means that the fetus inherits one allele (copy) of each gene and chromosome from the mother and one allele from the father. Therefore, the DNA blueprint of the fetus is comprised of an equal balance of paternally-derived and maternally-derived genetic information.

2. *Autosomal dominant inheritance*—The majority of hereditary cancer syndromes are dominantly inherited. In a genetic condition that is dominantly inherited, the presence of a single copy of the gene mutation is sufficient to have the disease (or predisposition to disease). Thus, an affected individual will have inherited a normal copy of the gene from one parent and an altered copy from the other parent. Pedigrees of dominantly inherited conditions typically show that the con-

dition is present on only one side of the family over at least two generations. Vertical transmission (an affected grandparent, parent, and child) is consistent with a dominantly inherited condition.

A parent with a dominantly inherited gene mutation has a 50% chance of passing on the mutation to *each* of his/her offspring. A mutation can also arise as a new genetic event (*de novo*) within the egg or sperm, a phenomenon that occurs more frequently in dominantly inherited disorders than recessive disorders. "Autosomal" refers to one of the numbered chromosomes (1–22) rather than one of the sex chromosomes (X or Y)

3. *Autosomal recessive inheritance*—In a genetic condition that is recessively inherited, both copies of the gene contain mutations. Thus, an affected individual has inherited an altered copy of the gene from one parent and an altered copy from the other parent. Parents who have one altered copy and one normal copy of the gene are called carriers or heterozygotes. Heterozygotes do not usually have any symptoms or problems related to their carrier status.

Parents may only learn of their carrier status after the birth of an affected child. Certain recessive conditions occur more frequently in specific ethnic groups, and carrier screening may be offered before or during pregnancy. Pedigrees of recessively inherited conditions may or may not reveal the presence of the condition. Horizontal transmission (unaffected parents and two or more affected siblings) is consistent with a recessively inherited condition.

APPENDIX B REVIEW OF BASIC PEDIGREE SYMBOLS

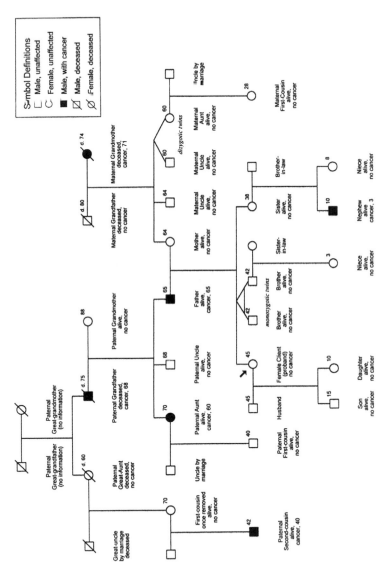

FIGURE B-1. This figure illustrates a mock pedigree. The pedigree begins with the age and cancer history of the client (proband) who is designated by an arrow. The 4-generation pedigree includes the following information on each relative: current status (alive or deceased), current age or age at death, and cancer history.

INDEX